Orthopedic Surgery and Injury Assessment

Orthopedic Surgery and Injury Assessment

Edited by Markus Wagner

hayle
medical

New York

Hayle Medical,
750 Third Avenue, 9th Floor,
New York, NY 10017, USA

Visit us on the World Wide Web at:
www.haylemedical.com

ISBN: 978-1-63241-538-7

Cataloging-in-Publication Data

Orthopedic surgery and injury assessment / edited by Markus Wagner.
    p. cm.
Includes bibliographical references and index.
ISBN 978-1-63241-538-7
1. Orthopedic surgery. 2. Musculoskeletal system--Wounds and injuries.
3. Orthopedics--Diagnosis. 4. Orthopedics. 5. Orthopedics--Treatment. I. Wagner, Markus.
RD731 .O78 2019
617.47--dc23

Table of Contents

Preface

The main aim of this book is to educate learners and enhance their research focus by presenting diverse topics covering this vast field. This is an advanced book which compiles significant studies by distinguished experts in the area of analysis. This book addresses successive solutions to the challenges arising in the area of application, along with it; the book provides scope for future developments.

Orthopedic surgery is a branch of surgery that is concerned with the treatment of conditions involving the musculoskeletal system. Both surgical and nonsurgical methods are used to treat sports injuries, bone tumors, congenital limb deformities or degenerative diseases. Fractures and major trauma can be dealt with from the specialized domains of trauma surgery and traumatology. The damage caused to skeletal systems or muscular systems because of a strenuous activity is known as musculoskeletal injury. Carpel tunnel syndrome, back pain, hand-arm vibration syndrome, tendinitis, etc. are some common examples of such injuries. This book contains some path-breaking studies in the field of orthopedic surgery and injury assessment. It discusses the fundamentals as well as modern approaches of orthopedics. Those in search of information to further their knowledge will be greatly assisted by this book.

It was a great honour to edit this book, though there were challenges, as it involved a lot of communication and networking between me and the editorial team. However, the end result was this all-inclusive book covering diverse themes in the field.

Finally, it is important to acknowledge the efforts of the contributors for their excellent chapters, through which a wide variety of issues have been addressed. I would also like to thank my colleagues for their valuable feedback during the making of this book.

Editor

Arthroscopic treatment of focal osteochondral lesions of the first metatarsophalangeal joint

Ersin Kuyucu[1]*, Harun Mutlu[2], Serhat Mutlu[3], Baris Gülenç[1] and Mehmet Erdil[1]

Abstract

Background: Although arthroscopic surgical treatment of the first metatarsophalangeal (MTP) joint involves painful sesamoid excision, synovectomy, debridement, and partial cheilectomy, no gold standard treatment technique has been defined in the literature for hallux rigidus and focal osteochondral lesions. This study aimed to assess the arthroscopic treatment for early grade focal osteochondral lesions of the first MTP joint and to determine the impact of arthroscopic microhole drill surgery on foot function and activities of daily living in a group of patients who failed conservative treatment.

Methods: This prospective study included 14 patients with hallux rigidus and focal osteochondral lesions of the first MTP joint who underwent surgery in 2014 and were followed on a regular basis thereafter.

Results: The patients had mean preoperative VPS (visual pain score) and AOFAS (American Orthopedic Foot and ankle Society)-Hallux scores of 8.14 ± 0.86 SD and 48.64 ± 4.27, respectively; the corresponding postoperative values of both scores were 1.86 ± 0.66 SD and 87.00 ± 3.70. Both VPS and AOFAS-Hallux scores changed significantly.

Discussion: In this prospective study, we explored the impact of arthroscopic microhole drill surgery on foot function and activities of daily living in patients with focal osteochondral lesions of the first MTP joint. Our results showed significant improvements in VPS and AOFAS scores with this treatment.

Conclusions: An arthroscopic microhole drill technique can be used with impressive functional scores and without any complications in patients who failed conservative therapy for hallux rigidus with focal chondral injury.

Keywords: Metatarsophalangeal joint, Hallux rigidus, Arthroscopy

Background

First defined by Watanabe in 1972 [1, 2], arthroscopic treatment of the first metatarsophalangeal (MTP) joint was later detailed by Barlett in 1988 [3]. Thanks to advancements in arthroscopic techniques and technology, arthroscopy of the first MTP joint is now used for both diagnosis and treatment of a variety of clinical conditions, such as hallux valgus, gout, and hallux rigidus [4]. Although arthroscopic surgical treatment of the first MTP joint involves painful sesamoid excision, synovectomy, debridement, and partial cheilectomy, no gold standard treatment technique has been defined

in the literature for hallux rigidus and focal osteochondral lesions.

This study aimed to assess arthroscopic treatment, one of the surgical treatment options for early grade focal osteochondral lesions of the first MTP joint, and determine the impact of arthroscopic microhole drill surgery on foot function and activities of daily living in a group of patients who failed conservative treatment.

Methods

This prospective study included 14 patients with hallux rigidus and focal osteochondral lesions of the first MTP joint who underwent surgery in 2014 and were followed on a regular basis thereafter. An initial recommendation for conservative treatment composed of footwear modification, analgesic use, and physical therapy for at least

* Correspondence: ersinkuyucu@yahoo.com.tr
[1]Orthopedics and Traumatology, Istanbul Medipol University, Istanbul, Turkey
Full list of author information is available at the end of the article

6 months was offered to all patients. Patients who failed this conservative therapy, had pain, showed full-thickness cartilage injury on magnetic resonance imaging (MRI), and were followed on a regular basis participated in the study after providing written informed consent. Patients with Coughlin-Shurnas Grade-4 hallux rigidus, osteochondral kissing lesions, or an indication for osteotomy and/or cheilectomy apart from arthroscopy were excluded, as were those who did not attend regular follow-up visits. Patients were also excluded if they underwent any foot operation or had another foot deformity such as flat foot, excessive foot pronation, or moderate or severe hallux valgus. All patients were operated on by surgeons (M.E, E.K) experienced in their field. The mean postoperative follow-up period was 16.43 ± 1.86 SD months. Eight (57.1%) patients were female and 6 (42.9%) were male. The median age of the patients was 44.07 years (range, 38–49).

Coughlin and Shurnas Classification [5] was used to determine the hallux rigidus grade; Outerbridge Classification [6] was used to grade cartilage lesions. Foot function before and after surgery was assessed by the American Orthopedic Foot and Ankle Society Score (AOFAS) [7]. Visual pain scale (VPS) was used for rating pain [8]. All patients were informed about the study and provided written informed consent.

Statistical analysis

Statistical analyses were done with the NCSS 2007 (Number Cruncher Statistical System, Kaysville, Utah, USA) software package. Descriptive statistics included mean, standard deviation, median, frequency, ratio, minimum, and maximum. Intra-group comparison of non-normal distribution parameters was done with the Friedman Test, and post hoc paired comparisons were done with the Wilcoxon signed-rank test. A p value of less than 0.01 was considered statistically significant.

Surgical technique

Patients were administered spinal anesthesia and placed in a supine position. An arthroscopic intra-articular water pressure system with pump was considered sufficient for hemostasis, and thus, no pneumatic tourniquet was used. A non-invasive joint distraction technique was applied. Before marking arthroscope entry points, 2–3 cc isotonic saline was administered intra-articularly to ensure capsule retention. Standard dorsolateral and dorsomedial portals were established 2–4 mm medial and lateral to the extensor hallucis longus tendon, and no additional portals were required. First, the dorsomedial portal site at the level of the joint was determined with the help of a needle. Following skin incision using a No. 15 scalpel, the joint was accessed by blunt soft tissue dissection using a hemostat, and it was visualized with a

2.0-mm 30° oblique arthroscope (Fig. 1). The dorsolateral portal was prepared with the same technique, and the arthroscope and manual devices were alternatively used through both portals. A 2.0 shaver, probe, and a straight punch were used as the manual devices. A synovectomy was done first to have a better view of the surgical field (Figs. 1 and 2). The cartilage was examined with the probe, and the joint was irrigated with abundant isotonic saline. After measuring the lesion size, the cartilage was intervened using the microhole drill method (Figs. 3 and 4). After ensuring adequate bleeding, the procedure was terminated, and the entry portals were sutured with 3/0 rapid suture.

Postoperative joint loading was permitted to the maximum tolerated point. Active and passive joint movements were not restricted on the first postoperative day. All patients were discharged 1 day after surgery. Control examinations were performed at 3 and 6 weeks and at 3, 6, 12, and 18 months.

Results

This study included 27 patients with hallux rigidus and osteochondral injury of the first MTP joint who underwent arthroscopic surgical treatment of the first MTP joint. Five patients had Coughlin-Shurnas Grade-4 hallux rigidus and were excluded from the study, five patients were excluded due to having an osteochondral kissing lesion, and three patients were excluded for not having attended regular follow-up after the third month. After excluding the above patients, the study was completed with 14 patients. Six patients were male, and eight were female. The mean age was 44.07 ± 3.40 years. The mean follow-up duration was 16.43 ± 1.86 months. All patients were operated on by two experienced surgeons (M.E., E.K.).

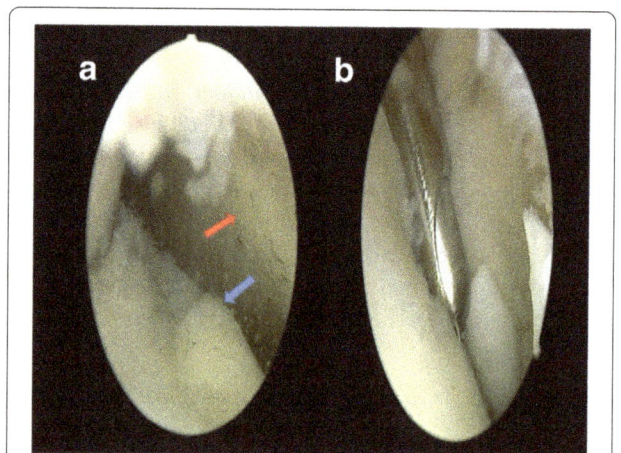

Fig. 1 a First view of the MTP joint by the 30° scope. *Blue arrow* is the metatarsal head. *Red arrow* is the proximal phalangeal joint surface. **b** Synovectomy and debridement of the joint by the shaver

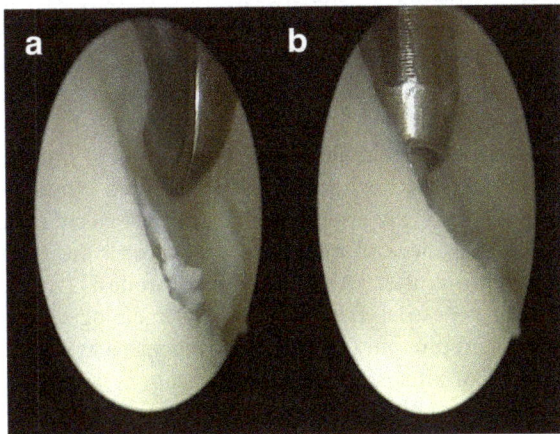

Fig. 2 a Curettage of the chondral lesion. b Microhole drill of the chondral lesion

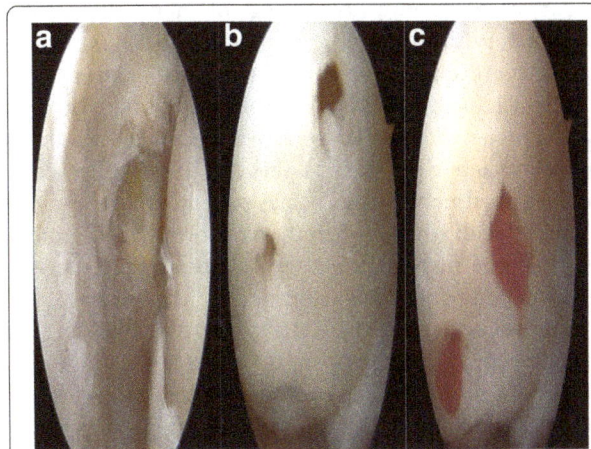

Fig. 4 a Chondral defect. b Chondral surface after the microhole drill. c Migration of the blood from the tunnels

The mean hallux valgus angle was 13.29° ± 1.93 SD, and the mean intermetatarsal angle was 9.14° ± 0.86 SD. Apart from joint arthroscopy, no soft tissue procedure or any procedure requiring osteotomy was done on any patient. The median operative duration was 27.8 min (range, 19–56). While nine patients had Coughlin-Shurnas Grade-2 hallux rigidus with moderate pain and joint flattening affecting less than 50% of the joint, five patients had Grade-3 hallux rigidus with severe pain and joint stiffness. Arthroscopically, all patients had Outerbridge Grade 4 full-thickness cartilage injury. Only one patient had diabetes mellitus controlled with oral antidiabetic medication.

The patients had mean preoperative VPS and AOFAS-Hallux scores of 8.14 ± 0.86 SD and 48.64 ± 4.27, respectively; the corresponding postoperative values of both scores were 1.86 ± 0.66 SD and 87.00 ± 3.70. Both VPS and AOFAS-Hallux scores changed statistically significantly ($p < 0.01$).

None of the patients developed postoperative complications.

Discussion

In this prospective study, we explored the impact of arthroscopic microhole drill surgery on foot functions and activities of daily living in patients with focal osteochondral lesions of the first MTP joint (Fig. 5). Our results indicated significant improvements in VPS and AOFAS scores with this treatment.

Hallux rigidus is the most common first-line pathology of the foot after hallux valgus [9]. This condition affects people at a younger age than hallux valgus, and the primary complaints are pain and movement limitations [9, 10]. Pain is usually the first symptom in the initial stages of hallux rigidus. At this stage,

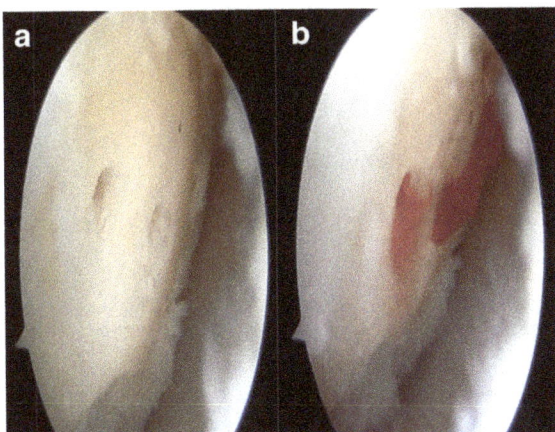

Fig. 3 a Chondral surface after the microhole drill. b Migration of the blood from the tunnels

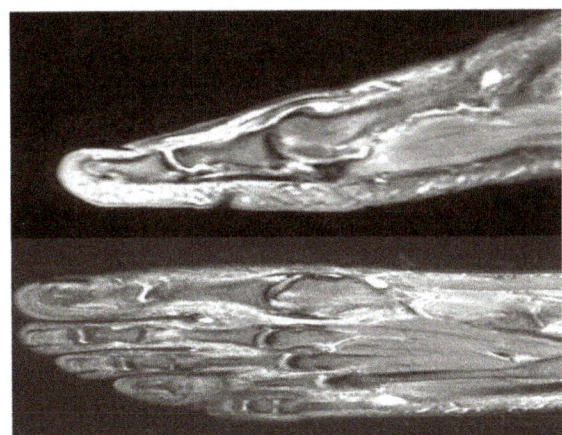

Fig. 5 MRI of the 39-year-old man right foot, sagittal and axial view of the MTP joint

conservative therapy consisting of nonsteroid anti-inflammatory drug (NSAID) use and footwear modification aims to suppress synovitis and joint inflammation and reduce pain [10–12]. However, surgical treatment may be preferred when conservative therapy fails in these young and active patients [11–14]. We first applied conservative treatment in the whole patient group, and we proceeded with surgery when that treatment failed. Hallux valgus can be managed via open or arthroscopic surgery, depending on patient characteristics and disease stage [14, 15] Derner and Aldo showed that arthroscopic surgery was more beneficial than open surgery by being minimally invasive, having a shorter recovery period, requiring no special rehabilitation program, and allowing patients to return to daily activities quickly [16–18]. We achieved fast return to work with the arthroscopic approach in suitable patients since this approach caused no complications and allowed joint loading with as much weight as tolerated on the same day of surgery as mentioned in the literature [16, 17]. Pain reduction is another important marker for treatment. Our study demonstrated significantly lowered VPS scores at both first month follow-up and the last control visit compared to the preoperative period in a homogenous patient population involving only patients with hallux rigidus.

Arthroscopic treatment of the MTP joint is used alone or in conjunction with metatarsal osteotomies for the treatment of a wide array of conditions such as synovitis, hallux rigidus, gout, and degenerative hallux valgus [16]. However, there is still insufficient information about the principles of the evaluation and treatment of these patients. Whereas, three patients in Anh's study [17] and five patients in the series published by Van Dijk [18] had this condition, no study to date has specifically addressed it. Moreover, there is no study that addresses patients having hallux rigidus with only focal osteochondral lesions.

Satisfactory improvement of hallux rigidus has been reported with arthroscopic cheilectomy and debridement without a need for revision [19]. However, the goal of this technique is to remove and clear only the injured part that restricts motion, but not to treat other intra-articular pathologies. As the potential for spontaneous healing is slim in the case of chondral injury, treatment with either the microfracture or microhole drill techniques should be considered. The microhole drill technique we used in this study is based on the principle of opening 4–6-mm-long tunnels to enable stem cells to migrate to the injured area and achieve healing with differentiation in full-thickness chondral injuries with exposed subchondral bone [20, 21]. As it was previously reported that the thickness and quality of the newly formed cartilage are better with the microhole drill technique than with the microfracture technique [21], we chose the former technique. The most

notable indication of the success of this surgical technique was the ability of the patient to use his/her foot with comfort in daily activities; likewise, we demonstrated significant increases in AOFAS scores following surgery.

Postoperative complications are another problem. While a secondary surgery may be required after open surgeries, especially when cheilectomy is selected [22], complications necessitating additional surgery may occur at a rate of 6% after arthroplasty or arthrodesis [23]. Lin and Murphy's trial reporting clinical-radiological progression and numbness in the first web space at a rate as high as 40% after cheilectomy in a patient group with hallux rigidus indicates the fact that surgical procedures that appear simple may not be as innocuous as perceived [24]. No minor or major complications occurred at early or late periods with our arthroscopic microhole drill technique; rather, there occurred a rapid relief of pain and a quick return to daily activities.

The strongest aspects of our study are its prospective cohort study design and a homogenous study sample. Our most notable limitations, on the other hand, are the lack of a comparison group with hallux rigidus managed by either open surgery or conservative therapy, as well as a short follow-up period. Another limitation of our study is its small sample size.

Conclusions

In conclusion, an arthroscopic microhole drill technique can be applied with impressive functional scores and without any complications in persons who failed conservative therapy for hallux rigidus with focal chondral injury. There is a need for comparative studies with long-term follow-up in this patient population.

Abbreviations
AOFAS: American Orthopedic Foot and Ankle Society Score;
MTP: Metatarsophalangeal; NSAID: Nonsteroidal anti-inflammatory drug;
VPS: Visual pain scale

Acknowledgements
No funding resources or acknowledgements.

Authors' contributions
EK organized the study and writing. HM and SM carried out the writing. ME organized the surgeries. BG analyzed the data. All authors read and approved the final manuscript.

Competing interests
The authors declare that they have no competing interests.

Author details

[1]Orthopedics and Traumatology, Istanbul Medipol University, Istanbul, Turkey. [2]Orthopedics and Traumatology, Taksim Ilkyardım Training and Education Hospital, Istanbul, Turkey. [3]Orthopedics and Traumatology, Kanuni Sultan Süleyman Training and Education Hospital, TEM Avrupa Otoyolu Göztepe Çıkışı No:1, Bağcilar, Istanbul, Turkey.

References

1. Lucas DE, Hunt KJ. Hallux rigidus: relevant anatomy and pathophysiology. Foot Ankle Clin. 2015;20(3):381–9.
2. Watanabe M. Selfoc-Arthroscope (Watanabe no. 24 arthroscope). Monograph. Tokyo: Teishin Hospital; 1972. p. 46–53.
3. Bartlett DH. Arthroscopic management of osteochondritis dissecans of the firstmetatarsal head. Arthroscopy. 1988;4(1):51–4.
4. Siclari A, Piras M. Hallux metatarsophalangeal arthroscopy: indications and techniques. Foot Ankle Clin. 2015;20(1):109–22. doi:10.1016/j.fcl.2014.10.012. Epub 2014 Dec 29.
5. Coughlin MJ, Shurnas PS. Hallux rigidus. Grading and long-term results of operative treatment. J Bone Joint Surg Am. 2003;85-A(11):2072–88.
6. Cameron ML, Briggs KK, Steadman JR. Reproducibility and reliability of the outerbridge classification for grading chondral lesions of the knee arthroscopically. Am J Sports Med. 2003;31(1):83–6.
7. Malviya A, Makwana N, Laing P. Correlation of the AOFAS scores with a generic health QUALY score in foot and ankle surgery. Foot Ankle Int. 2007;28(4):494–8.
8. Jensen MP, Chen C, Brugger AM. Interpretation of visual analog scale ratings and change scores: a reanalysis of two clinical trials of postoperative pain. J Pain. 2003;4(7):407–14.
9. Beeson P, Phillips C, Corr S. Hallux rigidus: a cross-sectional study to evaluate clinical parameters. Foot (Edinb). 2009;19(2):80–92. doi:10.1016/j.foot.2008.12.001. Epub 2009 Apr 17.
10. Haddad SL. Hallux rigidus. In: Kelikian AS, editor. Operative Treatment of the Foot and Ankle. Connecticut: Appleton & Lange; 1999. p. 127–46.
11. Camasta CA. Hallux limitus and hallux rigidus. Clinical examination, radiographic findings, and natural history. Clin Podiatr Med Surg. 1996;13(3):423–48.
12. Kunnasegaran R, Thevendran G. Hallux rigidus: nonoperative treatment and orthotics. Foot Ankle Clin. 2015;20(3):401–12. doi:10.1016/j.fcl.2015.04.003. Epub 2015 Jun.
13. Delman C, Kreulen C, Sullivan M, Giza E. Proximal phalanx hemiarthroplasty for the treatment of advanced hallux rigidus. Foot Ankle Clin. 2015;20(3):503–12. doi:10.1016/j.fcl.2015.05.002.
14. Ferguson CM, Ellington JK. Operative technique: interposition arthroplasty and biological augmentation of hallux rigidus surgery. Foot Ankle Clin. 2015;20(3):513–24. doi:10.1016/j.fcl.2015.05.003.
15. Rajczy RM, McDonald PR, Shapiro HS, Boc SF. First metatarsophalangeal joint arthrodesis. Clin Podiatr Med Surg. 2012;29(1):41–9. doi:10.1016/j.cpm.2011.11.001.
16. Derner R, Naldo J. Small joint arthroscopy of the foot. Clin Podiatr Med Surg. 2011;28:551–60. doi:10.1016/j.cpm.2011.05.004.
17. Ahn JH, Choy WS, Lee KW. Arthroscopy of the first metatarsophalangeal joint in 59 consecutive cases. J Foot Ankle Surg. 2012;51:161–7.
18. van Dijk N, Veenstra KM, Nuesch BC. Arthroscopic surgery of the metatarsophalangeal first joint arthroscopy. J Arthrosc Relat Surg. 1998;14(8):851–5.
19. Iqbal MJ, Chana GS. Arthroscopic cheilectomy for hallux rigidus. Arthroscopy. 1998;14(3):307–10.
20. Chen H, Chevrier A, Hoemann CD, et al. Characterization of subchondral bone repair for marrow-stimulated chondral defects and its relationship to articular cartilage resurfacing. Am J Sports Med. 2011;39:1731.
21. Chen H, Hoemann CD, Sun J, et al. Depth of subchondral perforation influences the outcome of bone marrow stimulation cartilage repair. J Orthop Res. 2011.
22. O'Malley MJ, Basran HS, Gu Y, et al. Treatment of advanced grades of hallux rigidus with cheilectomy and phalangeal osteotomy. J Bone Joint Surg Am. 2013;95(7):606–10. doi:10.2106/JBJS.K.00904.
23. Kennedy JG, Chow FY, Dines J, et al. Outcomes after interposition arthroplasty for treatment of hallux rigidus. Clin Orthop Relat Res. 2006;445:210–5.
24. Lin J, Murphy GA. Treatment of hallux rigidus with cheilectomy using a dorsolateral approach. Foot Ankle Int. 2009;30(2):115–9. doi:10.3113/FAI.2009.0115.

2

Isolated talonavicular arthrodesis and talonavicular-cuneiform arthrodesis for the Müller-Weiss disease

Hong-hui Cao[1], Wei-zhong Lu[2] and Kang-lai Tang[1]*

Abstract

Background: The study aimed to introduce the isolated talonavicular and talonavicular-cuneiform arthrodesis for the stage III and IV Müller-Weiss disease and analyze their clinical outcomes.

Methods: Thirty patients of stage III and IV Müller-Weiss disease were divided into the talonavicular (TN) arthrodesis group and the talonavicular-cuneiform (TNC) arthrodesis group according to the perinavicular osteoarthritis by MRI scans. For the isolated talonavicular arthrodesis group, 16 patients underwent talonavicular arthrodesis with two 4. 0 mm hollow headless compression screws. For the TNC arthrodesis group, 14 patients were received the TNC arthrodesis with reverse "V" shape osteotomy and autoallergic iliac bone graft. All patients were followed up at 3, 6, 9, and 12 months, and per 6 months after 1 year, by the AOFAS ankle-midfoot scores, and evaluated by radiographic measurements.

Results: All of them were followed up in two groups and all patients were satisfied with their clinical results. At the TN arthrodesis group, the patients' mean was 39.8 months (range, 11–66 months) follow-up. The mean AOFAS ankle and hindfoot scores had improved from 38.3 ± 5.1 preoperatively to 88.9 ± 1.9 at the last postoperative assessment. At the TNC arthrodesis group, the mean follow-up was 51.7 months (range, 12–90 months). The mean AOFAS ankle and hindfoot scores were 40.1 ± 7.9 preoperatively to 90.1 ± 2.0 at the last postoperative. All of the cases were solid fusion on the radiograph.

Conclusions: According to MRI evaluation, either TN or TNC arthrodesis for stage III or IV Müller-Weiss disease have the good clinical outcomes with solid fusion rate and obvious improvement of the quality of life of patients.

Keywords: Müller-Weiss disease, Autoallergic iliac bone graft, Arthrodesis, Osteotomy

Background

Müller-Weiss disease is a primary osteonecrosis of the tarsal navicular of unknown etiology [1]. Several theories have been proposed, including primary osteonecrosis [2], traumatic or biomechanical causes, congenital malformation, navicular osteoarthritis [3], and abnormal evolution of Kohler's disease [4], but the delayed ossification of the tarsal navicular and an abnormal force distribution pattern have been the most accepted [5]. Most of the patients complain of chronic dorsomedial midfoot pain on weightbearing midfoot pain resulting in perinavicular osteoarthritis.

Maceira [5] classified the patients into five stages according to lateral X-rays: stage 1 shows minimal changes, whereas stage 5 is defined by complete extrusion of the navicular, stages 2–4 showed different degree of the compression of the navicular and the lowering of the longitudinal arch height. But Maceira admitted that the severity of the symptoms may not correspond with the radiological destruction of navicular bone or the stage of the disease.

When prolonged conservative treatment fails, surgery may be indicated. We describe arthrodesis of talonavicular or talonavicular-cuneiform joint according to the perinavicular osteoarthritis by MRI scans for the stage III and IV Müller-Weiss disease. We believe the individualization arthrodesis can restore the length of the medial column

* Correspondence: tangkanglai@hotmail.com
[1]Department of Orthopaedic Surgery, Southwest Hospital, The Third Military Medical University, Gaotanyan Str. 30, Chongqing 400038, People's Republic of China
Full list of author information is available at the end of the article

and relieve the pain caused by removal between the fragments or osteoarthritis.

Methods

At the isolated talonavicular arthrodesis group, we records 16 patients since 2008 of the Southwest Hospital, Chongqing, China. Sixteen feet in 16 patients (2 men and 14 women) with MWD disease were identified. The average age of the patients at the time of surgery was 50.3 ± 8.4 years (range, 35 to 62 years). According to the Maceira classifications, there are 11 stage III and 5 stage IV. The compression of the navicular and the severe talonavicular joints arthritis were proved be processing in all cases by MRI (Fig. 1). But none of these patients showed obvious arthritic change in the calcaneocuboid or subtalar joint.

At the TNC group, we recorded 14 patients since 2008 at the same hospital. There involved 14 patients (4 men and 10 women) with the stage III MWD disease. The average age of the patients at the time of surgery was 49.2 years (range, 32 to 69 years). All patients complained of midfoot pain on standing and walking and had gradually collapsed of the medical longitudinal arch, with the arthritic change of talonavicular-cuneiform joint by MRI (Fig. 2).

In both groups, the patients were treated conservatively with insoles and physiotherapy for at least 6 months. None of them had trauma history, rheumatoid arthritis, renal failure, or lupus erythematosus. The patient, who accompanied with multiple arthritis or infection, obvious deformity in hindfoot, was excluded.

The surgical technique

For the isolated talonavicular arthrodesis group, all patients underwent surgical intervention by the two senior authors (HH Cao and KL Tang) in our hospital. After

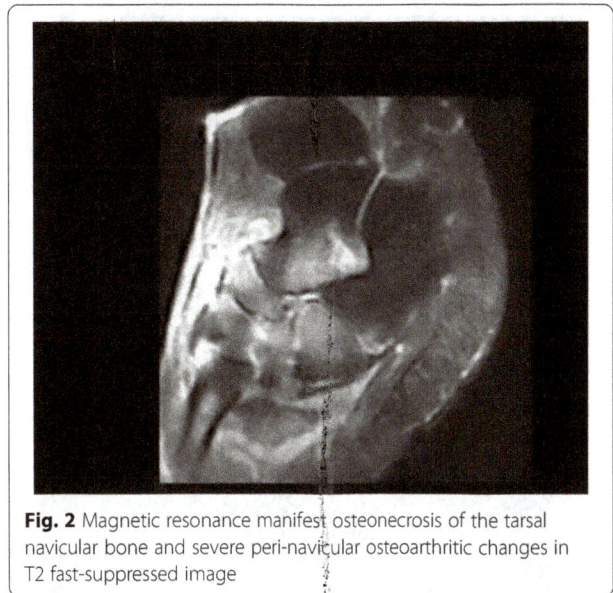

Fig. 1 The necrosis of navicular and severe talonavicular joints arthritis in T2 fast-suppressed image of MRI scans

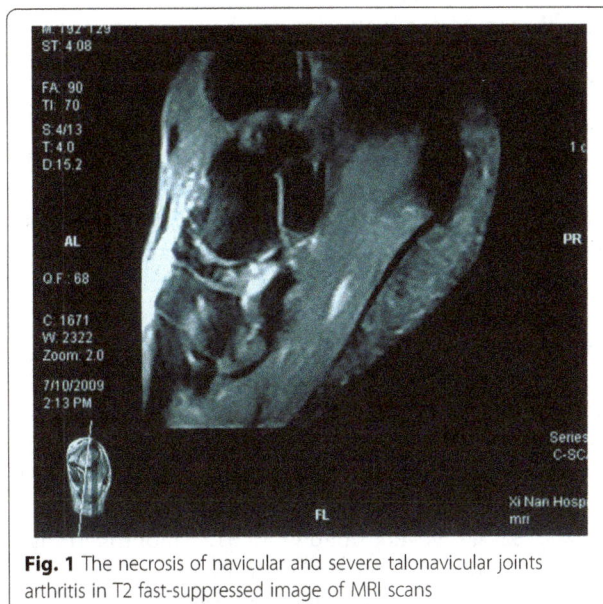

Fig. 2 Magnetic resonance manifest osteonecrosis of the tarsal navicular bone and severe peri-navicular osteoarthritic changes in T2 fast-suppressed image

general anesthesia, the procedure was performed in the supine position with a thigh tourniquet to stanch bleeding. An incision of about 4 cm was made between the anterior tibial tendon and the extensor hallucis longus to expose the talonavicular joint. The dorsolateral protruding necrotic navicular bone was excised and all residual cartilage was removed from the talonavicular joint. For the stage III cases, two 4.0 mm hollow headless compression screws (Newdeal, USA) were implanted through the talonavicular joint by vertically the articular surfaces (Fig. 3). The reverse "V" shape osteotomy of talonavicular joint to restore the medial arch height and autoallergic iliac bone graft were applied additionally for the stage IV cases.

For the TNC arthrodesis group, the Prof. Tang performed all operations as the former description by us [6]. After removed the cartilage of the talonavicular-cuneiform articular surfaces, the talonavicular joint was osteotomied by reversed "V" shape to restore the height of medial longitudinal arch (Fig. 4a). And then, an about 3 cm × 1.5 cm × 0.5 cm rectangle bed is carved on the dorsal side of talonavicular-cuneiform. A tricortical autogenous graft of same size and shape as above described is obtained from the iliac crest and is inserted in the practiced bed with the aid of plantarflexion of the foot (Fig. 4b). Two or three cannulated titanium screws of 4.0 mm (Newdeal, USA) were implanted through the autogenous iliac bone into the triple bones across the talonavicular-cuneiform fusion interface (Fig. 5).

Fluoroscopic control was used throughout to ensure optimal placement of the hardware in the two groups.

Postoperative management and evaluation

At the end of the surgery, a short leg cast was applied postoperatively for 6 weeks. The negative pressure wound

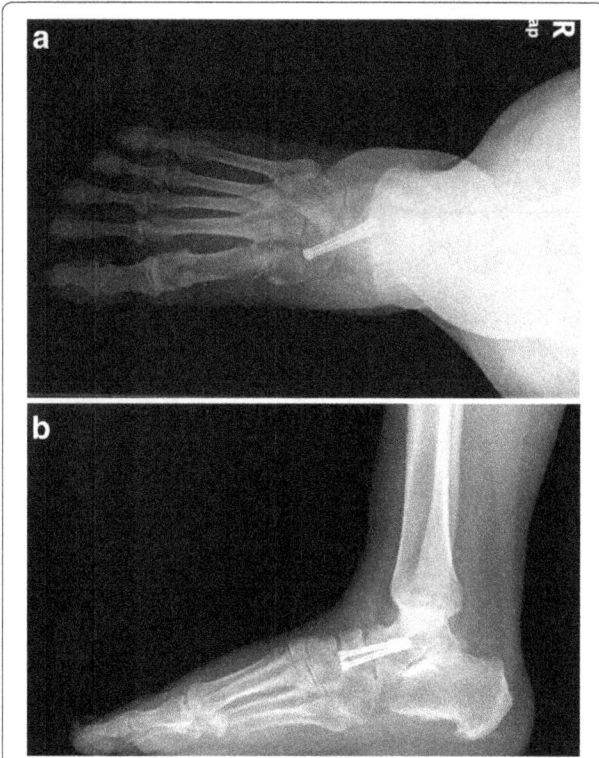

Fig. 3 a, b Two 4.0 mm hollow headless compression screws were implanted through the talonavicular joint by vertically the articular surfaces

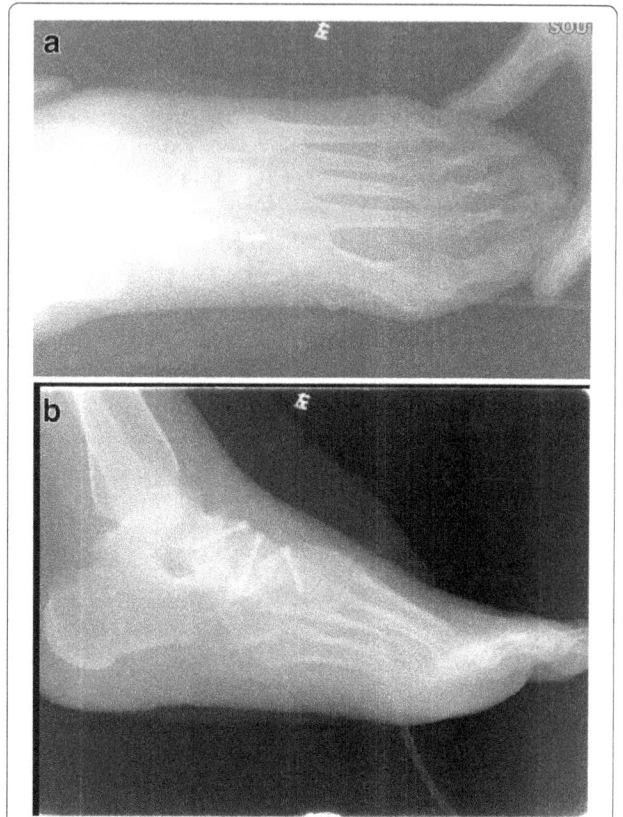

Fig. 5 a, b Three cannulated titanium screws of 4.0 mm were implanted through the autogenous iliac bone into the triple bones across the talonavicular-cuneiform fusion interface

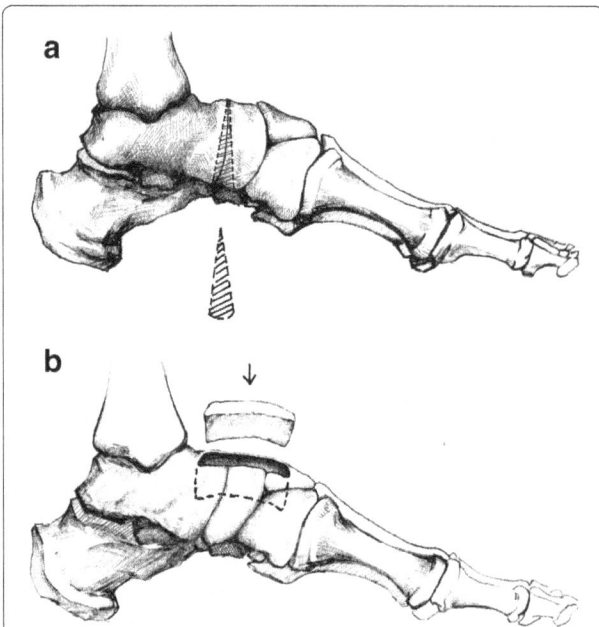

Fig. 4 a, b The talonavicular joint was osteotomied by reversed "V" shape to restore the height of medial longitudinal arch (**a**). A tricortical autogenous graft was inserted in the rectangle bed which was carved on the dorsal side of talonavicular-cuneiform (**b**)

drainage tube was removed within 48–72 h. Gradual protected weight bearing was allowed 6 weeks after surgery; walk with full weight bearing 3 months after surgery following radiographic evidence of consolidation.

The lateral and AP weight-bearing radiographs of foot were measured for evaluating the bone healing. All patients were evaluated pre-operatively, at 3, 6, 9, and 12 months, and per 6 months after 1 year by clinical examination with AOFAS ankle-hindfoot scores. The protocol of the foot pain, onset and deformity, and complications in or after surgery, were recorded exactly.

All the data was treated with SPSS 13.0, independent sample paired t test, and definite statistical difference as $p < 0.05$, significant statistical difference as $p < 0.01$.

Results

All of them were followed up in two groups: 16 TN arthrodesis [age at the intervention, 50.3 years (range, 35–60years); follow-up, 39.8 months (range, 11–66 months); Maceira classifications, 12 stage III and 4 stage IV and 14 TNC arthrodesis [age at intervention, 49.2 years (range, 32–69 years); follow-up, 51.7 months (range, 12–90 months); Maceira classifications, 14 stage III] (NS on all items between the two groups).

All patients were satisfied with their clinical results and were able to walk long distances 6 months after surgery in two groups. Only four patients in TNC arthrodesis complained the slight pain after long distance walking and can be ceased after rest or oral antiinflammatory medication. The mean AOFAS ankle and hindfoot scores had improved from 38.1 ± 5.0 preoperatively to 88.1 ± 2.7 at the last postoperative assessment in the TN arthrodesis group (Table 1) and the TNC arthrodesis group is 40.1 ± 7.7 preoperatively to 90.2 ± 2.0 at the last postoperative (Table 2). All of two groups were significantly different between preoperative and postoperative. There is nothing significantly different between the two groups at the last postoperative assessment.

Radiographically, All the operated feet fused solidly at 3 or 6 months after surgery without screw break or loosening; 9/16 in the TN arthrodesis group and 7/14 in the TNC arthrodesis group have removed the inter fixation (Figs. 6 and 7). All the operated feet fused solidly at 3 or 6 months after surgery without screw break or loosening. These results revealed improvements in terms of pain and mobility obtained by these surgical procedures.

Discussion

Müller-Weiss disease is primary osteonecrosis of the tarsal navicular bone in adult and a rare pathology of unclear etiology in middle age population [1]. The diagnosis of MWD can usually be made with plain radiographs. Maceira [5] further describes the disease by developing a five-stage classification system using lateral weightbearing radiograph, showing a progressive collapse of the medial arch and compression and splitting of the tarsal navicular. It should be distinguished from Köhler's disease [4], which occurs osteochondrosis of the tarsal navicular in children, and from secondary to systemic diseases (rheumatoid arthritis, SLE, renal failure, diabetes) or trauma [7].

It was reported that the therapy of MWD disease was described in the different stage [8]. For early MWD (stage I or stage II) with symptoms, initial conservative therapy includes ankle foot orthoses and oral antiinflammatory medication. If conservative treatment failure, simple excision or drilling decompression is enough [9]. For moderate stage MWD (stage III or stage IV), isolated talonavicular arthrodesis and talonavicular-cuneiform (TNC) arthrodesis were reliable. MWD (stage V) with marked deformity, the surgical treatment should be double fusion or triple arthrodesis [8–10]. There is no gold standard surgical technique that is effective and safe for the treatment of MWD disease. But early diagnosis and proper treatment are essential for patients' recovery [7]. Traditionally, the standard tools for the diagnosis of MWD disease and judgment of the stage are weightbearing plain radiographs of the foot. But it is difficult to show the minimal changes of adjacent joints. MRI scans may show loss of signal intensity of the navicular on theT1-weighted images and hyperintense diffuse marrow edema and periarticular fluid on the T2-weighted images [11]. In these two groups, we choose the isolated talonavicular arthrodesis and talonavicular-

Table 1 Demographic description of the TN Arthrodesis patients

Patient No	Sex	Age	Stage	Side	Bone graft	Osteotomy	AOFAS Score	
							Preoperatively	Postoperatively
1	F	39	III	Left	no	no	35	80
2	M	39	III	Left	no	no	37	89
3	F	58	III	Left	no	no	33	88
4	F	54	III	Left	no	no	39	90
5	M	52	III	Left	no	no	32	90
6	F	41	IV	Left	yes	yes	39	87
7	F	60	IV	Left	yes	yes	34	89
8	F	57	III	Left	no	no	33	82
9	F	44	III	Left	no	no	47	87
10	F	62	IV	Left	yes	yes	35	90
11	F	50	III	Left	no	no	32	95
12	F	35	III	Left	no	no	55	89
13	F	69	IV	Left	yes	yes	41	92
14	F	37	III	Left	no	no	47	90
15	F	58	IV	Right	yes	yes	35	87
16	F	50	III	Right	no	no	35	84
Mean	—	50.3 ± 8.4	—	—	—	—	38.1 ± 5.0	88.1 ± 2.7

Table 2 Demographic description of the TNC Arthrodesis patients

Patient No	Sex	Age	Stage	Side	AOFAS Score	
					Preoperatively	Postoperatively
1	F	46	III	Left	55	92
2	F	52	III	Right	49	94
3	F	41	III	Right	26	88
4	M	58	III	Left	27	90
5	F	49	III	Left	32	86
6	F	37	III	Left	50	87
7	F	60	III	Left	34	89
8	M	47	III	Left	44	89
9	M	32	III	Right	44	90
10	F	62	III	Left	32	95
11	F	34	III	Left	50	89
12	F	50	III	Right	38	92
13	F	69	III	Left	40	90
14	M	52	III	Left	35	82
mean	—	49.2 ± 8.4	—	—	40.1 ± 7.7	90.2 ± 2.0

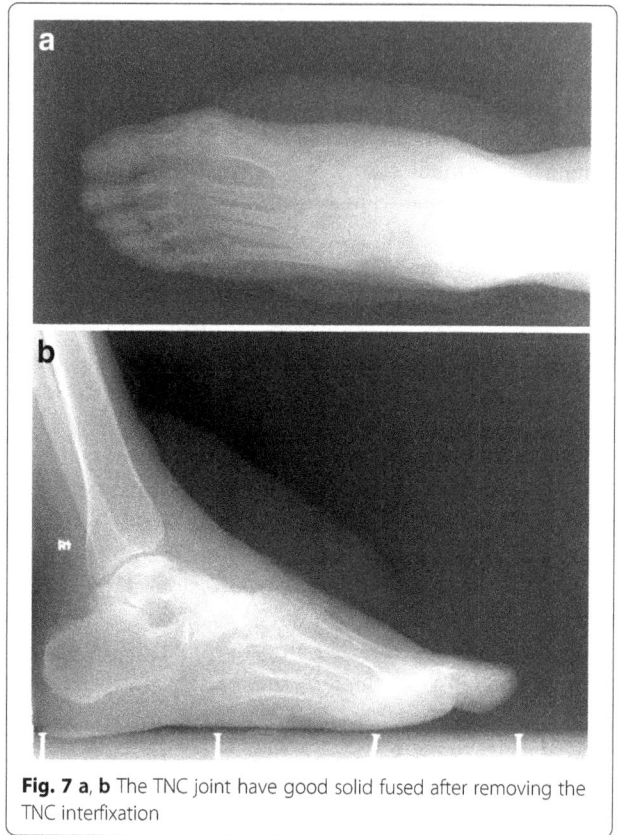

Fig. 7 a, b The TNC joint have good solid fused after removing the TNC interfixation

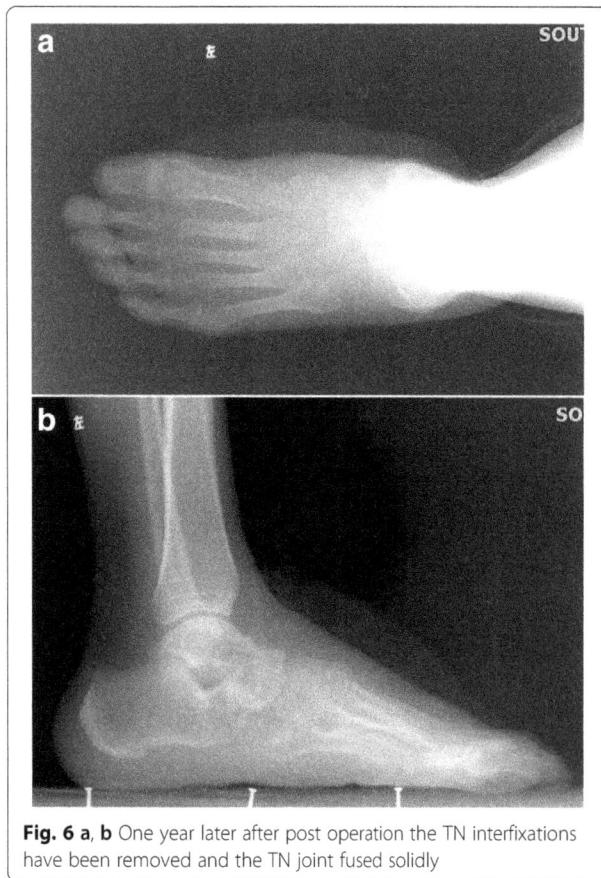

Fig. 6 a, b One year later after post operation the TN interfixations have been removed and the TN joint fused solidly

cuneiform (TNC) arthrodesis for the moderate MWD (stage III and IV) depending on the adjacent joints arthritic change by MRI scans. For the stage III or IV MWD disease, the isolated talonavicular arthrodesis is enough if the osteoarthrosis only exit in talonavicular joint. Talonavicular-cuneiform (TNC) arthrodesis is an advocated technique for the stage III MWD disease with alleviating the pain and excellent results in consolidation if osteoarthrosis in the joints around navicular. Reverse "V" shape osteotomy of the talonavicular joint can increase the medial longitudinal arch and avoid the secondary pain caused by flatfoot. We selected an allograft of tricortical iliac crest for reconstruction the excised navicular fragment [6].

The arthrodesis of peri-navicular could get the satisfaction clinic results. Lui [12] reported that of 6 patients with Müller-Weiss disease were treated with arthroscopic triple arthrodesis, at 43.5 months follow-up, the AOFAS ankle-hindfoot score increase 43.8 points (from 37.7 points preoperatively to 81.5 points postoperatively). CK Lu [11] reported that 13 feet of 13 patients with patients with Müller-Weiss disease with a mean age of 55.6 years were received the isolated talonavicular arthrodesis. The average modified American Orthopaedic Foot and Ankle Society (AOFAS) ankle-hindfoot score improved from 48.5 points preoperatively to 87.2 points at final follow-up (mean 51 months, range 10–114 months). Three cases were nonunion. In our study, either the isolated talonavicular arthrodesis or talonavicular-cuneiform (TNC) arthrodesis was gained the good clinic results and the solid fusion.

Conclusions

Throughout, the main limitation of the current study is the small number of cases; either TN or TNC arthrodesis for stage III or IV Müller-Weiss disease according to MRI evaluation have the good clinical outcomes with solid fusion rate and obvious improvement of the quality of life of patients. A large sample size and long-term clinical follow-up studies are required to evaluate the efficacy and safety of these methods.

Acknowledgements
We acknowledge the assistance of investigators and all subjects for participants in this study.

Funding
This study was supported by the Science Foundation of Southwest Hospital (No. SWH2016DCX1014).

Authors' contributions
All surgical procedures were carried out by K-LT. K-LT applied this study. H-HC participated in the patient selection, investigation on the outpatient clinic, and radiographic assessment, literature search, data monitoring, and manuscript writing. W-ZL carried out the statistical analysis. All authors have read and approved the final manuscript.

Competing interests
The authors declare that they have no competing interests.

Author details
[1]Department of Orthopaedic Surgery, Southwest Hospital, The Third Military Medical University, Gaotanyan Str. 30, Chongqing 400038, People's Republic of China. [2]Department of Orthopaedic Surgery, The Traditional Medical Hospital of Chongqing, China, The Brach 4th Panxi Road, Jiangbei, Chongqing 400021, People's Republic of China.

References
1. El-Karef E, Nairn D. The Müller-Weiss syndrome: spontaneous osteonecrosis of the tarsal navicular bone. Foot. 1999;9:153–5.
2. Reade B, Atlas G, Distazio J, Kruljac S. Müller-Weiss syndrome: an uncommon cause of midfoot pain. J Foot Ankle Surg. 1998;37(6):535–9.
3. Viladot A, Rochera R, Viladot Jr A. Necrosis of the navicular bone. Bull Hosp Joint Dis Orthop Inst. 1987;47(2):285–93.
4. Rochera R, Macule F, Diaz E, Sans JR. Aportacion al conocimiento de la escafoiditis tarsiana [An approach to the knowledge of tarsal scaphoiditis]. Chir del Piede. 1981;5(1):23–32.
5. Maceira E, Rochera R. Müller-Weiss disease: clinical and biomechanical features. Foot Ankle Clin N Am. 2004;9:105–25.
6. Cao HH, Tang KL, Xu JZ. Peri-navicular arthrodesis for the stage III Mu ̈ ller–Weiss disease. Foot Ankle Int. 2012;33(6):475–8.
7. Tosun B, Al F, Tosun A. Spontaneous osteonecrosis of the tarsal navicular in an adult: Mueller-Weiss syndrome. J Foot Ankle Surg. 2011;50:221–4.
8. Taimur M, Toby J, Dev D. Müller –Weiss disease- Review of current knowledge. Foot and Ankle Surgery. 2014;20:79–84.
9. Fernández de Retana P, Maceira E, Fernández-Valencia JA, Suso S. Arthrodesis of the talonavicular-cuneiform joints in Müller-Weiss disease. Foot Ankle Clin. 2004;9:65–72.
10. Zhang H, Li J, Qiao Y, et al. Open triple fusion versus TNC arthrodesis in the treatment of Mueller-Weiss disease. J Orthop Surg Res. 2017;12(1):13. doi:10.1186/s13018-017-0513-3.
11. Lu CK, Fu YC, Cheng YM, Huang PJ. Isolated talonavicular arthrodesis for Müller-Weiss disease. Kaohsiung J Med Sci. 2014;30:471–6.
12. Lui TH. Arthroscopic triple arthrodesis in patients with Müller-Weiss disease. Foot Ankle Surg. 2009;15:119–22.

3

Differences in placement of calcium phosphate-hybridized tendon grafts within the femoral bone tunnel during ACL reconstruction do not influence tendon-to-bone healing

Hirotaka Mutsuzaki[1]*, Hiromi Nakajima[2], Shunsuke Nomura[2] and Masataka Sakane[3]

Abstract

Background: Calcium phosphate (CaP)-hybridization of tendon grafts has been shown to improve tendon-to-bone healing. The purpose of this study was to clarify the influence of different tendon graft placement methods on tendon-to-bone healing using CaP-hybridized tendon grafts in anterior cruciate ligament (ACL) reconstructions in rabbits.

Methods: We compared two methods of tendon graft placement within the femoral bone tunnel: suspension of the tendon graft within the bone tunnel (suspension group) and implantation of the tendon graft coherent with the bone socket (coherence group). CaP-hybridized tendon grafts were used in both groups. Fifty-six male Japanese white rabbits were used for this study. The results of biomechanical tests ($n = 9$) and histological analyses ($n = 5$) were evaluated at 2 and 4 weeks after surgery.

Results: The ultimate failure load, stiffness, stress, soft tissue remaining in bone tunnel after biomechanical testing, and direct bonding area at tendon–bone interface did not differ significantly between the suspension and coherence groups at either 2 or 4 weeks after surgery ($p > 0.05$). In both groups, the ultimate failure load, stress, soft tissue remaining in the bone tunnel, and direct bonding area at interface at 4 weeks after surgery were significantly greater than those at 2 weeks after surgery ($p < 0.05$).

Conclusions: Tendon-to-bone healing in both groups progressed until the endpoint of 4 weeks. There was no influence of the CaP-hybridized tendon graft placement method on tendon-to-bone healing at 4 weeks after ACL reconstruction in rabbits. Thus, the CaP-hybridized tendon grafts were unaffected by differences in their placement within the bone tunnel and became equally anchored to the bone tunnel during the early postoperative period. The tendon graft placement method may not influence tendon-to-bone healing in ACL reconstruction when CaP-hybridized tendon grafts are used.

Keywords: Calcium phosphate hybridization, Tendon-to-bone healing, Tendon graft placement, Anterior cruciate ligament reconstruction, Alternate soaking process

* Correspondence: mutsuzaki@ipu.ac.jp
[1]Department of Orthopaedic Surgery, Ibaraki Prefectural University of Health Sciences, 4669-2 Ami, Inashiki-gun, Ibaraki 300-0394, Japan
Full list of author information is available at the end of the article

Background

We have previously developed a novel technique to improve tendon-to-bone healing that used an alternating soaking process to hybridize calcium phosphate (CaP) to tendon grafts [1]. The microstructure of the CaP-hybridized tendon grafts contained low-crystalline apatite and type I collagen, and thus resembled the microstructure of the bone [2, 3]. The use of our technique prior to tendon graft implantation stimulated osteogenesis, and areas of direct bonding were observed between CaP-hybridized tendon grafts and a newly formed bone at 2–3 weeks after implantation in a rabbit anterior cruciate ligament (ACL) reconstruction model [2, 3]. In contrast, indirect bonding with fibrous connective tissue was observed after implantation of untreated tendon grafts within bone tunnels during ACL reconstruction in rabbits [2–4]. In a goat model, ACL reconstruction with CaP-hybridized tendon grafts resulted in better anterior stability and greater in situ forces under applied anterior tibial loads using a robotic-universal force/moment sensor system at 1 year after surgery compared to those with ACL reconstruction using untreated tendon grafts [5]. Furthermore, in a recent clinical trial, use of CaP-hybridized tendon grafts improved anterior knee stability and clinical scores at 2 years after surgery and reduced the percentage of bone tunnel enlargement at 1 year after surgery, relative to the outcomes with untreated tendon grafts during ACL reconstruction [6].

There are two methods for tendon graft placement within the femoral bone tunnel during ACL reconstruction. In the first method, the implanted tendon is suspended within the femoral tunnel, and its tip does not make contact with the bone socket [7]. In the second method, the implanted tendon is coherent with the bone socket [8] and its tip makes contact with the bottom of the bone socket. It is unclear whether the differences between these two tendon graft placement methods influence tendon-to-bone healing when CaP-hybridized tendon grafts are used for ACL reconstruction. Because CaP hybridization of tendon grafts enhances new bone formation in the bone tunnel [2, 3, 5], we hypothesized that CaP-hybridized tendon grafts will be unaffected by the tendon graft placement method and will become equally anchored in the bone tunnel with both methods. The present study was performed to test the above hypothesis and clarify the influence of the tendon graft placement method on tendon-to-bone healing using CaP-hybridized tendon grafts for ACL reconstruction in rabbits.

Methods

Graft preparation

Fifty-six skeletally immature male Japanese white rabbits (weight range 2.5–3.0 kg; age 14 weeks) were used in this study. The flexor digitorum longus tendons were obtained from the right limb of each rabbit. A doubled 25-mm-long tendon graft with a diameter of 4.2 mm was prepared, and the tibial ends of the graft were secured to each other using a 2-0 nonabsorbable suture. At the looped femoral end of the graft, a 2-0 nonabsorbable suture was tied over a stainless-steel button and passed through the loop formed by the doubled-over tendon. The CaP hybridization method was the same as that described in our previous reports [2, 3, 5, 6]. Briefly, the grafts were soaked in 100 mL of Ca solution for 30 s, and then soaked in 100 mL of $NaHPO_4$ solution for 30 s, and this soaking cycle was repeated 10 times.

Graft placement during ACL reconstruction

During surgery, the ACL was completely resected in the right knee, and a 4.2-mm-diameter femoral bone tunnel was created from the medial aspect of the lateral femoral condyle. In the suspension group, the 4.2-mm-diameter femoral bone tunnel was extended to penetrate the lateral cortex of the lateral femoral condyle. In the coherence group, the 4.2-mm-diameter femoral bone tunnel was created to a length of 5.0 mm. In the coherence group, an additional 1.2-mm-diameter bone tunnel was created from the bottom of the bone socket to the lateral cortex of the distal femur for passing of a suture during implantation of the tendon graft. Next, in both groups, a 4.2-mm-diameter tibial bone tunnel was created from the center of the tibial insertion of the ACL to the medial cortex of the proximal tibia. In the suspension group, the 5.0-mm tip of the tendon graft was passed through the femoral bone tunnel (Fig. 1a), and then secured on the femoral side with a stainless-steel button. In the coherence group, the tendon graft was passed through the femoral bone tunnel until the tip of the tendon graft made contact with the bottom of the bone socket (Fig. 1b), and then secured on the femoral side with a stainless-steel button. In both groups, the tibial end of the graft was placed in the tibial bone tunnel (Fig. 1c) and secured to the tibia with a stainless-steel button. The incision was closed with a 2-0 nonabsorbable suture. After surgery, the animals were allowed to move freely in their cages and did not receive antibiotics. At 2 and 4 weeks after surgery, nine animals in each group were euthanized by deep anesthesia for biomechanical testing, and five animals in each group were euthanized by deep anesthesia for histological analysis. These time points were selected for evaluation based on previous studies in goats and rabbits. Specifically, the biomechanical data in a CaP group and an untreated group were equal at 6 weeks after ACL reconstruction in goats [9], while tendon-to-bone healing progressed up to 4 weeks after surgery in rabbits [2, 3]. The specimens for biomechanical testing were immediately stored at −80 °C until analysis.

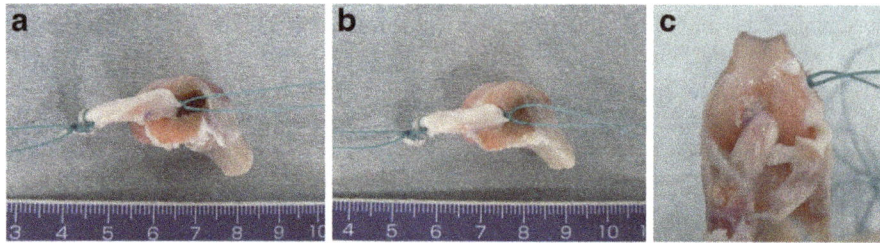

Fig. 1 Surgical procedures shown in the *left knee* of a rabbit cadaver. **a** Suspension group: the tip of the tendon graft was placed 5.0 mm into the femoral bone tunnel. **b** Coherence group: the tendon graft was passed through the femoral bone tunnel until the tip of the tendon graft made contact with the bottom of the 5.0-mm bone socket. **c** ACL reconstruction

Biomechanical analysis

Before biomechanical testing, each specimen was thawed for 24 h at room temperature, and the tibia was removed from the tendon graft. The cross-sectional area of the tendon graft at the joint line was measured using an apparatus specifically designed for measuring ligament cross-sectional areas (Jintai Danmenseki Sokuteiki, MEIRA Corporation, Nagoya, Japan). For biomechanical testing, each experimental femur-ACL graft complex was fixed to a custom-designed clamp that allowed tensile loading along the long axis of the graft on a single column materials-testing machine (TENSILON; STB-1225S; A&D Company Ltd., Tokyo, Japan). To ensure that we were determining the tensile properties of the graft and its interface within the tunnels, the stainless-steel button was removed. Load-to-failure testing at an elongation rate of 30 mm/min was performed, and the ultimate failure load (N) of the experimental femur-ACL graft complex was recorded. Stiffness (N/mm) was calculated from the slope of the linear region of the stress-strain curve. The ultimate failure load was divided by the cross-sectional area of the graft at the joint line to determine the stress (N/mm^2) for each specimen.

Histological analysis

After the biomechanical testing, the specimens were fixed in 10% neutral-buffered formalin, decalcified, and embedded in paraffin. Hematoxylin and eosin (H-E) staining was performed, and the stained specimens were examined by light microscopy after staining. Using Mac Scope software (Mitani Co., Fukii, Japan), we measured the area of the soft tissue, comprising the tendon graft, and the fibrous connective tissue remaining in the bone tunnel after the biomechanical testing (Fig. 2a). The area of the soft tissue remaining in the bone tunnel was divided by the length of the bone tunnel to yield a corrected value for the remaining tendon graft. The histological failure mode for each graft (pulled out with no tendon graft remaining or midsubstance rupture with tendon graft remaining) was recorded.

The other specimens were used for histological evaluation only. After collection, the femur-ACL grafts were fixed in 10% neutral-buffered formalin, decalcified, and embedded in paraffin. H-E staining and safranin-O staining were performed prior to examination by light microscopy. The total length of direct bonding between the tendon graft and bone (the region containing cartilaginous tissue at the tendon–bone interface) was measured using Mac Scope software (Fig. 2b and c). The total length of the direct bonding interface was divided by the length of the tendon graft within the bone tunnel to determine the rate of direct bonding area at the tendon–bone interface. The area of red safranin-O-stained glycosaminoglycan (GAG) in the cartilage layer at the interface was measured using Mac Scope software (Fig. 2d). Each GAG-stained area was divided by the length of the tendon graft in the bone tunnel to give a corrected value as a width.

The ligament tissue maturation index (LTMI) described by Murray et al. [10] was used to evaluate the maturation of the tendon grafts according to the following three criteria: (1) cellular aspects including cell density, nuclear shape, and orientation; (2) extracellular matrix characteristics including crimping; and (3) vascular features including blood vessel density and maturity. The total possible score was 28 points.

Statistical analysis

Normality of variances of the data was tested by the Shapiro–Wilk normality test. Homogeneity of variances was tested by Levene's test when the group variances showed normality. Subsequently, group mean values were compared by Student's t test when the homogeneity of variances was equal, by Welch's t test when the homogeneity of variances was unequal, and by the Mann–Whitney U test when the group variances did not show normality. Differences were considered significant for values of $p < 0.05$. Analyses were conducted using SPSS statistical package (version 22.0; IBM Corp., Armonk, NY).

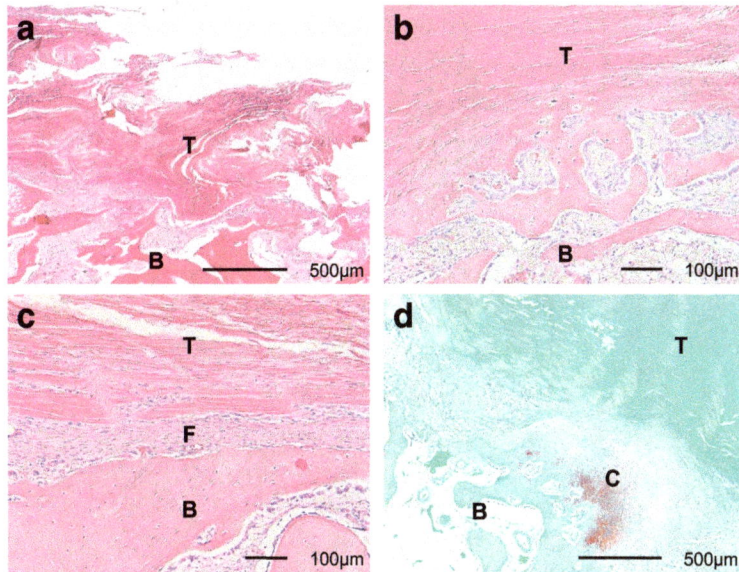

Fig. 2 Histological sections of the tendon graft–bone interface at 4 weeks after ACL reconstruction using CaP-hybridized tendon grafts in rabbits. **a** Soft tissue remaining in the bone tunnel after biomechanical testing (H-E staining; ×40). **b** Direct bonding area at the tendon graft–bone interface (H-E staining; ×100). **c** Indirect bonding area at the tendon graft–bone interface (H-E staining; ×100). Fibrous connective tissue is visible between the tendon graft and the bone. **d** Area of *red* safranin-O-stained GAGs in the cartilage layer at the tendon graft–bone interface (×40). *T* tendon graft, *B* bone, *F* fibrous connective tissue, *C* cartilage layer

Results

Biomechanical testing

The results of the biomechanical testing are summarized in Table 1. There were no significant differences in the ultimate failure load between the suspension group and the coherence group at 2 weeks ($p = 0.290$) or 4 weeks ($p = 0.566$) after surgery. Within each group, the ultimate failure load at 4 weeks was significantly greater than that at 2 weeks (suspension group, $p = 0.005$; coherence group, $p = 0.006$).

Table 1 Biomechanical testing

	Ultimate failure load (N)	
	Suspension group ($n = 9$)	Coherence group ($n = 9$)
2 weeks	$6.2 \pm 3.7^+$	$4.5 \pm 3.0^+$
4 weeks	$21.6 \pm 15.1^+$	$17.2 \pm 10.4^+$
	Stiffness (N/mm)	
	Suspension group ($n = 9$)	Coherence group ($n = 9$)
2 weeks	10.0 ± 8.1	7.5 ± 6.6
4 weeks	15.6 ± 7.1	14.5 ± 7.0
	Stress (N/mm^2)	
	Suspension group ($n = 9$)	Coherence group ($n = 9$)
2 weeks	$0.67 \pm 0.43^+$	$0.48 \pm 0.30^+$
4 weeks	$2.35 \pm 1.28^+$	$1.86 \pm 1.35^+$

Results are shown as mean ± SD
*:Significant difference between groups in the same week ($p < 0.05$)
+:Significant difference between weeks in the same group ($p < 0.05$)

There were no significant differences in stiffness between the suspension group and the coherence group at 2 weeks ($p = 0.484$) or 4 weeks ($p = 0.627$) after surgery. Within each group, there was no significant difference in stiffness between 2 and 4 weeks after surgery (suspension group, $p = 0.058$; coherence group, $p = 0.052$).

There were no significant differences in stress between the suspension group and the coherence group at 2 weeks ($p = 0.310$) or 4 weeks ($p = 0.438$) after surgery. Within each group, the stress at 4 weeks was significantly greater than that at 2 weeks (suspension group, $p = 0.003$; coherence group, $p < 0.001$).

Histological analysis

The results of the histological analysis are summarized in Table 2. The corrected values for the soft tissue remaining within the bone tunnel after the biomechanical testing did not differ significantly between the suspension group and the coherence group at 2 weeks ($p = 0.464$) or 4 weeks ($p = 0.691$) after surgery. In each group, the corrected value for the soft tissue remaining within the bone tunnel at 4 weeks was significantly greater than that at 2 weeks (suspension group, $p = 0.029$; coherence group, $p = 0.001$).

The failure mode did not differ significantly between the suspension group and the coherence group at 2 weeks ($p = 1.000$) or 4 weeks ($p = 1.000$) after surgery. At 2 weeks, seven of the nine specimens in each group failed at the tendon midsubstance, while in the

Table 2 Histological analysis

| | Failure mode (number) | |
	Suspension group (n = 9)	Coherence group (n = 9)
2 weeks	PO: 2/MS: 7	PO: 2/MS: 7
4 weeks	PO: 0/MS: 9	PO: 0/MS: 9
	Soft tissue remaining within the bone tunnel after biomechanical testing (μm²/μm)	
	Suspension group (n = 9)	Coherence group (n = 9)
2 weeks	$77.2 \pm 49.3^+$	$104.0 \pm 95.5^+$
4 weeks	$596.4 \pm 586.7^+$	$434.6 \pm 280.5^+$
	Direct bonding area (%)	
	Suspensor group (n = 5)	Coherence group (n = 5)
2 weeks	$32.1 \pm 12.5^+$	$30.2 \pm 9.9^+$
4 weeks	$51.4 \pm 7.4^+$	$50.9 \pm 7.0^+$
	Width of GAG-stained area (μm²/μm)	
	Suspension group (n = 5)	Coherence group (n = 5)
2 weeks	96.1 ± 12.2	76.2 ± 50.4
4 weeks	143.1 ± 90.3	124.3 ± 33.4
	LTMI score (points)	
	Suspension group (n = 5)	Coherence group (n = 5)
2 weeks	14.4 ± 1.3	14.4 ± 0.9
4 weeks	14.8 ± 1.8	14.2 ± 0.8

Results are shown as mean ± SD
PO pull out, MS tendon midsubstance, LTMI ligament tissue maturation index, GAG glycosaminoglycan
*:Significant difference between groups in the same week ($p < 0.05$)
+:Significant difference between weeks in the same group ($p < 0.05$)

remaining two specimens, the graft appeared to have pulled out of the femoral bone tunnel. At 4 weeks, all specimens in both groups failed at the tendon midsubstance.

The direct bonding area at the tendon–bone interface did not differ significantly between the suspension group and the coherence group at 2 weeks ($p = 0.796$) or 4 weeks ($p = 0.908$) after surgery. Within each group, the direct bonding area at the tendon–bone interface at 4 weeks was significantly greater than that at 2 weeks (suspension group, $p = 0.018$; coherence group, $p = 0.005$).

The width of the GAG-stained area at the tendon–bone interface did not differ significantly between the suspension group and the coherence group at 2 weeks ($p = 0.416$) or 4 weeks ($p = 0.675$) after surgery. Within each group, there was no significant difference in the width of the GAG-stained area at the tendon–bone interface between 2 and 4 weeks after surgery (suspension group, $p = 0.311$; coherence group, $p = 0.113$).

The LTMI scores did not differ significantly between the suspension group and the coherence group at 2 weeks ($p = 0.917$) or 4 weeks ($p = 0.516$) after surgery. The maturation of the tendon grafts was similar in the suspension and coherence groups at both 2 and 4 weeks

after surgery. Within each group, there was no significant difference in the LTMI scores between 2 and 4 weeks after surgery (suspension group, $p = 0.676$; coherence group, $p = 0.724$).

Discussion

In our study, the differences in placement of CaP-hybridized tendon grafts between the suspension and coherence groups did not influence the tendon-to-bone healing outcomes at 4 weeks after ACL reconstruction in rabbits. The results of the biomechanical testing and histological analysis did not differ significantly between the two groups at either 2 or 4 weeks after surgery. In rabbits, CaP-hybridized tendon grafts were shown to enhance new bone formation within the femoral bone tunnel in ACL reconstructions for up to 4 weeks after surgery [2, 3]. In the present study, CaP-hybridized tendon grafts bonded well to the femoral bone tunnel when implanted using both tendon graft placement methods examined. Yamazaki et al. [11] reported no significant effects of graft-tunnel diameter disparities of up to 2 mm on ultimate failure load at 3 or 6 weeks after ACL reconstruction in dogs. However, the conditions used in the present study were more severe than those used by Yamazaki et al. because of the shorter graft length in the bone tunnel and the shorter evaluation period.

In both groups, tendon-to-bone healing progressed until our final measurement point at 4 weeks after surgery. The ultimate failure load, stress, soft tissue remaining in the bone tunnel after biomechanical testing, and direct bonding area at the tendon–bone interface at 4 weeks after surgery were significantly greater than those at 2 weeks after surgery in both groups. The increases in the direct bonding area, ultimate failure load, and stress were likely related to the increased time after surgery. The increase in the amount of soft tissue remaining in the bone tunnel after mechanical testing can be considered to reflect the anchoring strength of the direct bond between the tendon graft and the bone, which exceeded the strength of the tendon graft. Previous studies reported the results of pull-out tests after implantation of untreated tendon grafts in the bone tunnels in rabbits and dogs [4, 12]. In these studies, the progressive increase in pull-out strength was correlated with tendon-to-bone healing [4, 12]. As the types of experimental animals and surgical methods in the previous studies differed from those in the present study, their results cannot be compared directly with our findings. However, the results of our study and the previous studies demonstrated that the tendon–bone interface progressively healed with time after graft implantation, regardless of whether untreated or CaP-hybridized tendon grafts were used.

While the width of the GAG-stained area at the tendon–bone interface and the stiffness at 4 weeks were larger than those at 2 weeks in both groups, there were no significant between-group differences in these values. The GAGs in the cartilage layers at ligamentous insertions mainly resist tensile and shear stresses [13–15]. In previous studies, CaP-hybridized tendon grafts promoted a more cartilaginous layer at the tendon–bone interface compared with the untreated group from 6 months to 2 years after ACL reconstruction in goats [5, 16–18]. A longer follow-up period is needed to evaluate the correlation between the formation of cartilaginous tissue and the stiffness at the tendon–bone interface in ACL reconstructions using CaP-hybridized tendon grafts.

The appearance of the grafted tendons was similar in the two groups. Therefore, the maturation of the CaP-hybridized tendon grafts after surgery was similar in the two groups. The tendon graft placement method also had no influence on the maturation of the CaP-hybridized tendon grafts at 4 weeks after ACL reconstruction in rabbits. The maturation of CaP-hybridized tendon grafts may continue to progress for more than 4 weeks after surgery. In addition, the grafts in two of the nine specimens in each group failed by pulling out

from the femoral bone tunnel histologically at 2 weeks postoperatively. At 4 weeks after surgery, all specimens in both groups failed in the tendon midsubstance histologically. In previous reports [4, 12], all tendon grafts failed macroscopically by pulling out of the bone tunnel from 2 to 8 weeks after surgery in dogs and at 3 weeks after surgery in rabbits. As we soaked the whole tendon grafts in the CaP solutions in this study, the CaP hybridization may influence the mechanical properties of the tendon grafts.

Clinically, our results suggest that when CaP-hybridized tendon grafts are used in ACL reconstruction, it is not necessary to change the postoperative rehabilitation protocols during the early postoperative period based on the tendon graft placement method because equal tendon-to-bone healing occurs regardless of the placement method used. In addition, mismatches between the tendon graft and the bone tunnel diameter may not influence tendon-to-bone healing when CaP-hybridized tendon grafts are used.

The present study had several limitations. Bonding of the tendon–bone interface may differ between animals and humans because of between-species differences in osteogenesis. In addition, postoperative evaluations were only performed in the early postoperative period after ACL reconstruction in this study. A longer follow-up time is needed to clarify the long-term effects of the tendon graft placement methods that we tested. We also did not compare the CaP-hybridized tendon grafts with untreated tendon grafts. However, the effectiveness of CaP-hybridized tendon grafts was previously demonstrated and compared with untreated grafts for up to 4 weeks after ACL reconstruction in rabbits [2, 3].

Conclusions

The tendon-to-bone healing in both groups progressed until the study endpoint at 4 weeks after surgery. There was no influence of the tendon graft placement method on the tendon-to-bone healing at 4 weeks after ACL reconstruction with CaP-hybridized tendon grafts in rabbits, as evaluated by biomechanical testing and histological analysis. The CaP-hybridized tendon grafts anchored equally in the bone tunnel after both placement methods, likely through enhancement of osteogenesis by the CaP hybridization. The tendon graft placement method may not influence tendon-to-bone healing in ACL reconstruction when CaP-hybridized tendon grafts are used.

Abbreviations
ACL: Anterior cruciate ligament; CaP: Calcium phosphate;
GAG: Glycosaminoglycan

Acknowledgements
None.

Funding

This work was supported by a Grant-in-Aid for Encouragement for Young Scientists from Ibaraki Prefectural University of Health Sciences, 2014.

Authors' contributions

HM, HN, and MS conceived the study and participated in its design and coordination. HM performed the animal experiments and mechanical testing and drafted the manuscript. HM, SN, and HN carried out the histological analyses. MS, SN, and HN interpreted the data and participated in drafting the text and figures. All authors read and approved the final manuscript.

Competing interests

The authors declare that they have no competing interests.

Author details

[1]Department of Orthopaedic Surgery, Ibaraki Prefectural University of Health Sciences, 4669-2 Ami, Inashiki-gun, Ibaraki 300-0394, Japan. [2]Department of Agriculture, Ibaraki University, 3-21-1 Chuo, Ami, Ibaraki 300-0393, Japan. [3]Department of Orthopaedic Surgery, Tsukuba Gakuen Hospital, 2573-1 Kamiyokoba, Tsukuba, Ibaraki 305-0854, Japan.

References

1. Taguchi T, Kishida A, Akashi M. Hydroxyapatite formation on/in hydrogels using a novel alternate soaking process. Chem Lett. 1998;8:711–2.
2. Mutsuzaki H, Sakane M, Nakajima H, Ito A, Hattori S, Miyanaga Y, Ochiai N, Tanaka J. Calcium-phosphate-hybridized tendon directly promotes regeneration of tendon-bone insertion. J Biomed Mater Res. 2004;70A:319–27.
3. Mutsuzaki H, Sakane M, Ito A, Nakajima H, Hattori S, Miyanaga Y, Tanaka J, Ochiai N. The interaction between osteoclast-like cells and osteoblasts mediated by nanophase calcium phosphate-hybridized tendons. Biomaterials. 2005;26:1027–34.
4. Grana WA, Egle DM, Mahnken R, Goodhart CW. An analysis of autograft fixation after anterior cruciate ligament reconstruction in a rabbit model. Am J Sports Med. 1994;22:344–51.
5. Mutsuzaki H, Sakane M, Fujie H, Hattori S, Kobayashi H, Ochiai N. Effect of calcium phosphate-hybridized tendon graft on biomechanical behavior in anterior cruciate ligament reconstruction in a goat model: novel technique for improving tendon-bone healing. Am J Sports Med. 2011;39:1059–66.
6. Mutsuzaki H, Kanamori A, Ikeda K, Hioki S, Kinugasa T, Sakane M. Effect of calcium phosphate-hybridized tendon graft in anterior cruciate ligament reconstruction: a randomized controlled trial. Am J Sports Med. 2012;40:1772–80.
7. Uchio Y, Ochi M, Sumen Y, Adachi N, Kawasaki K, Iwasa J, Katsube K. Mechanical properties of newly developed loop ligament for connection between the EndoButton and hamstring tendons: comparison with Ethibond sutures and Endobutton tape. J Biomed Mater Res. 2002;63:173–81.
8. Wardle NS, Haddad FS. Proximal anterior cruciate ligament avulsion treated with TightRope® fixation device. Ann R Coll Surg Engl. 2012;94:e96–8.
9. Mutsuzaki H, Sakane M, Hattori S, Kobayashi H, Ochiai N. Firm anchoring between a calcium phosphate-hybridized tendon and bone for anterior cruciate ligament reconstruction in a goat model. Biomed Mater. 2009;4:045013.
10. Murray MM, Spindler KP, Ballard P, Welch TP, Zurakowski D, Nanney LB. Enhanced histologic repair in a central wound in the anterior cruciate ligament with a collagen-platelet-rich plasma scaffold. J Orthop Res. 2007;25:1007–17.
11. Yamazaki S, Yasuda K, Tomita F, Minami A, Tohyama H. The effect of graft-tunnel diameter disparity on intraosseous healing of the flexor tendon graft in anterior cruciate ligament reconstruction. Am J Sports Med. 2002;30:498–505.
12. Rodeo SA, Arnoczky SP, Torzilli PA, Hidaka C, Warren RF. Tendon-healing in a bone tunnel. A biomechanical and histological study in the dog. J Bone Joint Surg Am. 1993;75:1795–803.
13. Woo SYL, Maynard J, Butler D, Lyon R, Torzilli P, Akeson W. Ligament, tendon, and joint capsule insertions to bone. In: Woo SLY, Buckwalter JA, editors. Injury and Repair of the Musculoskeletal Soft Tissues. Park Ridge: American Academy of Orthopaedic Surgeons; 1988. p. 133–66.
14. Benjamin M, Ralphs JR. Fibrocartilage in tendons and ligaments—an adaptation to compressive load. J Anat. 1998;193:481–94.
15. Setton LA, Zhu W, Mow VC. The biphasic poroviscoelastic behavior of articular cartilage: role of the surface zone in governing the compressive behavior. J Biomech. 1993;26:581–92.
16. Mutsuzaki H, Sakane M. Calcium phosphate-hybridized tendon graft to enhance tendon-bone healing two years after ACL reconstruction in goats. Sports Med Arthrosc Rehabil Ther Technol. 2011;3:31.
17. Mutsuzaki H, Sakane M, Nakajima H, Ochiai N. Calcium phosphate-hybridised tendon graft to reduce bone-tunnel enlargement after ACL reconstruction in goats. Knee. 2012;19:455–60.
18. Mutsuzaki H, Fujie H, Nakajima H, Fukagawa M, Nomura S, Sakane M. Effect of calcium phosphate hybridized tendon graft in anatomical single-bundle ACL reconstruction in goats. Orthop J Sports Med. 2016;4: 2325967116662653.

4

Clinical outcomes of arthroscopic surgery for external snapping hip

Amrit Shrestha[†], Peng Wu[†], Heng'an Ge and Biao Cheng[*]

Abstract

Background: Studies have reported on the arthroscopic technique for release of external snapping hip syndrome. However, no study with large sample size has been reported for arthroscopic surgery.

Methods: Patients with 229 bilateral and 19 unilateral external snapping hips were treated from January 2012 to June 2013. After locating the contracture position, arthroscopic surgery was performed accordingly. Preoperative and postoperative angles were compared.

Results: Comparing range of motion, all patients obtained higher adduction and flexion angles. At postoperative follow-up of 24 months, the adduction angle was improved from -14.4 ± 5.14 to 35.7 ± 4.21 for type I, from -31.2 ± 5.22 to 31.7 ± 2.84 for type II, from -49.0 ± 3.47 to 21.6 ± 3.43 for type III, and from -64.5 ± 4.65 to 18.3 ± 3.10 for type IV ($P < 0.001$). Similarly, the flexion angle was also significantly improved for all the four types ($P < 0.001$). Excellent ratio and satisfaction rate were good in types I and II. All the clinical features were cured after arthroscopic surgery.

Conclusions: Arthroscopic surgery could be an effective procedure for external snapping hip, due to less operating time, small scar, fast postoperative recovery, and complete contracture release.

Keywords: External snapping hip (ESH), Arthroscopy, Classification, Outcome

Background

Snapping hip syndrome (SHS) is characterized with an audible or palpable snap when flexing or extending the hip and sometimes can be associated with pain [1, 2]. Based on the causes, it can be divided into two types, intra-articular or extra-articular [3]. Intra-articular is mainly referred to the lesion in the joint itself, including synovial chondromatosis, labral tears, and fracture fragments or loose bodies. Extra-articular is the most common form of snapping hip that affects structures including the proximal hamstring tendon, the iliotibial band (ITB), the fascia lata, or the gluteus maximus (GM). Extra-articular is further classified into two types, internal and external snapping hip (ESH). ESH usually occurs with flexion and extension of the hip during exercise when the thick taut posterior border of the ITB moves over the great trochanter (GT) [4, 5].

Commonly, the first step of management of ESH is conservative. This consists of rest, avoiding movements that provoke snapping, stretching exercise, non-steroidal anti-inflammatory drugs (NSAID), and injections of steroid into the trochantric bursa [6, 7]. Once conservative treatment is useless for the contracture, surgical release is necessary. Various open procedures of ITB release have been described, such as Z-plasty, N-plasty with trochanteric bursectomy, ellipsoid resection of the tract over the trochanter, cruciate incision with sutured flaps to the tract, and resection of the posterior half of the tract at the GM insertion [6, 8, 9]. Each of these procedures has had varying degrees of success in the contracture release. Besides, extensive surgical trauma, hematoma formation, wound complication, and slow postoperative recoveries are the drawbacks of these traditional open surgeries (Fig. 1) [10].

Recently, arthroscopic technique to release the ITB in patients with ESH was introduced with excellent contracture release and fast recovery [3, 11]. In 2006, Ilizaliturri et al. [12] was the first to report

* Correspondence: dr_biaocheng@163.com
[†]Equal contributors
Department of Orthopedics, Shanghai Tenth People's Hospital, Tongji University School of Medicine, No. 301 Yanchang Middle Road, Jing'an District, Shanghai 200072, China

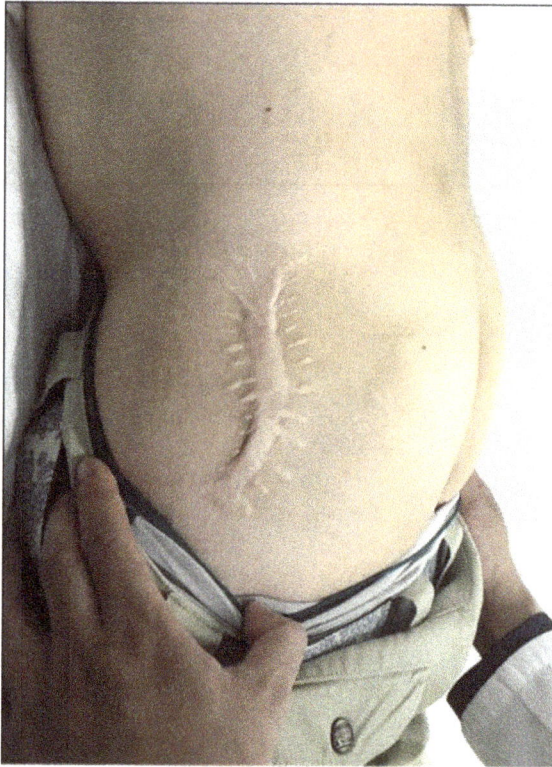

Fig. 1 Patient with hypertropic scar after open surgery. This patient came to our hospital for arthroscopic surgery after failure of open surgery. The huge scarring in the incision can also been seen

Therefore, we conducted this study with large sample size to assess the outcomes for the treatment of ESH patients with different severity according to different types of ESH.

Methods

This study was approved by the Institutional Review Board of Shanghai Tenth People's Hospital affiliated to Tongji University. Each subject provided his or her written informed consent.

Between January 2012 and June 2013, a total of 248 patients (99 male and 149 female) with ESH syndrome treated in our hospital by arthroscopic surgery were included in this study, based on the inclusion criteria. Patients mainly presented themselves with complaints of snapping, clicking or popping sound heard when squatting from the standing position or during jugging at the lateral upper thigh over the area of GT, sometimes accompanied by pain. Furthermore, all patients experienced this disorder from repeated injection on hip during their childhood. Inclusion criteria were set as follows: (1) all patients diagnosed with ESH by history and physical examination, (2) all patients aged between 16 and 40 years old, (3) all patients received the contracture release under arthroscopy, (4) a minimum of 2-year follow-up, and (5) available data for hip assessment. Exclusion criteria were (1) the presence of intra-articular disease, (2) the presence of bony deformities, and (3) the patients with chronic disease or infections.

All patients experienced failed conservative treatment which is used for each patient for a period of at least 3 months before surgery. Passive and active stretching was applied to increase muscle length. Eccentric control is trained to modify neuromuscular control to allow muscle lengthening. Modification of movement patterns (gains) and consistent stretching

arthroscopy surgery for ESH. Since then, various methods of arthroscopy have been reported to treat ESH, and it depends on surgeon's preference and the pathology being treated. With reviewing the published literature online, we found there is no article of arthroscopy to treat ESH in which sample size was more than 100. The exact outcomes for the treatment of ESH under arthroscopy remain unclear.

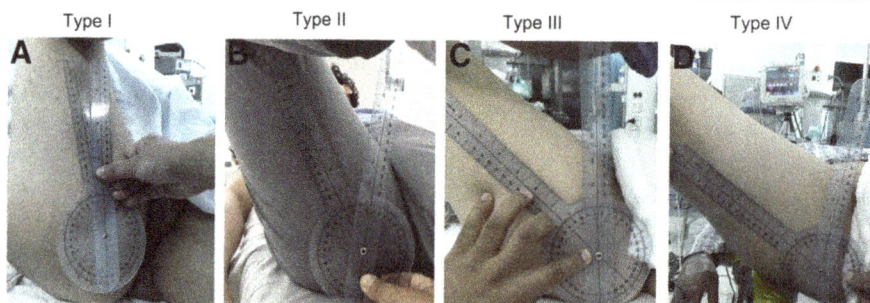

Fig. 2 Range of motions of different types of ESH. **a** Adduction angle is −10° with hip and knee joint in 90° for type I patient. **b** Adduction angle is −35° with hip and knee joint in 90° for type II patient. **c** Adduction angle is −45° with hip and knee joint in 90° for type III patient. **d** Adduction angle is −60° with hip and knee joint in 90° for type IV patient

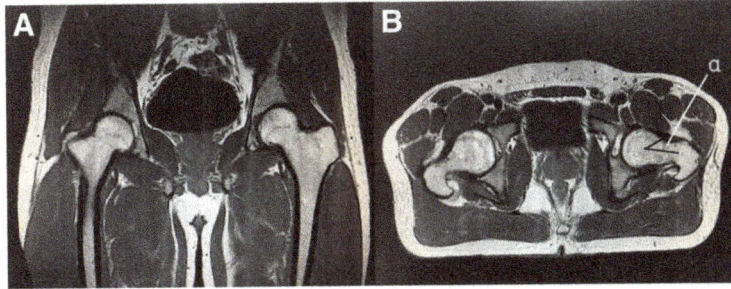

Fig. 3 Differential diagnosis of intra-articular pathologies in MRI images. **a** Normal hip in coronal section. **b** Normal angle *a* showed in transverse section

can be helpful to prevent recurrence. Rest, icing, and anti-inflammatories were advocated to avoid inflammation of tissues.

Before surgery, we performed the preoperative evaluation including physical and radiographic examinations. Preoperative range of motion of hip was measured (Fig. 2). A hip MRI was taken to identify if any bony abnormalities, calcifications, avulsion of GT, loss of joint space, pincer lesions, acetabular dysplasia, or other pathologies were existed (Fig. 3). Based on the angle of adduction with flexion of hip in 90°, patients were graded into four types (Table 1).

All the arthroscopy operations were performed under general anesthesia. Patient was placed in lateral decubitus position on a standard operating table. The hip being flexed, adducted, and internally rotated to the maximum possible degree without traction was the position of the operation. Standard sterile draping was done. Two portals were approximately 3–4 cm apart and were marked over the GT. For portals, oblique incision of 3 mm in size was made on the skin and subcutaneous tissue. A standard 30° scope with a diameter of 4 mm was inserted through proximal portal at a 30° angle (Fig. 4). For good vision of the peritrochanteric space, 40 ml of normal saline was pumped at low pressure during surgery. Through inserting the distal portal saver, the fat and fibrous tissues were cleaned in the operating space. Shaver was removed and radiofrequency

device was inserted through the same distal portal. ITB (Fig. 5) was initially cut partially from both anterior and posterior sides. Only after final exploration was done, the remaining part of ITB was cut completely whereas contractures of GM and tensor fascia lata (TFL) bands were cut completely at once. After the contractures were removed, the leg was slowly moved to through a full range of motion (ROM) of the hip to confirm no clicking sounded. The sciatic nerve should be considered to avoid its injury when operating. In presence of any bleeding point, cautery can be used. Once the surgeon was satisfied, fluid was aspirated and the skin was sutured to close the portals. A similar process was done on the other side. The total duration of operation was approximately 15–20 min.

After surgery, non-steroidal anti-inflammatory drugs and ice therapy were used for pain release for just 3 days postoperatively. The patients were encouraged to flex the hip and knee joint and cross the legs. The rehabilitation program was suggested to achieve rapid recovery until 6 months postoperatively. Postoperative rehabilitation was same for each patient. Patients were evaluated preoperatively and at 3, 6, 12, and 24 months postoperatively. At each follow-up, physical examination and questionnaire were performed. If subjects could obtain completely recovered, they were identified as excellent for type I or an adduction angle of hip that increased >30° for type II, 45° for type III, and 60° for type IV.

All statistical analyses were performed using SPSS 19.0 software. All preoperative and postoperative indices were compared by a paired t test. For ratio comparison, chi-square was performed. A P value <0.05 was considered statistically significant.

Table 1 Classification for the location of contraction of external snapping hip

Type	Angle of hip
I	Hip adduction −5° to −20° with hip and knee joint flexion in 90°
II	Hip adduction −20° to −40° with hip and knee joint flexion in 90°
III	Hip adduction −40° to −60° with hip and knee joint flexion in 90°
IV	Hip adduction >−60° with hip and knee joint flexion in 90°

Results

In this study, there were 248 patients who received arthroscopic surgery to treat ESH (Table 2). The mean

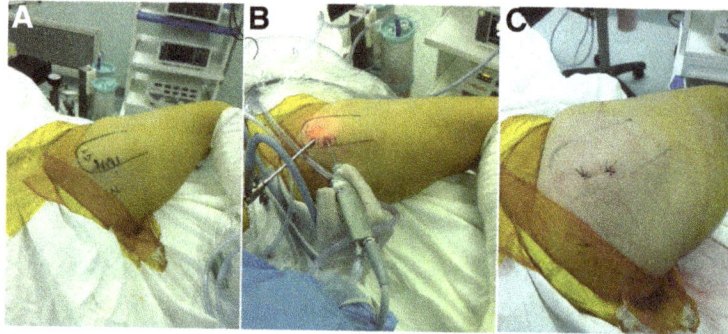

Fig. 4 Operative position and portals. **a** Clinical photograph showing important landmarks: *GT* (greater trochanter), *SN* (sciatic nerve), and position of the two portals. Proximal and distal portals are marked 3–4 cm apart on GT. **b** Standard 30° scope is inserted through the proximal portal in 30° angle. Shaver and radiofrequency device is inserted through the distal portal. **c** After the surgery was completed, the portals are closed

age of the patient was 26 years old (range 8–38 years old) with an average body mass index (BMI) being 22 kg/m^2 (range 17.7–29). Median duration of symptom was 10 years (range 1 month–30 years). Among the 248 patients, 76 were diagnosed with type I, 83 with type II, 55 with type III, and 34 with type IV.

With regard to ROM, compared with preoperative examination, all patients obtained higher adduction and flexion angles (Table 3). At postoperative follow-up of 24 months, the adduction angle and flexion angle were improved for each type of ESH (Fig. 6). We had also compared ROM between males and females; however, there is no difference between different genders (Table 4).

After surgery, no long-term postoperative complications were found in this study, including permanent muscle weakness, neural injury (sciatic nerve), and vascular injury. No infections occurred in the series. Moreover, there was no major swelling, hematomas, and wound dehiscence in these cases. All patients could sit with their legs crossed (Fig. 7). Neither out-toe gait nor Ober's sign was observed, and there were no recurrent contracture of hip abductors, no snapping, and no residual hip pain or gluteal muscle wasting were seen. There are 15 patients with associated knee pain. After surgery, knee pains of these patients were released.

The outcome of surgery in type I and type II were significantly higher than in type III and IV patients ($P < 0.05$) (Table 5). The excellent ratio in type I [76/76 (100%)] and type II [83/83 (100%)] was higher than in type III [51/55 (92.7%)] and type IV [25/34 (73.5%)]. The satisfaction rate was higher in types II [67/69 (97.1%)] and III [53/55 (96.4%)] than in type I [73/76 (96.1%)]. Although the satisfaction

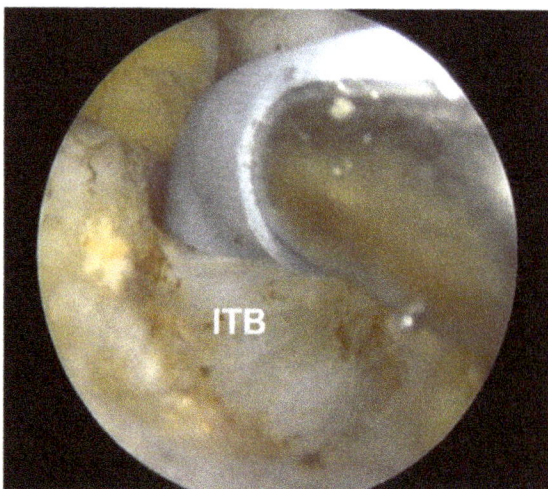

Fig. 5 Intraoperative view. The picture suggests the intraoperative view under arthroscopy showing radiofrequency device cutting the iliotibial band (*ITB*)

Table 2 Baseline characteristics of the included patients

Variables	
No. of patients	248
Age, mean (range)	26 (8–38)
Gender (M/F)	99/149 (40%/60%)
Symptoms	
Knee pain	15 (6.0%)
Snapping	248 (100%)
Duration of symptoms, median (range)	10 years (1 month–30 years)
Total days in hospital, days, mean (range)	6 [1–19]
Length of postoperative hospital stay, days, mean (range)	3 [1–9]
BMI, median (range)	22.0 (17.7–29.0)

M/F, male/female

Table 3 Comparison of pre-operation and post-operation in range of motion

	Adduction		P value	Flexion		P value
	Pre-op	Post-24		Pre-op	Post-24	
Type I	−14.4 ± 5.14	35.7 ± 4.21	<0.001	104.5 ± 9.84	129.5 ± 6.72	<0.001
Type II	−31.2 ± 5.22	31.7 ± 2.84	<0.001	99 ± 5.03	125.6 ± 5.89	<0.001
Type III	−49.0 ± 3.47	21.6 ± 3.43	<0.001	82.9 ± 6.60	122.5 ± 5.12	<0.001
Type IV	−64.5 ± 4.65	18.3 ± 3.10	<0.001	68.1 ± 8.02	114.5 ± 5.75	<0.001

Pre-op pre-operation, *post-24* 24 months follow-up postoperatively

rate of type IV [32/34 (94.1%)] is comparatively lower than in other three types, patient compliance were very good and happy with the results.

Discussion

In the current study, we included a total of 248 patients to investigate the outcomes of treatment of ESH under arthroscopy. After surgery, we found all patients received the contracture released. Although outcomes in types I and II are significantly higher than those in types III and IV, there is no difference with the patients' satisfaction in four types.

ESH syndrome was first reported by Valderrama in 1969 [13]. Although multiple factors played roles in the development of ESH, the most common factor was a history of repeated injections in the buttocks, based on the previous reports [14, 15]. ESH is described as hip snapping during moving the hip, mainly due to the thickening of the posterior part of ITB or the anterior border of the GM sliding over the GT [4]. It is commonly seen in athletes like ballet dancers, runners, and soccer players [4]. The pathological changes result in limitation of hip movement with abnormal gait [10, 16, 17]. In some cases, anatomical deformities like oblique pelvis, compensatory scoliosis, and bilateral dislocation of the hip joints are seen [15, 18, 19]. Other impairments of daily activities include being unable to sit with the legs crossed, difficulty in tying shoe laces, and, for some, difficulty in driving. Inflammation of the underlying bursa caused by sliding of the ITB over the GT results in painful snapping to the patient [4, 9].

Commonly, a program of conservative management for systematic ESH is applied first. In case that conservative therapy failed to treat with ESH, a variety of surgical techniques are attempted with variable success. Zoltan et al. [20] performed open procedure with significantly improved or relieved symptoms. Zhao et al. [21] also used an open surgical technique to treat with ESH. After follow-up, they showed that operative management was effective in patients at all levels and suggested that either conservative or operative management should be conducted as early as possible. White et al. [2] reported open procedure for ESH in 16 patients with improvement of the pain and snapping in 14 patients. Therefore, open surgery for ESH could obtain good release of symptom for ESH.

However, there are many complications for open techniques, including large scar, wound complication, and

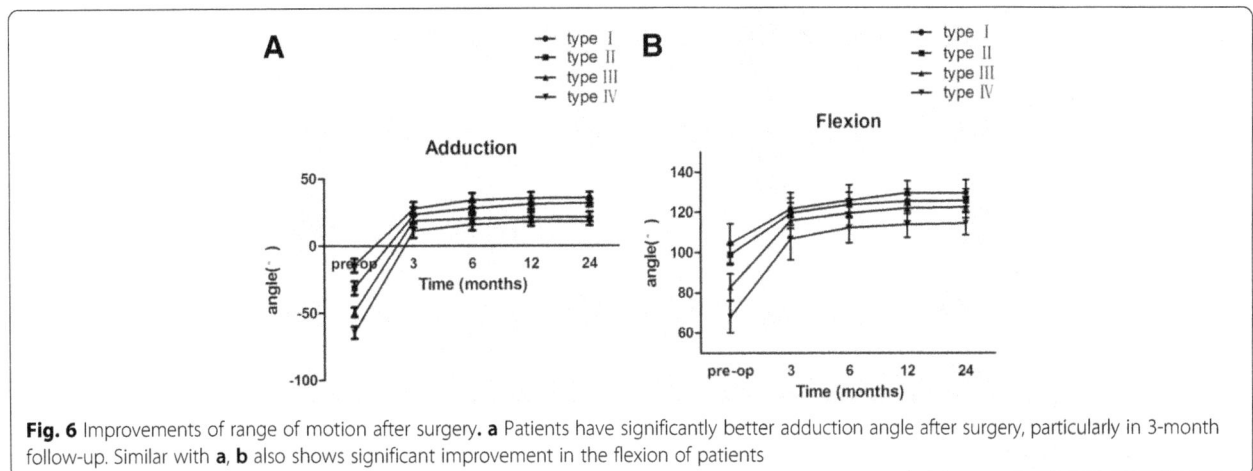

Fig. 6 Improvements of range of motion after surgery. **a** Patients have significantly better adduction angle after surgery, particularly in 3-month follow-up. Similar with **a**, **b** also shows significant improvement in the flexion of patients

Table 4 Comparison of range of motion post-operatively according to gender

	Adduction		P-value	Flexion		P-value
	Male	Female		Male	Female	
Type I	35.2 ± 4.23	35.8 ± 4.20	> 0.05	130.5 ± 7.74	128.9 ± 6.43	> 0.05
Type II	32.3 ± 2.92	31.4 ± 2.76	> 0.05	124.8 ± 5.72	126.7 ± 5.99	> 0.05
Type III	21.9 ± 3.42	21.5 ± 3.49	> 0.05	121.5 ± 5.21	123.6 ± 5.08	> 0.05
Type IV	18.6 ± 3.35	18.2 ± 3.02	> 0.05	113.8 ± 6.02	114.7 ± 5.69	> 0.05

slow recovery. Arthroscopic release of the ESH has become more common. Ilizaliturri et al. [22] reported that a total of 6 patients obtained complete resolution of symptoms after arthroscopic release of the iliopsoas tendon. Flanum et al. [23] showed that 6 patients with arthroscopic release at the lesser trochanter received 100% resolution of symptoms. El Bitar et al. [24], in their study with 55 patients, showed that 82% patients had excellent results. Although these studies showed good results in arthroscopic release for ESH, small sample size cannot be ignored as shortages for these articles. Therefore, we perform this study with over 200 patients to investigate the role of arthroscopic surgery for ESH. And the result of the current study was comparable to that of the surgical procedures in the previous studies.

Some limitations should be mentioned. First, inherent bias of retrospective analysis might be inevitable. Moreover, a lack of effective assessment for ESH resulted in difficulty in comparison with other studies. Finally, comparison between open and arthroscopic surgery was not performed in this study.

Conclusions

In the present study, arthroscopic surgery could be an effective procedure for ESH, due to less operating time, small scar, fast postoperative recovery, and complete contracture release. These promising results of arthroscopic treatment of ESH need randomized trial to compare with open procedures.

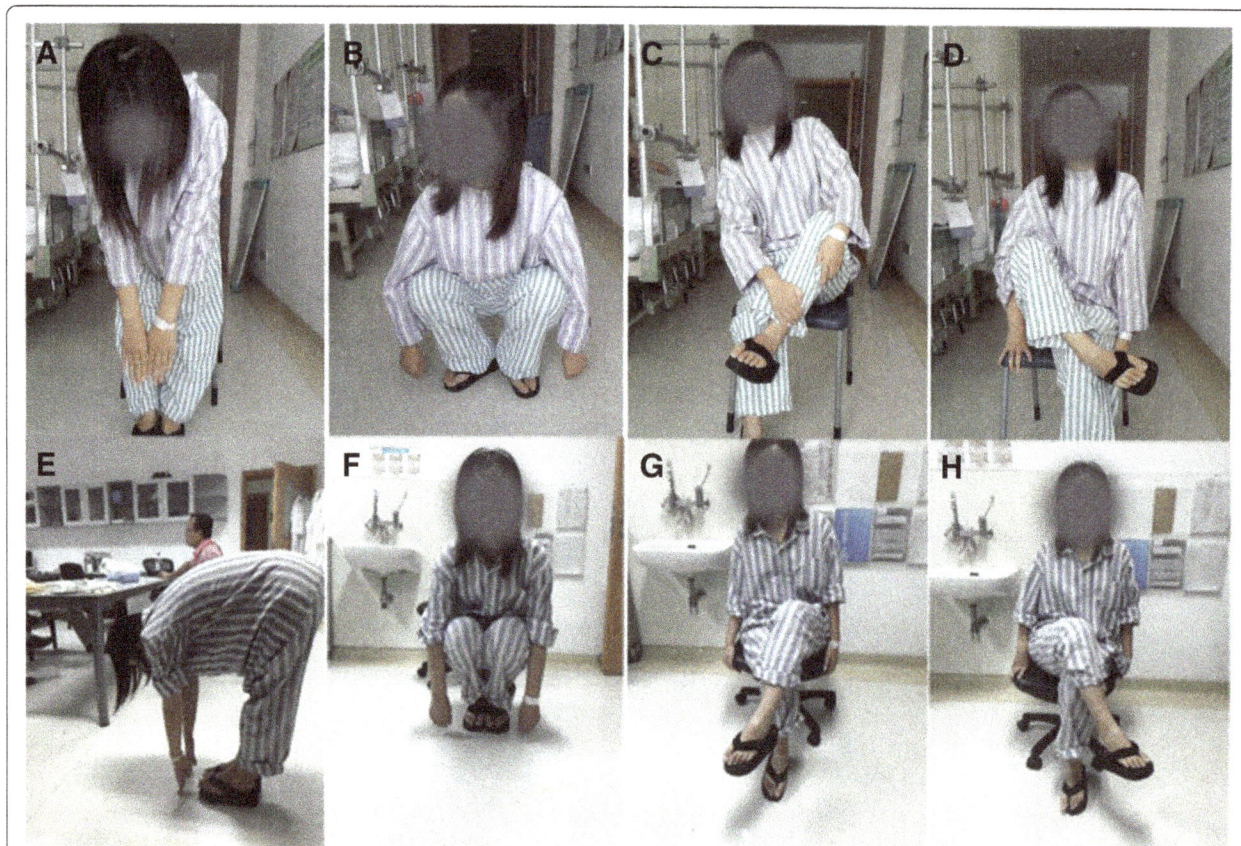

Fig. 7 Comparison of range of motion between preoperative and postoperative management. **a** Before surgery, the patient is unable to touch the big toe while flexing the spine with the knee straight. **b** Fixed hip abduction and external rotation are seen during crouching leading to frog leg position. **c**, **d** The patient is unable to sit with her legs crossed. **e** After arthroscopic surgery, the patient is able to touch the big toe while flexing the spine with the knee straight. **f** Frog leg deformity is corrected; the patient can crouch with the both knees together. **g**, **h** The patient is able to sit with her legs crossed

Abbreviations

BMI: Body mass index; ESH: External snapping hip; GM: Gluteus maximus; GT: Great trochanter; ITB: Iliotibial band; NSAID: Non-steroidal anti-inflammatory drugs; ROM: Range of motion; SHS: Snapping hip syndrome

Acknowledgements

We thank Dr. Jie Hua for editing the manuscript.

Funding

The study was supported by the grants from the Natural Science Foundation of China (Nos. 81372005 and 81401851) and Scientific Research Project supported by the Shanghai Committee of Science and Technology (No. 13DZ194808).

Authors' contributions

AS collected the clinical data, performed the statistical analysis, and drafted the manuscript. PW helped in collecting the clinical data and participated in the design of the study. HG participated in the statistical analysis. BC conceived of the study and participated in its design. All authors read and approved the final manuscript.

Competing interests

The authors declare that they have no competing interests.

References

1. Polesello GC, Queiroz MC, Domb BG, Ono NK, Honda EK. Surgical technique: endoscopic gluteus maximus tendon release for external snapping hip syndrome. Clin Orthop Relat Res. 2013;471:2471–6.
2. White RA, Hughes MS, Burd T, Hamann J, Allen WC. A new operative approach in the correction of external coxa saltans: the snapping hip. Am J Sports Med. 2004;32:1504–8.
3. Kunac N, Trsek D, Medancic N, Starcevic D, Haspl M. Endoscopic treatment of the external snapping hip syndrome: surgical technique and report of two cases. Acta Clin Croat. 2012;51:661–6.
4. Allen WC, Cope R. Coxa saltans: the snapping hip revisited. J Am Acad Orthop Surg. 1995;3:303–8.
5. Kotha VK, Reddy R, Reddy MV, Moorthy RS, Kishan TV. Congenital gluteus maximus contracture syndrome—a case report with review of imaging findings. J Radiol Case Rep. 2014;8:32–7.
6. Provencher MT, Hofmeister EP, Muldoon MP. The surgical treatment of external coxa saltans (the snapping hip) by Z-plasty of the iliotibial band. Am J Sports Med. 2004;32:470–6.
7. Idjadi J, Meislin R. Symptomatic snapping hip: targeted treatment for maximum pain relief. Phys Sportsmed. 2004;32:25–31.
8. Brignall CG, Stainsby GD. The snapping hip. Treatment by Z-plasty. J Bone Joint Surg (Br). 1991;73:253–4.
9. Larsen E, Johansen J. Snapping hip. Acta Orthop Scand. 1986;57:168–70.
10. Liu G, Du J, Yang S, Zheng Q, Li J. A retrospective analysis of the gluteal muscles contracture and discussion of the relative problems. J Tongji Med Univ. 2000;20:70–1.
11. Ilizaliturri Jr VM, Camacho-Galindo J. Endoscopic treatment of snapping hips, iliotibial band, and iliopsoas tendon. Sports Med Arthrosc. 2010;18:120–7.
12. Ilizaliturri Jr VM, Martinez-Escalante FA, Chaidez PA, Camacho-Galindo J. Endoscopic iliotibial band release for external snapping hip syndrome. Arthroscopy. 2006;22:505–10.
13. Fernandez de Valderrama JA, Esteve de Miguel R. Fibrosis of the gluteus maximus: a cause of limited flexion and adduction of the hip in children. Clin Orthop Relat Res. 1981;(156):67-78.
14. Mehta MH. Bilateral congenital contracture of the ilio-tibial tract. J Bone Joint Surg (Br). 1972;54:532–4.
15. Cai JH, Gan LF, Zheng HL, Li H. Iliac hyperdense line: a new radiographic sign of gluteal muscle contracture. Pediatr Radiol. 2005;35:995–7.
16. Gao GX. Idiopathic contracture of the gluteus maximus muscle in children. Arch Orthop Trauma Surg. 1988;107:277–9.
17. Liu G, Yang S, Du J, Zheng Q, Shao Z, Yang C. Treatment of severe gluteal muscle contracture in children. J Huazhong Univ Sci Technolog Med Sci. 2008;28:171–3.
18. Dini GM, Ferreira LM. Capsular contracture in gluteal implant patients. Plast Reconstr Surg. 2006;117:1070–1.
19. Ni B, Li M. The effect of children's gluteal muscle contracture on skeleton development. Sichuan Da Xue Xue Bao Yi Xue Ban. 2007;38:657–9. 677.
20. Zoltan DJ, Clancy Jr WG, Keene JS. A new operative approach to snapping hip and refractory trochanteric bursitis in athletes. Am J Sports Med. 1986;14:201–4.
21. Zhao CG, He XJ, Lu B, Li HP, Wang D, Zhu ZZ. Classification of gluteal muscle contracture in children and outcome of different treatments. BMC Musculoskelet Disord. 2009;10:34.
22. Ilizaliturri Jr VM, Villalobos Jr FE, Chaidez PA, Valero FS, Aguilera JM. Internal snapping hip syndrome: treatment by endoscopic release of the iliopsoas tendon. Arthroscopy. 2005;21:1375–80.
23. Flanum ME, Keene JS, Blankenbaker DG, Desmet AA. Arthroscopic treatment of the painful "internal" snapping hip: results of a new endoscopic technique and imaging protocol. Am J Sports Med. 2007;35:770–9.
24. El Bitar YF, Stake CE, Dunne KF, Botser IB, Domb BG. Arthroscopic iliopsoas fractional lengthening for internal snapping of the hip: clinical outcomes with a minimum 2-year follow-up. Am J Sports Med. 2014;42:1696–703.

Open surgical implantation of a viable cryopreserved placental membrane after decompression and neurolysis of common peroneal nerve

E. Rodriguez-Collazo[1] and Y. Tamire[2*]

Abstract

Background: The purpose of this study is to report on the rehabilitative outcomes associated with common peroneal nerve (CPN) decompression and neurolysis revision when performed with open surgical implantation of a viable cryopreserved placental membrane (vCPM).

Methods: Seven patients who underwent secondary CPN decompression and neurolysis with open surgical implantation of a viable cryopreserved placental membrane (vCPM) after previously failed surgery without vCPM utilization were identified through a retrospective medical record review and outcomes were analyzed. Primary mechanism of injury, severity of symptoms at time of referral, pre-operative and post-operative evaluations on edema with ultrasound, Medical Research Council (MRC) scale for motor strength, range of motion, nerve conduction velocity (NCV), and electromyography (EMG) were analyzed.

Results: Five patients (71.4%) achieved full recovery of motor function MRC grade 5/5, and the remaining two patients achieved MRC grade 4/5. At the 7-month follow-up visit, NCV tests indicated improved conduction velocity and normal amplitude for all 7 patients, and all patients demonstrated proper gait pattern with a return to normal activities of daily living. There were no vCPM-related adverse events.

Conclusions: The use of vCPM wrap as an adjunct to surgical repairs of CPN injuries may contribute to positive clinical outcomes.

Keywords: Common peroneal nerve injury, Placental membranes, Surgical nerve repair, Foot drop

Background

The common peroneal nerve (CPN) is the most frequently injured peripheral nerve in the lower extremity [1–4]. Due to its superficial position on the lateral aspect of the knee and its direct contact with the fibular neck, CPN is vulnerable to injuries secondary to blunt or penetrating trauma, internal or external compression, stretch, contusion, fracture of adjacent bones, lacerations, or other medical conditions [1–4]. CPN neuropathy typically presents with foot drop, motor function deficit, and sensory symptoms, such as pain and paresthesia [3, 5, 6].

Majority of these symptoms can resolve spontaneously or through conservative rehabilitative therapy, however, surgical interventions such as decompression, nerve suture, nerve grafting, and nerve or tendon transfer may be necessary to restore nerve and muscle functions [4, 7, 8].

Although surgical decompression is typically successful, there is a risk of re-entrapment and the development of neuropathy and chronic pain that can contribute to life-long morbidity. The purpose of this report is to examine, through a case review, the rehabilitative outcomes associated with CPN decompression and neurolysis revision when performed with open surgical implantation of a viable cryopreserved placental membrane (vCPM) (Grafix®-PRIME, Osiris Therapeutics, Inc., Columbia, MD).

* Correspondence: ytamire@osiris.com
[2]Medical Science Liaison, Osiris Therapeutics, Inc., 7015 Albert Einstein Drive, Columbia, MD 21046, USA
Full list of author information is available at the end of the article

Methods

Population

Following expedited institutional review board approval, Saint Joseph Hospital Protocol #2016-30, data were obtained through a retrospective medical record review of patients who underwent secondary CPN decompression and neurolysis by a single surgeon at the Department of Surgery at Chicago Foot & Ankle Deformity Corrections Center. A total of seven subjects (four males, three females) who had undergone previously failed CPN decompression were identified for analysis. The collection of de-identified data sets included the primary mechanism of injury, severity of symptoms at time of referral, pre-operative and post-operative evaluations on edema with ultrasound, Medical Research Council (MRC) scale for motor strength, range of motion, nerve conduction velocity (NCV), and electromyography (EMG). Descriptive statistics (mean, standard deviation, etc) were used for data analysis.

Description of viable cryopreserved placental allograft

vCPM is a point-of-care allograft that retains an intact extracellular matrix, resident growth factors, and endogenous neonatal mesenchymal stem cells, fibroblasts, and epithelial cells native to the fresh tissue through a proprietary cryopreservation method [9–11]. vCPM is fully tested according to FDA and AATB requirements and has a 2-year shelf life at −80 °C [12]. vCPMs are ~100-μM-thin membranes that are conforming and self-adherent to other tissues. Human placental membranes have been reported to support natural tissue repair and to reduce inflammation, pain, and scar formation [13, 14]. These properties, make them attractive for various soft tissue reconstructive procedures including microsurgical CPN repairs where minimizing postoperative inflammation, pain, and adhesion formation are critical for successful clinical outcome (Fig. 1a).

Surgical technique

All procedures were carried out after induction of general anesthesia with surgeon's utilization of 3.5 loupe magnification for appropriate field visualization. The patients were positioned in lateral decubitus with the affected limb flexed at approximately 35°. After site preparation and draping, a 3-cm lazy "S" shaped transverse incision was made 3 cm distally and 2 cm medially to the fibular head with a 10-blade scalpel. Using Metzenbaum scissors, the incision was carried down to the subcutaneous tissue while protecting vital structures and nerves. Careful blunt dissection by Metzenbaum scissors was performed to separate the muscular fascia and expose the CPN. The CPN was traced around the fibular neck while excising the fascia of the anterior and lateral compartments to decompress the deep peroneal and superficial nerves. A portable nerve stimulator (Checkpoint®; NDI Medical), set at 0.02–2 mA for 2–3 s, was used to locate areas of severe nerve scarring. Microsurgical instruments were used to perform longitudinal and circumferential epineurotomy. Internal and external neurolysis was performed until the bands of Fontana were observed in the fascicles. Over the area of fascicular damage, vCPM allograft was applied (Fig. 1a). Then, the CPN was wrapped with a collagen nerve conduit (Fig. 1b) (NeuraGen®; LifeSciences Corporation). Additional nerve stimulation was performed to ensure no compression was caused by the graft or the conduit. The conduit was transposed laterally and was sutured to the adjacent lateral subcutaneous tissue. The subcutaneous tissue was reapproximated in a layered fashion using a 3-0 Vicryl sutures, and the skin was closed using skin staples. A semicompressive dressing was applied over the incision site, and affected lower extremity was placed in surgical shoe. Patients were placed into immobilization of the affected lower extremity and were provided with post-operative instructions for gradual progression into full weight-bearing ambulation as tolerated.

Results

Seven patients, three females and four males, were included in this study. The average patient age at the time of surgery was 48 years (range 38–59) (Table 1). Patients

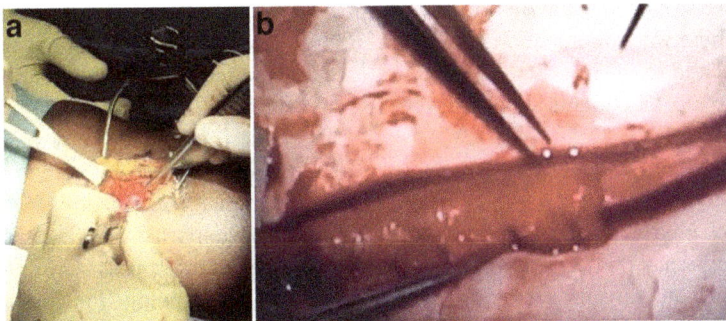

Fig. 1 a Placement of vCPM around the CPN prior to nerve wrap. **b** Nerve wrap placement after superficial PN internal neurolysis

Table 1 Mechanism of injury and treatment outcome summary

Patient	Mechanism of injury	Pre-op disposition	Pre-op		Post-op	
			ROM	MRC grade	ROM	MRC grade
1	Sprained foot	- Neurapraxia - Latency - Foot drop	DF: 5 PF:15	1/5	DF: 10 PF:20	5/5
2	Sprained foot	- Neurapraxia - Latency - Foot drop	DF: 8 PF:15	1/5	DF: 13 PF:20	4/5
3	TKA	- Neurapraxia - Latency - Foot drop	DF: 3 PF:10	1/5	DF: 8 PF:15	5/5
4	Trauma to knee	- Neurapraxia - Latency - Foot drop	DF:10 PF:15	1/5	DF:15 PF:20	5/5
5	TKA	- Neurapraxia - Latency - Foot drop	DF: 7 PF:15	1/5	DF: 12 PF:20	4/5
6	Sprained foot and ankle	- Neurapraxia - Latency - Foot drop	DF: 7 PF: 5	1/5	DF: 12 PF: 10	5/5
7	Sprained foot and ankle	- Neurapraxia - Latency - Foot drop	DF: 5 PF:10	1/5	DF: 10 PF:15	5/5
Mean ± SD	N/A	N/A	DF: 6.43 ± 2.30 PF: 12.14 ± 3.93	1	DF: 11.43 ± 2.30 PF: 17.14 ± 3.93	4.71 ± 0.49

ROM range of motion, *TKA* total knee arthroplasty, *MRC* Medical Research Council, *DF* dorsiflexion, *PF* plantar flexion, *pre-op* pre-operative, *post-op* post-operative, *SD* standard deviation, *N/A* not applicable

presented with foot drop, neurapraxia, and decreased latency. Initial CPN decompressions were attributed to foot and ankle sprain ($n = 4$), total knee arthroplasty ($n = 2$), and trauma to the knee ($n = 1$). Preoperatively, all patients had muscle weakness (MRC grade 1/5). After the revision surgery, 5 (71.4%) of the 7 patients had 100% recovered motor function, MRC grade 5/5, and 2 patients achieved MRC grade of 4/5 (80% recovery) in a mean time of 7 months. Additionally, active range of motion showed a 5-degree increase for both dorsiflexion and plantarflexion in all patients compared to pre-operative assessment. Perineural edema at presentation was resolved by week 12, postoperatively. NCV indicated improved conduction velocity and normal amplitude in each of the cases. All patients resumed proper gait pattern with a return to activity levels of daily living demonstrated prior to injurious event. There were no infections or other adverse events reported related to the use of vCPM. At an average of 16-month follow-up, all patients showed no recurrence of symptoms.

Discussion

Although majority of CPN injuries can resolve spontaneously, surgical interventions may be necessary to resolve debilitating motor dysfunction, sensory loss, and pain. Surgical manipulation of peripheral nerves, however, is frequently followed by extraneural scar formation and epineural thickening that may lead to chronic compression [15, 16]. The presence of perineural and intraneural scarring and fibrotic adhesions causes physiological obstruction to nerve conduction with subsequent edema and hemorrhage that may interfere with functional recovery of the nerve [15–19]. Furthermore, compared to the outcomes of other peripheral nerves, surgical outcomes of CPN injuries are discouraging [20, 21]. After assessing 28 studies, George et al. reported that functional outcomes of M4 or M5 were obtained in 80% of patients undergoing neurolysis [22]. A 32-year retrospective analysis of 318 patients with knee-level common peroneal nerve lesions by Kim et al. reported that external CPN neurolysis was carried out in 121 (38%) of their patients of which 88% experienced functional outcomes of grade 3 or higher [15]. Seidel et al. also reported that a functionally useful result (M ≥ 4) was produced in 72% of the cases having either external or internal neurolysis and in 28% of the cases with nerve graft [23].

Prevention or reduction of scar and adhesion formation by minimizing postoperative fibrosis is imperative for optimal functional recovery [5, 16, 18, 19]. Various animal models have reported significantly less perineural adhesions and fibrosis in nerves wrapped in human amniotic membrane following neurorrhapy in comparison to control [13, 14]. Based on anti-inflammatory, angiogenic, antimicrobial, and anti-fibrotic properties of placental membranes that may contribute to minimizing postoperative inflammation, pain, and adhesion formation, vCPM allograft was selected for evaluation as an adjunct to augment CPN decompression and neurolysis revision [16–19]. The present study reported the rehabilitative outcomes associated with CPN decompression and neurolysis revision when performed with open surgical implantation of a viable cryopreserved placental membrane. Compared to the outcomes of the previous surgical interventions in these patients, all patients achieved motor function improvement, nerve conduction velocity, and normal amplitude, along with full recovery from foot drop and returned to daily living activities when CPN decompression and neurolysis were in conjunction with the implantation of vCPM. These outcomes were observed in an average of 7 months with no recurrence of symptoms for an average of 16 months compared to unresolved foot drop, neurapraxia, and decreased latency for an average of 16 months after previous unsuccessful CPN decompression and neurolysis.

Limitations of this case series include its retrospective nature, small sample size, and lack of a control group.

Conclusions

Due to the risk of lifelong morbidity associated with common nerve repair procedures, the efficacy of surgical technique and careful selection and use of an accompanying allograft is paramount. The present study suggests that the use of vCPM wrap as an adjunct to CPN surgery can deliver encouraging results in the recovery of foot drop due to CPN injuries. vCPM may contribute to the natural process of nerve regeneration and repair, with clinical outcomes demonstrated by improved muscle function, nerve conduction velocity, recovery from foot drop, and return to normal activities of daily living in a shorter period.

Abbreviations
AATB: The American Association of Tissue Banks; CPN: Common peroneal nerve; DF: Dorsiflexion; EMG: Electromyography; FDA: Food and Drug Administration; MRC: Medical Research Council; NCV: Nerve conduction velocity; PF: Plantar flexion; Post-Op: Post-operative; Pre-Op: Pre-operative; ROM: Range of motion; SD: Standard deviation; TKA: Total knee arthroplasty; vCPM: Viable cryopreserved placental membrane

Acknowledgements
The authors would like to thank Alla Danilkovitch and Georgina Michael of Osiris Therapeutics, Inc., for their editorial support.

Funding
There was no funding required to do data collection, analysis, and writing of the manuscript.

Authors' contributions
ER performed data collection and analyzed and interpreted the patient data. YT performed back ground research for topic and prepared the manuscript for submission. Both ER and YT were major contributors in writing the manuscript. All authors read and approved the final manuscript.

Competing interests
Dr. Edgardo R Rodriguez-Collazo has declared no competing interest. Yeabsera G Tamire is a member of Medical Affairs at Osiris Therapeutics, Inc.

Author details
[1]Chicago Foot & Ankle Deformity Corrections Center, Department of Surgery Adults & Pediatric Ilizarov Correction, Microsurgical Limb Reconstruction, Presence Saint Joseph Hospital, Chicago, Illinois, USA. [2]Medical Science Liaison, Osiris Therapeutics, Inc., 7015 Albert Einstein Drive, Columbia, MD 21046, USA.

References
1. Wood MB. Peroneal nerve repair: surgical results. Clin Orthop Relat Res. 1991;267:206–10.
2. Lee SK, Wolfe SW. Peripheral nerve injury and repair. J Am Acad Orthop Surg. 1999;8:243–52. doi:10.1097/00006534-198804000-00086.
3. Kouyoumdjian JA. Peripheral nerve injuries: a retrospective survey of 456 cases. Muscle Nerve. 2006;34:785–8.
4. Giuffre JL, Bishop AT, Spinner RJ, Levy BA, Shin AY. Symposium: complex knee ligament surgery partial tibial nerve transfer to the tibialis anterior motor branch to treat peroneal nerve injury after knee trauma. 2011.
5. Grinsell D, Keating CP. Peripheral nerve reconstruction after injury: a review of clinical and experimental therapies. Biomed Res Int. 2014;2014.
6. Ramanan M, Chandran KN. Common peroneal nerve decompression. ANZ J Surg. 2011;81(10):707–12.
7. Emamhadi M, Bakhshayesh B, Andalib S. Surgical outcome of foot drop caused by common peroneal nerve injuries; is the glass half full or half empty? Acta Neurochir. 2016;158(6):1133–1138.
8. Baima J, Krivickas L. Evaluation and treatment of peroneal neuropathy. Curr Rev Musculoskelet Med. 2008;1:147–53. doi:10.1007/s12178-008-9023-6.
9. Duan-Arnold Y, Uveges TE, Gyurdieva A, Johnson A, Danilkovitch A. Angiogenic potential of cryopreserved amniotic membrane is enhanced through retention of all tissue components in their native state. Adv Wound Care (New Rochelle). 2015;4:513–22. doi:10.1089/wound.2015.0638.
10. Duan-Arnold Y, Gyurdieva A, Johnson A, Jacobstein DA, Danilkovitch A. Soluble factors released by endogenous viable cells enhance the antioxidant and chemoattractive activities of cryopreserved amniotic membrane. Adv Wound Care. 2015;4:329–38. doi:10.1089/wound.2015.0637.
11. Duan-Arnold Gyurdieva A, Johnson A, Uveges T, Jacobstein D, Danilkovitch AY. Retention of endogenous viable cells enhances the anti-inflammatory activity of cryopreserved amnion. Adv Wound care. 2015;4:523–33.
12. Grafix® GWG. A cryopreserved placental membrane, for the treatment of chronic/stalled wounds. Adv Wound Care. 2015;4:534–44. doi:10.1089/wound.2015.0647.
13. Liu J, Sheha H, Fu Y, Liang L, Tseng SC, Gruss JS, et al. Amniotic membrane: from structure and functions to clinical applications. Can Med Assoc J. 2009;349:1237–46. doi:10.1007/s00441-012-1424-6.
14. Niknejad H, Peirovi H, Jorjani M, Ahmadiani A, Ghanavi J, Seifalian AM. Properties of the amniotic membrane for potential use in tissue engineering. Eur Cell Mater. 2008;15:88–99. http://www.ncbi.nlm.nih.gov/pubmed/18446690.
15. Kim DH, Murovic JA, Tiel RL, Kline DG. Neurosurgery. 2004;54:1421–9. doi:10.1227/01.NEU.0000124752.40412.03.
16. Meng H, Li M, You F, Du J, Luo Z. Assessment of processed human amniotic membrane as a protective barrier in rat model of sciatic nerve injury. Neurosci Lett. 2011; 496(1):48–53.
17. Brown BA, Francisco S. Internal Neurolysis in Treatment of. 1969. p. 460–2.
18. Flores AJ, Lavernia CJ, Owens PW. Anatomy and physiology of peripheral nerve injury and repair. Am J Orthop MEAD. 2000;29:167–78. http://www.ncbi.nlm.nih.gov/pubmed/10746467.
19. Houschyar KS, Momeni A, Pyles MN, Cha JY, Maan ZN, Duscher D, et al. The role of current techniques and concepts in peripheral nerve repair. Plast Surg Int. 2016;2016:1–8. doi:10.1155/2016/4175293.
20. Ferraresi S, Garozzo D, Buffatti P. Common peroneal nerve injuries: results with one-stage nerve repair and tendon transfer. Neurosurg Rev. 2003;26:175–9. doi:10.1007/s10143-002-0247-4.

6

Does the location of placement of meniscal sutures have a clinical effect in the all-inside repair of meniscocapsular tears?

Uğur Tiftikçi and Sancar Serbest*

Abstract

Background: Meniscocapsular separation (MCS) is a lesion of the area which is attached from the peripheral section of the meniscus to the capsule and is seen less often than other meniscus injuries. The aim of this study was to investigate which of the different side applications of all-inside MCS repair of the meniscus was better in respect of clinical and functional results.

Methods: In this retrospective study, 53 patients with MCS pattern in their knee joints were treated with arthroscopic meniscus repair made with the all-inside method. The patients were separated into three groups according to the surface from which the fixation was applied: group 1, from the femoral joint surface of the meniscus ($n = 17$), group 2, from the tibial joint surface of the meniscus ($n = 21$) and group 3, from the femoral and tibial joint surfaces of the meniscus ($n = 15$). The participants were assessed using the subjective International Knee Documentation Committee Scoring (IKDC), Lysholm Knee Scale, Tegner Activity Level Scale, Barrett criteria and Kellgren–Lawrence classification after a 45 ± 12.1 months (range, 24–70 months) follow-up.

Results: Postoperatively, all the groups exhibited significantly increased subjective IKDC score, Lysholm score and Tegner activity score compared with their preoperative results ($p < 0.001$). At 6 months postoperatively, a statistically significant difference was determined between the groups in respect of the subjective IKDC score, Tegner activity score and Lysholm score with group 2 showing better results than the other groups ($p < 0.001$). At the final follow-up examination, no statistically significant difference was determined between the groups in respect of the subjective IKDC score, Tegner activity score or Lysholm score. A statistically significantly lower level of pulling and stress sensation was determined in group 2 ($p < 0.001$).

Conclusions: MCS repair made with the all-inside method is successful clinically and functionally and in respect of MRI findings. In addition, it was seen that the fixation method applied from the tibial surface of the meniscus does not disturb the anatomic position of the meniscus in MCS repair. The tibial joint surface is the most appropriate area for suturation in all-inside repair of MCS.

Level of evidence: Level IV.

Keywords: Meniscocapsular separation, Arthroscopi, Meniscus repair, All-inside method

* Correspondence: dr.sancarserbest@hotmail.com
Faculty of Medicine, Department of Orthopaedics and Traumatology, Kırıkkale University, Kırıkkale, Turkey

Background

Meniscocapsular separation (MCS) is a lesion of the area which is attached from the peripheral section of the meniscus to the capsule and is seen less often than other meniscus injuries [22, 25]. MCS is most often in the posterior horn section, is often a lesion in the meniscotibial ligament and accompanies microtrauma and anterior cruciate ligament (ACL) tears [1, 4, 13]. Several studies have reported a high rate of recovery after MCS repair [9, 10, 12]. As the blood circulation is good in the meniscocapsular region and in the peripheral third of the meniscus, studies have reported that the recovery rate is high and the re-operation risk is low [18, 19]. MCS is repaired with inside-out and all-inside methods. Each method has its own advantages and disadvantages. MCS inside-out repair is the gold standard in respect of biomechanical strength. However, the disadvantage is that posteromedial and posterolateral cuts are required [5, 16, 17, 20, 21]. Although inside-out techniques are the gold standard in MCS repair, current applications are all-inside suturation techniques. The most significant advantages of MCS repair with new all-inside devices are that it can be easily and quickly applied and that there is no need for an extra cut [8, 12]. Disadvantages are neurovascular injuries and that the anterior meniscus is not suitable for suturation. Another problem is caused by the elevation of the meniscus to the femoral side [27]. In these patients, there is a greater pulling and stress sensation, especially when the knee moves from the flexion to extension. This symptom can be caused by exposure to greater stress because of the change in the anatomic orientation in the function of dynamic stability of the meniscocapsular complex.

The primary aim of this study was to report the clinical and functional results of MCS all-inside repair. The secondary aim was to investigate which of the different side applications of all-inside repair of the meniscus was better in respect of the clinical and functional results.

Methods

The study included 111 patients with MCS pattern who underwent meniscus repair in the Orthopaedics and Traumatology Clinic between 2009 and 2014. Approval for the study was granted by the Local Ethics Committee (2014/23). A retrospective review was made of the patient files. Criteria for inclusion in the study were that patients were determined with MCS arthroscopically or with findings of MCS on magnetic resonance imaging (MRI) which were in the zones 3 and 4 posterior of the meniscus, had not benefitted from more than 3 months of physical therapy, were aged over 18 years and below 55 years and were followed up for at least 24 months. Patients excluded from the study for the reasons mentioned above were as follows: ACL reconstruction was applied (20 cases), microfracture surgery was applied (11 case), medial parapatellar plica excision was applied (12 cases), severe knee dislocation or a fracture around the knee (5 cases), aged below 18 years or over 55 years (fourteen cases), follow-up of less than 24 months (16 cases). Fifty three patients met the inclusion criteria and were therefore included in the study (Fig. 1).

The patients were separated into three groups according to the surface from which the suturation was applied: group 1 ($n = 17$), from the femoral joint surface of the meniscus, group 2 ($n = 21$), from the tibial joint surface of the meniscus and group 3 ($n = 15$), from the femoral and tibial joint surfaces of the meniscus (Fig. 1).

A record was made for all patients of symptoms (locking, pain, swelling, postoperative pulling sensation), age, gender, whether pain was acute (<3 months) or chronic (>3 months), MRI diagnosis, location of the meniscus tear, MCS length, number of sutures used, comorbidities, postoperative complications or side-effects, requirement for postoperative drainage, preoperative and postoperative (6 months and final 24 months follow-up examination) subjective International Knee Documentation Committee Scoring (IKDC), Lysholm Knee Scale [14], Tegner Activity Level Scale [26], Barrett criteria (joint area, effusion, McMurray test sensitivity) [2] and Kellgren–Lawrence classification for degenerative arthritis [11]. All the preoperative and postoperative MR images (Achieva 1.5T MRI system-Philips Medical Systems, Best, The Netherlands) were evaluated by a radiologist experienced in the musculoskeletal system.

Surgical technique

With the patient in the standard knee arthroscopy position, entry to the knee was made from the anterolateral and anteromedial portals. Meniscus tear was determined arthroscopically. The tear ends were cleaned in the meniscocapsular region with a shaver and rasp. All-inside meniscus repair was applied to all the patients with MCS lesion. The all-inside meniscal repair was made according to the options of application from the femoral, tibial and femoral-tibial surfaces of the meniscus (Fig. 2). The Omnispan Meniscal Repair System (Mitek, Norwood, MA, USA) all-inside suture device was used for meniscal repair. In arthroscopy, the size and location of the meniscus tear, the number of sutures used and the status of other anatomic structures (ACL injuries, cartilage injuries, parapatellar plica) in the knee were recorded.

Postoperative rehabilitation

All patients started early postoperative patellar mobilisation exercises with isometric quadriceps exercises, and walking was permitted with two crutches non-weight-bearing. Passive knee joint exercises up to 90° were applied for 2 weeks postoperatively, and after 2 weeks, full

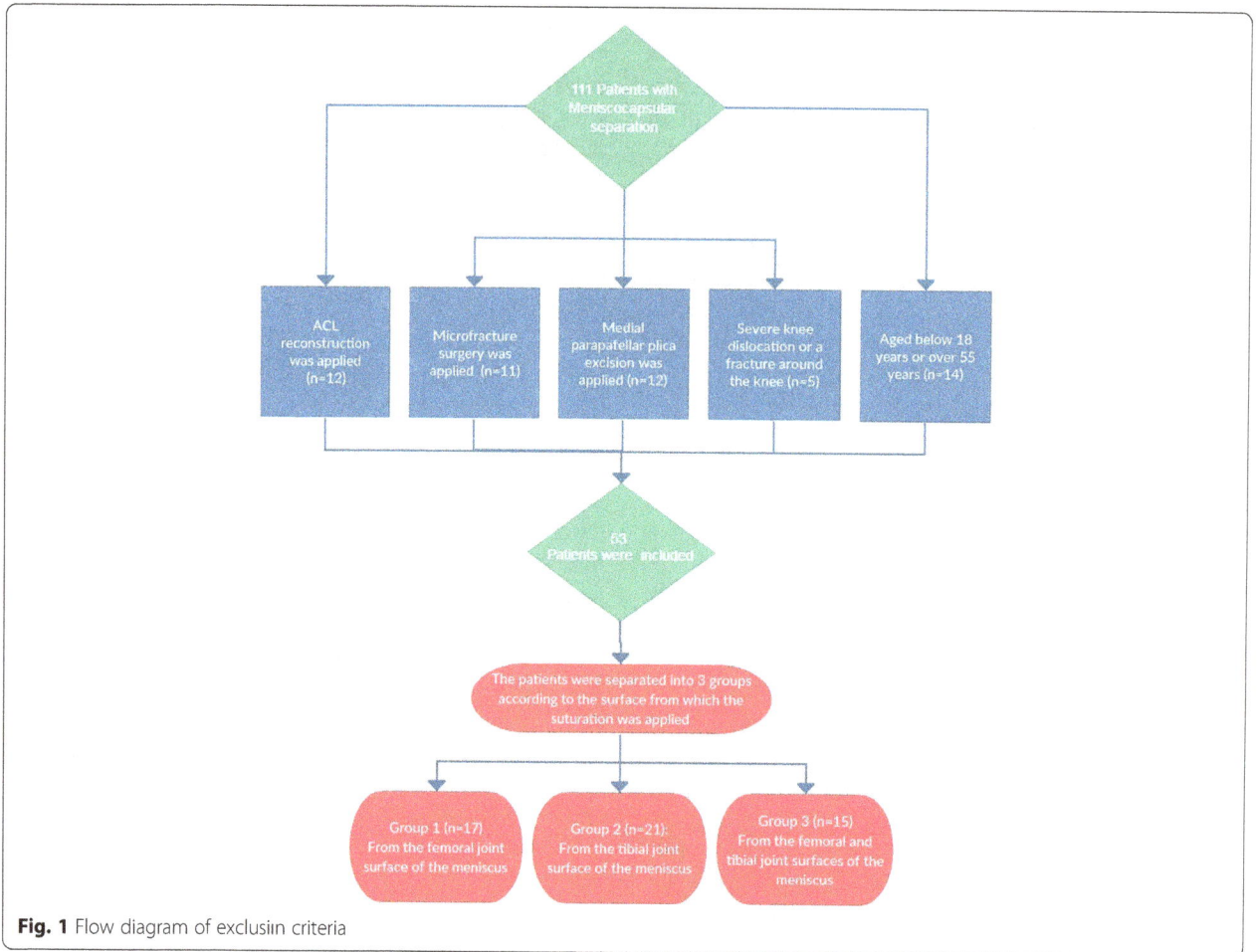

Fig. 1 Flow diagram of exclusiin criteria

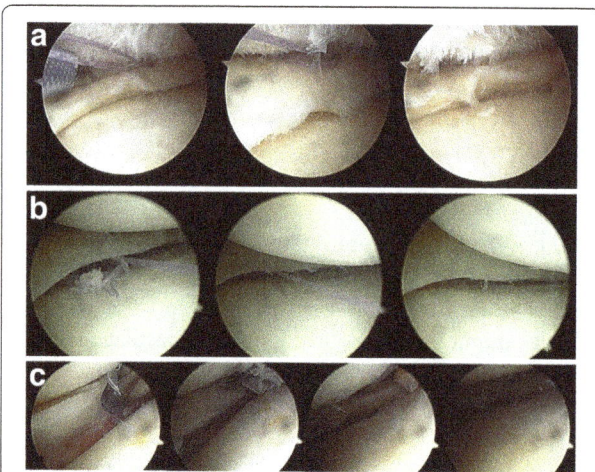

Fig. 2 The all-inside meniscal repair was made according to the options of application from the femoral joint surface of the meniscus (**a**), from the tibial joint surface of the meniscus (**b**) and from the femoral and tibial joint surfaces of the meniscus (**c**)

joint movement was permitted. After the fourth week, unassisted walking with weight-bearing as tolerated was permitted and full joint movement exercises were started. In posterior meniscus tears, active knee flexion over 90° and squatting and sitting on the floor were not permitted for up to 6 weeks. At 3 months after arthroscopy, patients with no knee complaints (swelling, pulling, locking, pain and negative McMurray test) were permitted to recommence active sports and high-level activities.

Statistical analysis

All statistical analyses were performed with SPSS ver. 16.0 (SPSS Inc., Chicago, IL, USA). A confidence interval (CI) of 95% and a two-tailed $p < 0.05$ were determined to be statistically significant for all of the analyses. The distance between the center of the talus and each landmark was expressed as mean and SD. One-way ANOVA with Turkey–Kramer test was used for the comparison among landmarks. Statistical significant was set at $p < 0.05$.

Results

The mean age of the total 53 patients was 37.6 ± 9.4 years (range, 20–55 years). Repair was made to the right knee of 28 patients, the left knee of 25 patients, in the medial meniscus in 47 cases, the lateral meniscus in 6 and to traumatic tears in 37 cases. The demographic characteristics and preoperative examination findings of the groups are shown in Table 1. The mean follow-up period was 45 ± 12.1 months (range, 24–70 months). Preoperatively, there were no findings of MCS in 14 cases. No major complication developed in any patient intra-operatively or in the early postoperative period. No statistically significant difference was determined functionally between the groups in respect of the pre-operative subjective IKDC score, Lysholm Knee Scale score and Tegner Activity Level Scale score. At 6 months postoperatively, a statistically significant difference was determined between the groups in respect of the subjective IKDC score, Lysholm Knee Scale score and Tegner Activity Level Scale score with group 2 (tibial side) showing better results than the other groups ($p < 0.001$). At the final 24 months follow-up examination, no statistically significant difference was determined between the groups in respect of the subjective IKDC score, Lysholm Knee Scale score and Tegner Activity Level Scale score (Table 2).

A pulling and stress sensation was present in 12 of the 17 patients in group 1 and continued for up to 6 months, in 3 of the 21 patients in group 2 and in 7 of the 15 patients in group 3. A statistically significantly lower level of pulling and stress sensation was determined in group 2 ($p < 0.001$).

Degeneration was classified according to the Kellgren–Lawrence grading system on the final radiographs. These were determined as grade 0 in 42, grade 1 in 8, grade 2 in 2 and grade 3 in the 0 knees (Table 3). No statistically significant difference was determined between the groups ($p > 0.05$). Insufficient recovery was determined postopertively in two patients. Clinically, there was no effusion in these two patients. In one, there was sensitivity in the joint line, and in the other, the Mc Murray test [15] was positive. As the symptoms were mild, re-operation was not considered for either patient.

In all the patients, a significant improvement was determined in the functional scores compared to the preoperative values. The feeling of pulling and stress was determined to be lower in group 2, where MCS repair was made from the tibial section of the meniscus. The functional scores of the knee in the early postoperative period were also seen to be better in group 2. No statistically significant difference was determined between the groups in respect of the other variables evaluated of age, gender, side, number of sutures, traumatic or chronic, size of the tear, ACL status or comorbidities.

Discussion

The most important point of MCS is that care must be taken during MRI and arthroscopy and the diagnosis should not be overlooked. In this study, the mid-term clinical results were extremely good and the anatomic and early clinical results of the application of all-inside suturing from the tibial side were better than those of the other groups.

MCS is a lesion separating the meniscus from the meniscus joint capsule, and as the severity of the trauma increases, a longitudinal tear pattern occurs. It generally accompanies microtrauma and ACL tears [1, 4, 13]. In MCS, the lesion is often in the meniscotibial ligament. The meniscotibial ligament attaches the medial meniscus to the tibia and plays an important role in static and dynamic stability of the knee. In a cadaver study by Dugas et al. [6] related to the contact of MCS lesion with biomechanics, no significant difference was found in the transfer of pressure. It was also determined that there was a tendency to return to normal after MCS repair; although, the knee was not tested at different flexion angles. That study demonstrated that the meniscocapsular complex played an important role more in dynamic stability. When the meniscotibial ligament is involved in the lesion, it cannot undertake the function of braking stabilisation on the femoral condyle and thus causes instability [3, 7, 24]. This is also one of the most significant causes of MCS lesion. Therefore, MCS lesion repair

Table 1 The demographic characteristics and preoperative examination findings of the groups

	Total (n = 53)	Group 1 (n = 17)	Grup 2 (n = 21)	Grup 3 (n = 15)
Age (mean ± SD)	37.6 ± 9.4	36.5 ± 10.1	36.5 ± 9.0	40.4 ± 9.4
Gender M/F	36/17	13/4	13/8	10/5
Extremity side–right/left	28/25	7/10	13/8	8/7
Meniscus side M/L	47/6	16/1	18/3	13/2
Follow-up (mean ± SD)	45.0 ± 12.1	50.7 ± 11.8	42.3 ± 10.6	42.3 ± 12.3
MRI lesion present/absent	39/14	12/5	18/3	9/6
McMurray test	42	14	17	11
Effusion	27	9	11	7
Joint sensitivity	38	12	13	13

Table 2 Functional results

Evaluation method	Preoperative scores	Postoperative scores 6 months	Postoperative scores 24 months	Postoperative 6 months				Postoperative 24 months			
				p	p (1-2)	p (1-3)	p (2-3)	p	p (1-2)	p (1-3)	p (2-3)
Lysholm	61.19 ± 12.64	79.75 ± 7.56	90.92 ± 4.54	<0.001	<0.001	>0.05	<0.001	<0.001	>0.05	>0.05	>0.05
Group 1	59.24 ± 11.37	77.12 ± 6.56	89.94 ± 5.64								
Group 2	61.71 ± 12.75	84.95 ± 4.89	91.76 ± 4.02								
Group 3	62.67 ± 14.37	75.47 ± 7.76	90.87 ± 3.88								
Tegner	3.43 ± 1.43	4.92 ± 1.28	6.23 ± 1.52	<0.001	<0.001	>0.05	<0.001	<0.001	>0.05	>0.05	>0.05
Group 1	3.18 ± 1.38	4.76 ± 1.20	6.59 ± 1.80								
Group 2	3.86 ± 1.42	5.43 ± 1.28	6.19 ± 1.43								
Group 3	3.13 ± 1.45	4.40 ± 1.18	5.87 ± 1.30								
IKDC	50.45 ± 10.06	78.98 ± 5.78	91.93 ± 4.90	<0.001	<0.001	>0.05	<0.001	<0.001	>0.05	>0.05	>0.05
Group 1	50.35 ± 8.27	75.18 ± 6.64	88.09 ± 4.33								
Group 2	50.68 ± 5.20	82.18 ± 3.30	95.65 ± 2.80								
Group 3	55.77 ± 8.33	78.82 ± 5.00	91.06 ± 4.14								

plays an important role in knee stability. In parallel with this knowledge, it is possible to place the sutures from the tibial side in the all-inside method of meniscotibial ligament repair in MCS lesion. In a repair made from the tibial side of the meniscus, the anatomical position of the meniscus is better [27].

There are very few studies in literature reporting repair with all-inside suture materials because of MCS [9, 10, 12]. Hirtler et al. reported that all-inside repair was a safe and advantageous treatment option in the repair of acute and chronic MCS in young athletes [10]. Li et al. reported satisfactory results in patients applied with ACL reconstruction and all-inside arthroscopic repair of MCS tear of the posterior horn of the meniscus [12]. In the current study, with the exception of two patients, good recovery was determined in all the other patients at the final follow-up examination according to the clinical scores, functional scores (IKDC, Lysholm score) and MRI. In the patients of the current study where repair was applied from the femoral surface of the meniscus, the postoperative congruence was less satisfactory and the knee functions were seen to improve later.

If the MCS lesion is <5 mm, it may not be able to be diagnosed on MRI and diagnosis can be made arthroscopically in these patients. The history, physical examination, chronic medial knee pain and careful arthroscopic viewing are very important in these patients [9]. In a study by

Sonnery et al., it was reported that occult lesions of the medial meniscus are extremely frequent and diagnosis can be made more easily with debridement of the synovial tissues in the meniscocapsular region [23]. In the current study, there were no findings of MCS on preoperative MRI in 14 (26%) patients. In 11 of these patients, there was ACL lesion and meniscocapsular separation was diagnosed during arthroscopy and then repaired. In the other eight patients, diagnosis was able to be made during arthroscopy applied because of persistent joint pain, degenerative joint and other lesions in the meniscus. In arthroscopy applied because of ACL lesion, the presence of MCS in particular must be investigated.

As reported in a study by Tiftikci and Serbest, in a repair made with an all-inside suture device, femoral elevation of the meniscus impairs the normal anatomic placement [27]. In these patients, there is a greater pulling and stress sensation in the area where suturation is applied. To the best of our knowledge, there are no studies in literature related to this pulling and stress sensation. In the postoperative follow-up of patients applied with all-inside repair of MCS, pulling and stress sensation is a significant clinical problem which causes discomfort to patients. In the current study, the pulling and stress sensation was observed more often in the group where repair was made from the femoral joint surface of the meniscus. The group where these symptoms were

Table 3 Preoperative and postoperative Kellgren–Lawrence OA classification scores

	Total (n = 53)		Group 1 (n = 17)		Grup 2 (n = 21)		Grup 3 (n = 15)	
	Preoperative scores	Postoperative scores 24 months	Preoperative scores	Postoperative scores 24 months	Preoperative scores	Postoperative scores 24 months	Preoperative scores	Postoperative scores 24 months
Kellgren–Lawrence grading								
Grade 0/1/2/3	47/6/0/0	42/8/2/1	15/2/0/0	12/3/1/1	19/2/0/0	17/3/1/0	13/2/0/0	13/2/0/0

observed the least was the group where repair was made from the tibial surface of the meniscus.

The most significant limitation of this study is that it was retrospective. Secondly, the number of patients was low. Thirdly, there was no comparison of the all-inside repair method with the inside-out or outside-in methods. Finally, the pulling and stress sensation in the knee could have been caused by incorrect placement related to the medial-lateral collateral ligament of the all-inside peak diameters.

Conclusions

The results of this study showed that MCS repair made with the all-inside method is successful clinically and functionally and in respect of MRI findings. In addition, it was seen that the suturation method applied from the tibial surface of the meniscus does not disturb the anatomic position of the meniscus in MCS repair. Furthermore, the optimum conditions are provided for the restoration of the functions of the meniscus and there is a lower rate of symptoms such as pulling and stress in the postoperative period. The tibial joint surface is the most appropriate area for suturation in all-inside repair of MCS.

Abbreviations
ACL: Anterior cruciate ligament; IKDC: International Knee Documentation Committee; MCS: Meniscocapsular separation; MRI: Magnetic resonance imaging

Acknowledgements
None.

Funding
None.

Authors' contributions
SS designed this study. SS and UT wrote the manuscript. SS and UT contributed to the discussion and reviewed/edited the manuscript and researched data. SS and UT helped to draft the manuscript. SS and UT researched data and contributed to discussion. All radiological and clinical outcome evaluation was made by SS and UT. The statistical analysis was made by SS. Both authors read and approved the final manuscript.

Competing interests
The authors declare that they have no competing interests.

References
1. Ahn JH, Bae TS, Kang KS, Kang SY, Lee SH. Longitudinal tear of the medial meniscus posterior horn in the anterior cruciate ligament-deficient knee significantly influences anterior stability. Am J Sports Med. 2011;39:2187–93.
2. Barrett GR, Field MH, Treacy SH, Ruff CG. Clinical results of meniscus repair in patients 40 years and older. Arthroscopy. 1988;14:824–9.
3. Beltran J, Matityahu A, Hwang K, Jbara M, Maimon R, Padron M, et al. The distal semimembranosus complex: normal MR anatomy, variants, biomechanics and pathology. Skelet Radiol. 2003;32(8):435–45.
4. Bollen SR. Posteromedial meniscocapsular injury associated with rupture of the anterior cruciate ligament: a previously unrecognised association. J Bone Joint Surg (Br). 2010;92:222–3.
5. DeHaven KE. Meniscus repair. Am J Sports Med. 1999;27:242–50.
6. Dugas JR, Barrett AM, Beason DP, Plymale MF, Fleisig GS. Tibiofemoral contact biomechanics following meniscocapsular separation and repair. Int J Sports Med. 2015;36(6):498–502.
7. El-Khoury GY, Usta HY, Berger RA. Meniscotibial (coronary) ligament tears. Skelet Radiol. 1984;11(3):191–6.
8. Espejo-Baena A, Figueroa-Mata A, Serrano-Fernández J, de la Torre-Solís F. All-inside suture technique using anterior portals in posterior horn tears of lateral meniscus. Arthroscopy. 2008;24:369.e1–4.
9. Hetsroni I, Lillemoe K, Marx RG. Small medial meniscocapsular separations: a potential cause of chronic medial-side knee pain. Arthroscopy. 2011;27(11):1536–42.
10. Hirtler L, Unger J, Weninger P. Acute and chronic menisco-capsular separation in the young athlete: diagnosis, treatment and results in thirty seven consecutive patients. Int Orthop. 2015;39(5):967–74.
11. Kellgren JH, Lawrence JS. Radiological assessment of osteo-arthrosis. Ann Rheum Dis. 1957;16(4):494–502.
12. Li WP, Chen Z, Song B, Yang R, Tan W. The FasT-Fix repair technique for ramp lesion of the medial meniscus. Knee Surg Relat Res. 2015;27(1):56–60.
13. Liu X, Feng H, Zhang H, Hong L, Wang XS, Zhang J. Arthroscopic prevalence of ramp lesion in 868 patients with anterior cruciate ligament injury. Am J Sports Med. 2011;39:832–7.
14. Lyscholm J, Gillquist J. Evaluation of the ligament surgery results with special emphasis on use of scoring scale. Am J Sports Med. 1982;10:150–4.
15. McMurray TP. The semilunar cartilages. Br J Surg. 1942;29:407–14.
16. Noyes FR, Barber-Westin SD. Repair of complex and avascular meniscal tears and meniscal transplantation. J Bone Joint Surg Am. 2010;92:1012–29.
17. Noyes FR, Barber-Westin SD. Management of meniscus tears that extend into the avascular region. Clin Sports Med. 2012;31:65–90.
18. Paxton ES, Stock MV, Brophy RH. Meniscal repair versus partial meniscectomy: a systematic review comparing reoperation rates and clinical outcomes. Arthroscopy. 2011;27:1275–88.
19. Popescu D, Sastre S, Garcia AI, Tomas X, Reategui D, Caballero M. MR-arthrography assessment after repair of chronic meniscal tears. Knee Surg Sports Traumatol Arthrosc. 2015;23(1):171–7.
20. Post WR, Akers SR, Kish V. Load to failure of common meniscal repair techniques: effects of suture technique and suture material. Arthroscopy. 1997;13:731–6.
21. Rimmer MG, Nawana NS, Keene GC, Pearcy MJ. Failure strengths of different meniscal suturing techniques. Arthroscopy. 1995;11:146–50.
22. Rubin DA, Britton CA, Towers JD, Harner CD. Are MR signs of meniscocapsular separation valid? Radiology. 1996;201:829–36.
23. Sonnery-Cottet B, Conteduca J, Thaunat M, Gunepin FX, Seil R. Hidden lesions of the posterior horn of the medial meniscus: a systematic arthroscopic exploration of the concealed portion of the knee. Am J Sports Med. 2014;42:921–6.
24. Stephen JM, Halewood C, Kittl C, Bollen SR, Williams A, Amis AA. Posteromedial meniscocapsular lesions increase tibi-ofemoral joint laxity with anterior cruciate ligament deficiency, and their repair reduces laxity. Am J Sports Med. 2016;44:400–8.
25. Stone RG. Peripheral detachment of the menisci of the knee: a preliminary report. Orthop Clin North Am. 1979;10:643–57.
26. Tegner Y, Lysholm J. Rating systems in evaluation of knee ligament injuries. Clin Orthop. 1985;198:43–9.
27. Tiftikci U, Serbest S. The optimal placement of sutures in all-inside meniscocapsular separation. Open Orthop J. 2016;10:89–93.

7

An anatomical-like triangular-vector ligament reconstruction for the medial collateral ligament and the posterior oblique ligament injury with single femoral tunnel

Hongtao Xu[1†], Kai Kang[1†], Jian Zhang[2], Dongmei Xin[3], Wei Liu[1], Guorong Jin[1], Jiangtao Dong[1*] and Shijun Gao[1]

Abstract

Background: The purpose of this study was to evaluate the clinical outcomes of anatomical-like triangular-vector ligament reconstruction (TLR) in treating the combined injury of medial collateral ligament (MCL) and posterior oblique ligament (POL).

Methods: During July 2013 to May 2014, 26 patients who received anatomical-like TLR were included into this study. All patients received clinical physical examination, imaging examination, and knee joint function score both preoperative and follow-up. The stability of the medial structure of the knee joint was examined by physical examination and imaging evaluation, including excessive knee medial opening (EKMO) and tibial external rotation angle (TERA). The function of the knee was evaluated by the subjective questionnaire, including Lysholm, Tegner, and IKDC score. SPSS software was used for statistics analysis.

Results: The mean follow-up time exceeds 24 months. Two patients occurred with serious heterotopic ossification, and one patient received revision because of screw breakage. EKMO over the contralateral state at 0° decreased from 9.76 ± 2.76 mm to 2.79 ± 1.02 mm with statistical significance ($P < .001$) and 10.32 ± 2.75 mm decreased to 3.13 ± 0.85 mm at 30° ($P < .001$). Meanwhile, TERA significantly decreased from $53.38 \pm 6.71°$ to $27.15 \pm 4.92°$ ($P < .001$). The postoperative Lysholm, Tegner, and IKDC score were superior to preoperative with statistical significance ($P < .001$).

Conclusions: Anatomical-like TLR can reconstruct the graft to cover the insertions which can regain anatomic form and function with a cramped space. Not only the valgus stability and rotational stability can be restored obviously at follow-up but also the usage of implantation can be reduced, decreasing the incidence rate of allergy and saving costs.

Keyword: Medial collateral ligament, Posterior oblique ligament, Anatomical reconstruction, External rotation stability

* Correspondence: hbsydongjiangtao@sina.com
†Equal contributors
[1]Department of Joint Surgery, The Third Hospital of Hebei Medical University,
NO. 139 Ziqiang Road, Shijiazhuang 050051, Hebei, People's Republic of
China
Full list of author information is available at the end of the article

Statement of clinical significance

This study provides evidence of the superiority of anatomical-like triangular-vector ligament reconstruction (TLR) in treating the combined injury of medial collateral ligament and posterior oblique ligament.

Background

The medial collateral ligament (MCL) is one of the most commonly injured ligamentous structures [1]. It serves as the primary medial static stabilizer against valgus stress, though along with the posteromedial corner provides resistance to external rotation forces applied to the lower extremity [2]. Those sports involve valgus knee loading, such as hockey, skiing, and football, have contributed to the frequent occurrence of MCL injuries [3]. Both MCL and posterior oblique ligament (POL) are two main static stabilizers [4]. And the combined injury could result in clinically significant valgus or rotational instability [5]. Michael et al. reported that Hughston's grade III MCL injury often result with a high risk up to 78% of concomitant ligament injury [6]. Of these cases, 95% involve with the ACL, may lead to chronic instability followed by disability [7, 8]. A better recovery of valgus and rotational stability was essential for massive MCL injury, let alone one who suffer with grade III MCL injury combine ACL injury.

Previous anatomical studies have demonstrated the relative position was unparalleled on different planes between MCL and POL [9, 10]. When the knee extended, the MCL runs parallel to the axis of the femur/tibia and the POL formed an angle of 25° with the axis of the femur/tibia. Since non-parallel, the extension lines of these two ligaments would intersect at one point at superior of femoral condyle.

This study shows the surgical procedure of an anatomical-like triangular-vector ligament reconstruction (TLR) technical of the MCL and POL which bring a satisfied result of medial knee stability.

Methods

Participants

The retrospective study (level of evidence 3) was conducted with the approval of the ethics committee of The Third Hospital of Hebei Medical University, Shijiazhuang, China. From July 2013 to May 2014, 47 patients suffered with unilateral MCL injury in our institute. The inclusion criteria were (1) simple injury of the MCL, (2) preoperative magnetic resonance imaging (MRI) that confirmed the MCL rupture, and radiographic stress position imaging showed the excessive knee medial opening over the contralateral state (EKMO) was more than 3 mm compared with contralateral knee [11, 12], (3) the valgus stress test was positive at 0° and 30° knee flexion, (4) no previous knee surgery, and (5) with whole clinical follow-up data.

The surgical indications for anatomical-like TLR were (1) chronic MCL injury; (2) Hughston grade III or above sub-acute or acute MCL injury with posterior-medial structure injury (the valgus stress tests showed both positive at 0° and 30° knee flexion) [12–14]. Six (12.8%) of them were excluded from the study because they combined with ACL injury which have an effect on the rotational instability. In total of 16 patients who suffered acute MCL injury were not suited in this study. However, five (19.2%) included patients whose injury to operation interval were fewer than 3 days because their EKMO over the contralateral state were more than 10 mm both at 0° and 30° knee flexion. This massive valgus laxity was considered as high grade MCL injury which needs to be treated with surgical repair or reconstruction. In addition, 17 (65.4%) chronic patients and 4 (15.4%) sub-acute patients were included into this study. So there were total 26 patients received anatomical-like TLR and be included into this study. General patient information is listed in Table 1.

Study procedures

The data were collected from the resident's admission note, physical examination, preoperative radiographic stress position imaging, operation records, and records of pre- and post-operative functional scores. Patients were evaluated using the Lysholm score, Tegner activity level, and International Knee Documentation Committee (IKDC) Knee Evaluation Form before the operation (Fig. 1). An average of 24.4-month follow-up, 26 patients returned to complete the same examination and evaluation as performed preoperatively.

Surgical technique

Physical examination and arthroscopic evaluation

After anesthesia, the medial structures were evaluated by a surgeon. To detect medial joint opening, EMKO was applied at 0° and 30° of knee flexion (Fig. 2). The estimation of knee rotation was assessed in comparison with the contralateral knee which profited from the author's

Table 1 Demographic characteristics and intraoperative data

Basic information		Data
Age, mean ± SD, years		27.42 ± 4.19
Sex, male:female, n		21/5
Side, left/right, n		11/15
BMI, mean ± SD, kg/m²		27.47 ± 6.20
Injury to operation interval, mean ± SD, days		35.88 ± 20.26
EKMO over the contralateral state, mean ± SD, millimeters	0°	9.76 ± 2.27
	30°	10.32 ± 2.76
TERA, Mean ± SD, degrees		53.38 ± 6.71
Follow-up, mean ± SD, months		24.38 ± 3.23

BMI body mass index, *EKMO* excessive knee medial opening, *TERA* tibial external rotation angle, *n* number

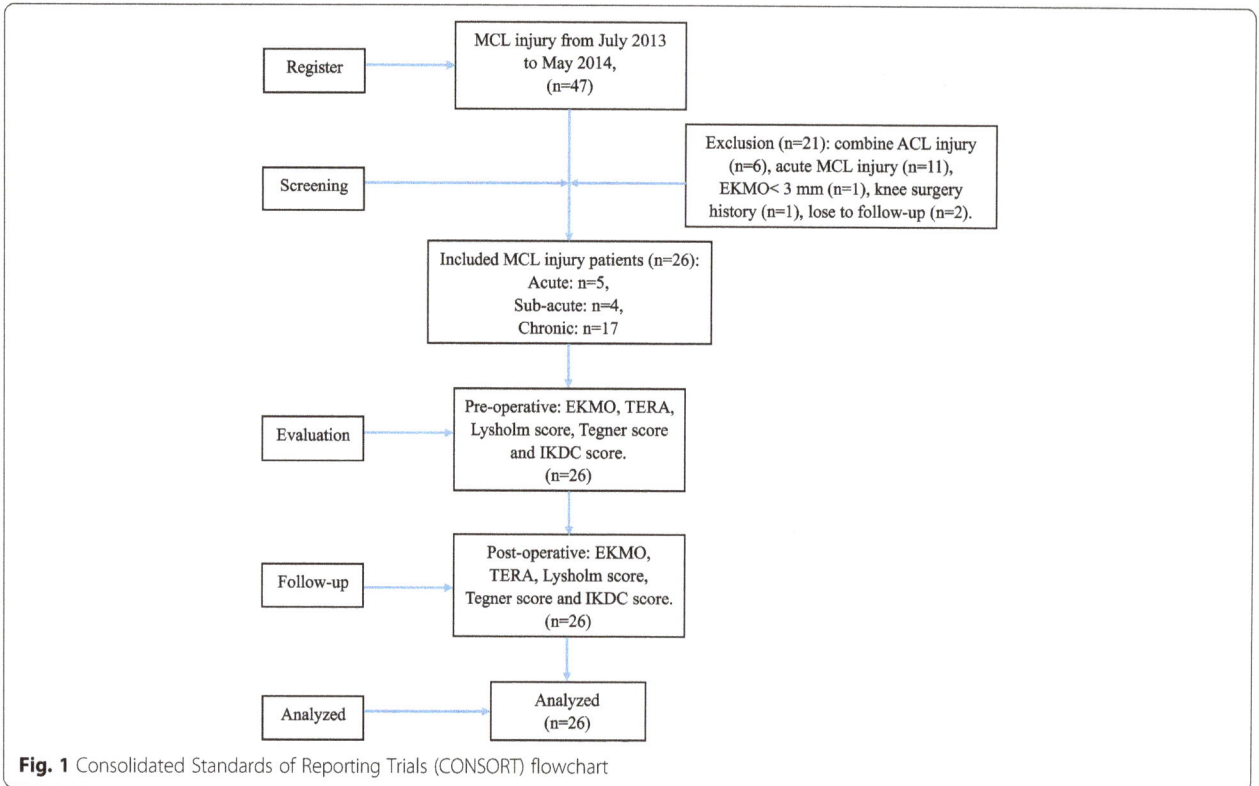

Fig. 1 Consolidated Standards of Reporting Trials (CONSORT) flowchart

patent called tibial external rotation angle (TERA) Measuring Instrument (201620091253.9) (Fig. 3). Whether other structure were injured or not, they should be eliminated and dealt with during arthroscopic evaluation. FasT-Fix was considered as the first choice to deal with meniscal lesion. If the meniscal tear type was difficult to suture, meniscectomy was performed.

Preparation of allograft

A thawed allograft should be soaked for 20 min. The graft was measured to make sure no less than 24 cm in length and 5 mm in diameter, meanwhile, the diameter of the combined ends was no less than 7 mm. Because

of the relevance between the graft length and tunnel depth, only one free end was braided with no. 2 Ethibond Excel Polyethylene non-absorbable sutures. Then a thread was passed through combined graft and was looped around which can guide the sutured end.

Reconstruction procedure of MCL–POL

Locating the insertions of MCL and POL A curved medial skin incision was directed from 1 cm above the adductor tubercle down to 6 cm beyond the joint line. Generally observing on the MCL and POL, then locating insertions respectively. The tibial MCL insertion was selected at the place 1 cm anterior the

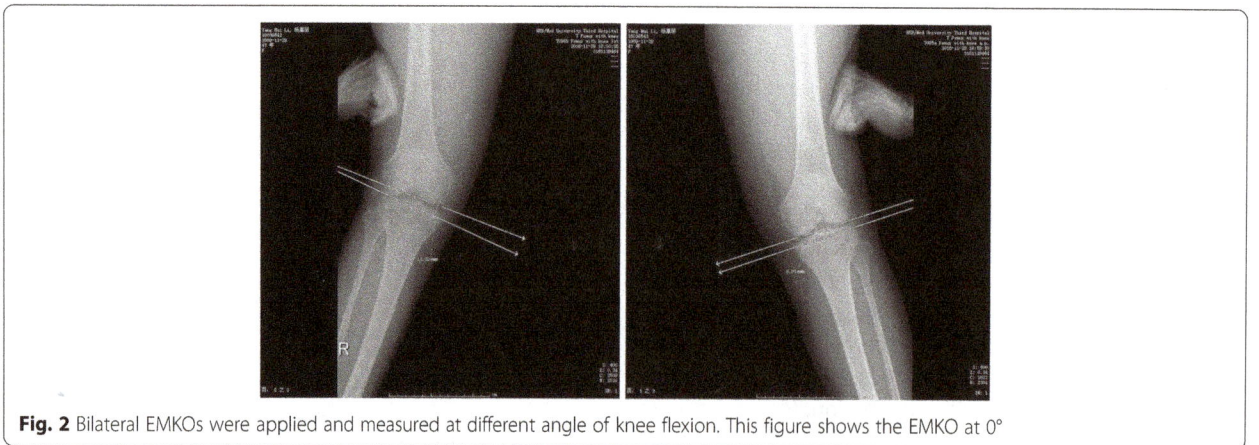

Fig. 2 Bilateral EMKOs were applied and measured at different angle of knee flexion. This figure shows the EMKO at 0°

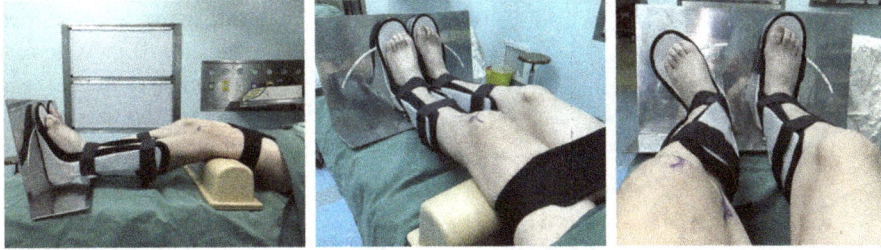

Fig. 3 The knee rotation angle was measured by the TERA

narrowing point of posterior tibial ridge and 4.5 cm below the tibia plateau. The tibial POL insertion is selected at 2 mm lateral of the medial tibia and 2 cm below the tibia plateau. After, the medial femoral epicondyle was exposed and both the femoral MCL and the POL insertion sites were identified. The femoral MCL insertion was approximately selected at the anterior inferior part of adductor tubercle of condyle of femur, 3 mm below the proximal medial epicondyle of femur and 5 mm anterior the posterior edge of medial epicondyle of femur. The femoral POL insertion was selected at 8 mm below the medial epicondyle of femur and 6 mm anterior the posterior edge of medial epicondyle of femur that is closed to the femoral anatomical attachment points of the MCL. Two Kirschner wires (K-wires) were used to locate and link the MCL and the POL insertions of tibia and femur, respectively. The two K-wires had an intersection point which was the drilling location of the femoral tunnel (Fig. 4).

Drilling tibial and femoral tunnel The tibial tunnel linked the center situs of two ligament insertions. A 2-mm guide pin was oriented by a guide apparatus which was used for cruciate ligament reconstruction (Fig. 5). And then the tibial tunnel was broadened by a 5-mm bone pin (Fig. 6). The sutured graft end was pulled through the tunnel by the previous guide pin.

The femoral drilling site had been located by the preceding K-wires' intersection point. Another guide pin was drilled into the intersection point along the epicondylar axis, which formed an angle of 30° with sagittal plane and came out at the lateral condyle of the femur. So the intercondylar notch could avoid from being crossed by the pin. A 7-mm bone pin was drilled approximately 2.5 cm in depth along with the previous guide pin which could accommodate the femoral attachments of the graft (Fig. 7). The graft was measured a second time after running through the tunnels. Then the non-sutured end could be sutured with an appropriate length (Fig. 8).

Graft passage and fixation The two free ends of the graft were pulled through the femoral tunnel, respectively, by guide pin. A tensile force was provided when the knee was kept at 30° flexion with varus stress and neutral rotation. A bio-interference screw with the same size as the femoral tunnel was screwed into the tunnel entrance where the graft was choked (Fig. 9). The graft was sutured to the surrounding soft tissue at the two tunnel exits in tibial which could prevent sliding and impact between the graft and bone tunnel.

Arthroscopic reexamination and stitching up Arthroscopic evaluation was performed again to confirm the intrinsic femur-tibia gap was no more expanded. Then the wound was thoroughly irrigated and sutured.

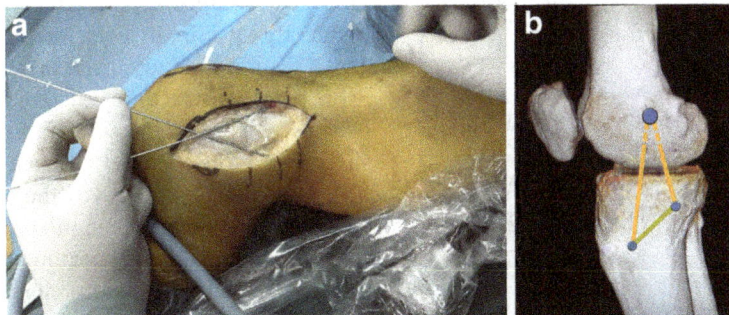

Fig. 4 a Two Kirschner wires (K-wires) were used to locate and link the MCL and the POL insertions of tibia and femur, respectively. **b** They had an intersection point which was the drilling location of the femoral tunnel

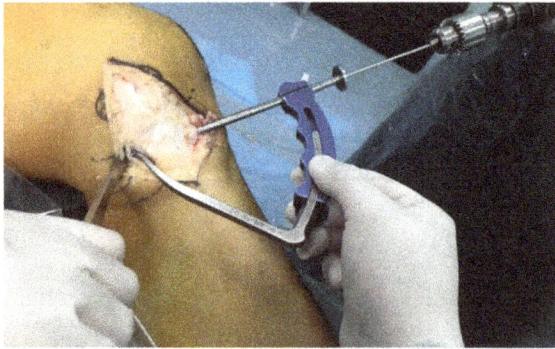

Fig. 5 A guide apparatus was used for drilling tunnel accurately

Postoperative treatment and rehabilitation

Patients were injected with cefazolin sodium pentahydrate every 6 h during the first 24 h. After the anesthetic effect dissipated, the patient needed to practice ankle pump as earlier as possible. Not only the swelling could be reduced but also the incidence rate of deep venous thrombosis could be declined.

The patient received a long hinged brace with no weight bearing for 6 weeks. Non-weight-bearing walking was encouraged, but the long hinged brace should keep equipped. During this period, range of motion (ROM) exercises were restricted from 0° to 90° of knee flexion. Six weeks later, knee flexion progressed to a full ROM and weight-bearing walking was allowed as tolerated and mobilization without brace protection was permitted. Patients could do further controlled activities after 3 months and contact sports after 6 months.

Follow-up

At follow-up, 26 patients were re-examined clinically using the EKMO over the contralateral state, TERA, Lysholm Score, Tegner Activity Level, and IKDC. The mean follow-up period was 24.38 ± 3.23 months.

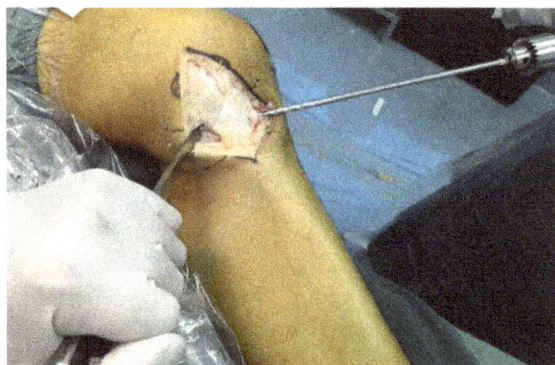

Fig. 6 The tibial tunnel was broadened by a bone pin of 5 mm in diameter

Statistical analysis

Data were analyzed using SPSS software for Windows (version 21.0; Chicago, IL). Wilcoxon matched-pairs signed-rank test (non-parametric) was used to compare the difference in the positive rate for the preoperative and follow-up data. The significance level was set at $P < .05$.

Results

A total of 26 patients (21 males and 5 females) with a mean age of 27.42 ± 4.19 years were analyzed in this study. Patient demographic data are listed in Table 1. There were 24 cases whose EKMO over the contralateral state widened up to 5 mm at 0°, and all 26 cases' EKMO over the contralateral state were widened up to 5 mm at 30°.

At a mean 24.4-month follow-up time, significant differences were observed between the preoperative and postoperative data for all of these measures ($P < .001$). EKMO over the contralateral state at 0° decreased from 9.76 ± 2.76 mm to 2.79 ± 1.02 mm with statistical significance ($P < .001$) and 10.32 ± 2.75 mm decreased to 3.13 ± 0.85 mm at 30° ($P < .001$). Meanwhile, TERA significantly decreased from 53.38 ± 6.71° to 27.15 ± 4.92° ($P < .001$). The subjective evaluation and activity level scores, included Lysholm, Tegner, and IKDC score, increased with statistical significance ($P < .001$). The data are listed in Table 2.

Complications

Two patients (7.7%) complained knee joint medial pain because heterotopic ossification occurred in the inlet of femoral tunnel (Fig. 10). Analgesic plaster was used for conservative treatment and no further complaint. One revision (3.8%) had failure of fixation in the femoral tunnel because of the screw breakage. There was no graft rejection and infection during follow-up.

Discussion

Currently, the treatment for the MCL and POL injury is a broad academic controversy. However, a significant proportion of surgeons reached a consensus that Hughston's grade III MCL injury, which were considered as a massive MCL and POL injury, need to be treated with surgical repair or reconstruction because there was a high risk of valgus and rotational instability [11, 12, 15]. This study elaborated the method of anatomical-like TLR of the MCL and POL and proved the better recovery of medial stability and clinical function.

Numerous surgical treatment procedures had been described with satisfactory clinical results [3, 13, 16–18, 19–22]. As the typical surgical methods for medial instability, Lind et al. [13], Yoshiya et al. [22], and Borden et al. [18] reported a double-bundle graft technique which

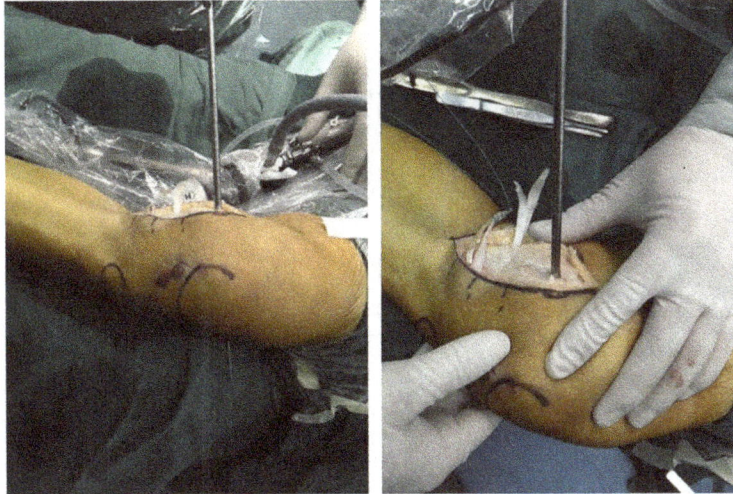

Fig. 7 A thick bone pin was drilled approximately 2.5 cm in depth

can restore critical medical valgus stability. However, there were limited data available to evaluate their effectiveness of such procedures in improving rotational stability. We speculated that these treatments might ignore the high grade MCL injury that could combine posterior-medial structure damage, especially that the POL plays a secondary structure in resisting external rotational stability [4, 5]. After comparing the anatomic ligament repair (ALR) and TLR in treating grade III MCL injury in earlier stage works, Dong et al. found that TLR offered better rotatory stability than ALR at final follow-up [23]. In our study, the TERA significantly decreased from $53.38 \pm 6.71°$ to $27.15 \pm 4.92°$ ($P < .001$) which proved the effectiveness of restoring rotational stability. Both at $0°$ and $30°$ knee flexion, the EKMO over the contralateral state decreased with significant difference ($P < .001$ both at $0°$ and $30°$ knee flexion). It also demonstrated that the anatomical-like TLR can obtain satisfactory results in respect of restoring valgus stability.

Even though most included patients (17/26, 65.4%) in our study were chronic injury, still 5 (19.2%) patients with acute injury received anatomical-like TLR. A great majority of surgeon supported that non-surgical treatment of acute injury and surgical repair or reconstruction of those

ineffective cases with chronic processing injury [14]. Because of the reliable self-healing ability, the injured MCL could attain satisfactory clinical results with proper rehabilitation [3, 16]. But high grade MCL injury was commonly held as a massive injury which often combined with POL or posterior-medial structure [5]. Because of the muscle atrophy, derangement, and scar healing, the high grade MCL injury could not gain a satisfactory clinical result as good as low grade MCL injury without concomitant structure injury [24]. So some authors advocated acute surgical repair or reconstruction for cases with grade III or above laxity [13, 16, 25]. Dong et al. put forward similar point that 3° MCL injury could hardly yield a satisfactory result if only with revision scarring and incomplete healing. Moreover, if MCL and ACL injuries are combined, the ACL and MCL surgical procedures could not be separated because the medial instability was harmful to the ACL tendon-bone healing and early stage rehabilitative exercises [14]. That is also a similar reason we adopted a more radical approach to the high grade MCL injury combined with posterior-medial structure injury. Because extensive posterior-medial structure injury leads to massive instability and isolated MCL self-healing was unsatisfactory.

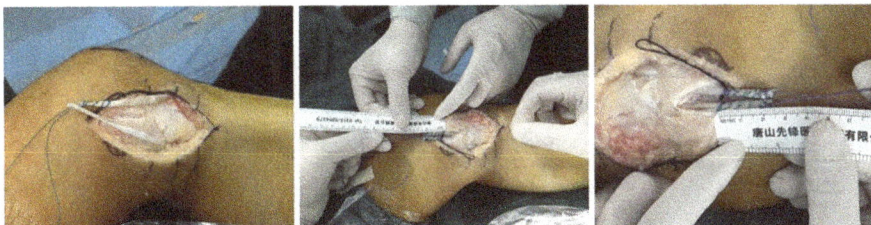

Fig. 8 The graft was measured again and then sutured the non-sutured end

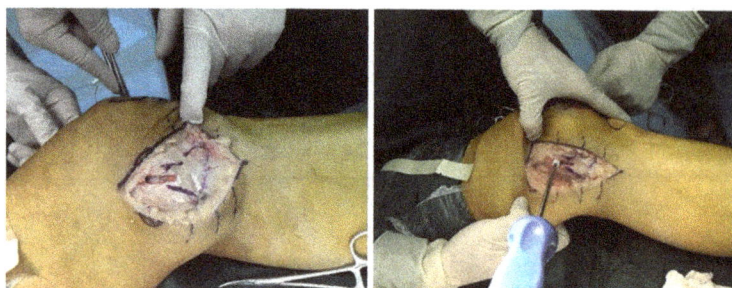

Fig. 9 A bio-interference screw was screwed into the tunnel entrance

Previous studies have confirmed that anatomical reconstructions better restore normal knee biomechanics than non-anatomical reconstructions [13]. Coobs et al. demonstrated that anatomical medial reconstruction of MCL-POL to their insertions resulted in nearly normal biomechanical knee stability and satisfying prognosis [26]. Many surgeons select drilling multi-tunnels into each of the insertions. Weimann et al. described a technique with two tibial tunnels which were located at the insertions of MCL and POL [27]. However, on the tibia two eyelet pins are drilled from medial to lateral. Even though the lateral tunnel export was set below the baseline which can reduce the damage rate of endangering the peroneal nerve, long tubular bone was not a nutritious place for tendon-bone healing. So the allograft fixation could not get a tendon-bone healing firm of long-term outcome after operation. Liu et al. reported a technique with two femoral tunnels which were also located at the insertions. But two anatomical femoral tunnels would be inappropriate [28]. The major reason was the cramped space cannot accommodate two anatomical tunnels with a 2-mm bone wall between them. At least 2 mm thickness of the bone wall between two tunnels was required to retain a safe reconstruction [29]. According to LaPrade et al. report, the location of the MCL and POL insertions, from the geometric point of view, the distance between the two insertions' center on the femur was approximately 5 mm [9]. If the 2-mm bone wall was kept entirely, there was only 1.5 mm left on each side. Generally, the diameter of the suitable size of bio-interference screw was 7 mm. If the center of the tunnel was located into the center of these two insertions, the 3.5-mm screw radius would definitely devour the bone wall. And worse, multi-tunnel had a high potential destroying accessory structures. Compared with the 7 mm screw, the single bundle allograft only had 5 mm in diameter. The graft grated with high-risk while screwing in. Dong et al. reported the original technique of triangular-vector reconstruction, who essentially abandoned the conception of anatomical reconstruction, especially the femoral tunnel was not selected at the anatomical insertion [30]. The femoral tunnel was located at the rotatory center of the knee that had been considered as isometric point. The anatomical reconstruction of the MCL was not taken into account, let alone reconstructed the function of POL. What truly matters is when the guide pin drilled paralleled with the joint line along the epicondylar axis, the intercondylar notch and the femoral insertion of PCL can be particularly vulnerable.

Table 2 EKMO over the contralateral state, TERA, subjective evaluation, and activity level scores before and after surgery

		Preoperative mean ± SD (95%CI)	Follow-up mean ± SD (95%CI)	Z	P
EKMO over the contralateral state	0°	9.76 ± 2.27 (8.84-10.67)	2.79 ± 1.02 (2.38-3.20)	−4.457	<.001[a]
	30°	10.32 ± 2.76 (9.21-11.44)	3.13 ± 0.85 (2.78-3.47)	−4.458	<.001[a]
TERA		53.38 ± 6.71 (50.68-56.09)	27.15 ± 4.92 (25.17-29.14)	−4.460	<.001[a]
Lysholm		49.42 ± 5.32 (47.28-51.57)	90.35 ± 4.55 (88.51-92.18)	−4.461	<.001[a]
Tegner		1.65 ± 0.56 (1.43-1.88)	5.77 ± 0.86 (5.42-6.12)	−4.498	<.001[a]
IKDC		47.85 ± 5.17 (45.76-49.93)	87.88 ± 3.62 (86.42-89.34)	−4.463	<.001[a]

EKMO excessive knee medial opening, *TERA* tibial external rotation angle, *IKDC* international knee documentation committee knee evaluation form, *CI* confidence interval
A Wilcoxon matched-pairs signed rank test (non-parametric) was used to compare the difference in the positive rate for the preoperative and follow-up data
[a]Statistically significant

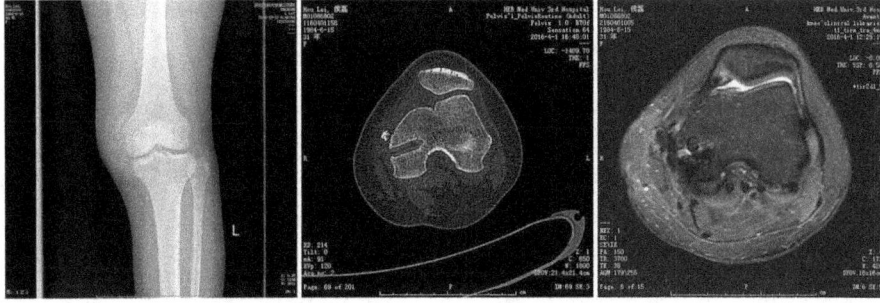

Fig. 10 Post-operative heterotopic ossification at the femoral tunnel can be diagnosed by X-ray, CT scan and MRI scan, respectively

The greatest benefit of our technical procedure was that the tunnel on the tibia can drill through the two centers of MCL and POL insertion without transfixion. The femoral intersection point was located as the drilling center of femoral tunnel. Not only the cramped space can be solved but also the graft would cover the insertions which can regain anatomical form and function. Thus it can be called an anatomical-like reconstruction. In our study, we found the subjective evaluation and activity level scores, including Lysholm, Tegner, and IKDC score, increased with statistical significance ($P < .001$). On the other side, it also proved that the anatomical-like TLR can gain good clinical function. Furthermore, reducing the usage of implantation can decrease the incidence rate of allergy and save costs.

Some studies have reported heterotopic ossification in the medial part of knee which could cause pain and tenderness [15, 31]. However, heterotopic ossification could not be distinguished whether it is caused by the MCL site injury or by the post-operative friction at bone-graft interface around the tunnels. Meanwhile, no study can explain the reason for pain or tenderness after a long post-operative period. Actually, the heterotopic ossification was probably due to medial chronic inflammation post-operatively. Dong et al. suggested the surgeon to suture the graft to the surrounding soft tissue in tibial to prevent sliding [14]. But in our study, we found that even though the screw had been fixed at the femoral tunnel, the friction and impact still occurred at the bone-graft interface which might lead to chronic inflammation as the knee moves from flexion to extension and causes heterotopic ossification. So according to our experience, we highly suggest that surgeons better suture both the femoral side and tibial side grafts with the surrounding soft tissue to diminish the friction and impact which might reduce the incidence rates of heterotopic ossification.

Limitation

The limitation includes three points. The first is the intersection point of those two K-wires could be located relatively high in some cases. The femoral insertion of medial patellofemoral ligament (MPFL) might be interfered by the bone drill. This is due to the distance of two femoral insertions is approximately 10 mm [32].While measuring, the K-wire which linked the POL insertions could be appropriately slopped a bit more because of the three separate arms of POL. The second limitation is that long-term outcomes need a minimum follow-up of 3 years which can prove the effectiveness of the modified technique. Moreover, the third limitation is that the superiority of anatomical-like TLR and non-anatomical site TLR needs to be researched.

Conclusions

Anatomical-like TLR can reconstruct the graft to cover the insertions which can regain anatomical form and function with a cramped space. Not only the valgus stability and rotational stability can be restored obviously at follow-up but also the usage of implantation can be reduced, decreasing the incidence rate of allergy and saving costs.

Abbreviations
ALR: Anatomic ligament repair; EKMO: Excessive knee medial opening; IKDC: International Knee Documentation Committee; MCL: Medial collateral ligament; MPFL: Medial patellofemoral ligament; POL: Posterior oblique ligament; TERA: Tibial external rotation angle; TLR: Triangular-vector ligament reconstruction

Acknowledgements
The authors wish to acknowledge Dr. Baicheng Chen for his help in scientific research instruction.

Funding
No funding or benefits have been received in the preparation of this manuscript.

Authors' contributions
HX and JD conceived or designed the study. JZ and DX performed the research. WL and GJ analyzed the data. SG contributed new methods or models. HX and KK wrote the paper. HX and KK contributed equally to this study. All authors read and approved the final manuscript.

Competing interests
The authors declare that they have no competing interests concerning this article.

Author details
[1]Department of Joint Surgery, The Third Hospital of Hebei Medical University, NO. 139 Ziqiang Road, Shijiazhuang 050051, Hebei, People's Republic of China. [2]People's Hospital of Ri Zhao, Taian Road, Rizhao 276800, Shandong, People's Republic of China. [3]Hospital of TCM, 35 Wanghai Road, Rizhao 276800, Shandong, People's Republic of China.

References
1. Narvani A, Mahmud T, Lavelle J, Williams A. Injury to the proximal deep medial collateral ligament: a problematical subgroup of injuries. Bone Joint J. 2010;92:949–53.
2. Warren LA, Marshall JL, Girgis F. The prime static stabilizer of the medical side of the knee. J Bone Joint Surg Am. 2013;56:137–44.
3. Azar FM. Evaluation and treatment of chronic medial collateral ligament injuries of the knee. Sports Med Arthrosc. 2006;14:84–90.
4. Madonna V, Screpis D, Condello V, Piovan G, Russo A, Guerriero M, Zorzi C. A novel technique for combined medial collateral ligament and posterior oblique ligament reconstruction: technical note. Knee Surg Sports Traumatol Arthrosc. 2015;23:1–6.
5. Griffith CJ, Wijdicks CA, Laprade RF, Armitage BM, Steinar J, Lars E. Force measurements on the posterior oblique ligament and superficial medial collateral ligament proximal and distal divisions to applied loads. Am J Sports Med. 2009;37:140–8.
6. Michael E, Johnson DL. Management of medial-sided knee injuries. Orthopedics. 2015;38:180–4.
7. Marchant MH, Tibor LM, Sekiya JK, Hardaker WT, Garrett WE, Taylor DC. Management of medial-sided knee injuries, part 1: medial collateral ligament. Am J Sports Med. 2011;39:1102–13.
8. Tibor LM, Marchant Jr MH, Taylor DC, Hardaker Jr WT, Garrett Jr WE, Sekiya JK. Management of medial-sided knee injuries, Part 2: posteromedial corner. Am J Sports Med. 2011;39:1332–40.
9. Laprade RF, Anders Hauge E, Ly TV, Steinar J, Wentorf FA, Lars E. The anatomy of the medial part of the knee. J Bone Joint Surg Am. 2007;89:2000–10.
10. Wijdicks CA, Griffith CJ, Johansen S, Sunderland A, Arendt E, Engebretsen L. Radiographic identification of the primary medial knee structures. J Bone Joint Surg Am. 2009;91:521–9.
11. Bollier M, Smith PA. Anterior cruciate ligament and medial collateral ligament injuries. J Knee Surg. 2014;27:359–68.
12. Laprade RF, Bernhardson AS, Griffith CJ, Macalena JA, Wijdicks CA. Correlation of valgus stress radiographs with medial knee ligament injuries: an in vitro biomechanical study. Am J Sports Med. 2010;38:330–8.
13. Lind M, Jakobsen BW, Lund B, Hansen MS, Abdallah O, Christiansen SE. Anatomical reconstruction of the medial collateral ligament and posteromedial corner of the knee in patients with chronic medial collateral ligament instability. Am J Sports Med. 2009;37:1116–22.
14. Dong JT, Chen BC, Men XQ, Wang F, Hao JD, Zhao JN, Wang XF, Zhang XY, Sun R. Application of triangular vector to functionally reconstruct the medial collateral ligament with double-bundle allograft technique. Arthroscopy. 2012;28:1445–53.
15. Hughston JC, Andrews JR, Cross MJ, Moschi A. Classification of knee ligament instabilities. Part I. The medial compartment and cruciate ligaments. J Bone Joint Surg Am. 1976;58:159–72.
16. Bin SI, Nam TS. Surgical outcome of 2-stage management of multiple knee ligament injuries after knee dislocation. Arthroscopy. 2007;23:1066–72.
17. Fanelli GC, Edson CJ. Arthroscopically assisted combined anterior and posterior cruciate ligament reconstruction in the multiple ligament injured knee: 2- to 10-year follow-up. Arthroscopy. 2002;18:703–14.
18. Borden PS, Kantaras AT, Caborn DN. Medial collateral ligament reconstruction with allograft using a double-bundle technique. Arthroscopy. 2002;18:E19.
19. Wahl CJ, Nicandri G. Single-Achilles allograft posterior cruciate ligament and medial collateral ligament reconstruction: A technique to avoid osseous tunnel intersection, improve construct stiffness, and save on allograft utilization. Arthroscopy. 2008;24:486–9.
20. Chen L, Kim PD, Ahmad CS, Levine WN. Medial collateral ligament injuries of the knee: current treatment concepts. Curr Rev Musculoskelet Med. 2008;1:108–3.
21. Cooper DE, Stewart D. Posterior cruciate ligament reconstruction using single-bundle patella tendon graft with tibial inlay fixation: 2- to 10-year follow-up. Am J Sports Med. 2004;32:346–60.
22. Yoshiya S, Kuroda R, Mizuno K, Yamamoto T, Kurosaka M. Medial collateral ligament reconstruction using autogenous hamstring tendons: Technique and results in initial cases. Am J Sports Med. 2005;33:1380–5.
23. Dong J, Xiao FW, Men X, Zhu J, Walker GN, Xiao ZZ, Jin BG, Chen B, Wang F, Zhang Y, Gao S. Surgical treatment of acute grade iii medial collateral ligament injury combined with anterior cruciate ligament injury: anatomic ligament repair versus triangular ligament reconstruction. Arthroscopy. 2015;31:1108–16.
24. Woo SL, Vogrin TM, Abramowitch SD. Healing and repair of ligament injuries in the knee. J Am Acad Orthop Surg. 2000;8:364–72.
25. Frolke JP, Oskam J, Vierhout PA. Primary reconstruction of the medial collateral ligament in combined injury of the medial collateral and anterior cruciate ligaments: short-term results. Knee Surg Sports Traumatol Arthrosc. 1998;6:103–6.
26. Coobs BR, Wijdicks CA, Armitage BM, Spiridonov SI, Westerhaus BD, Johansen S, Engebretsen L, Laprade RF. An in vitro analysis of an anatomical medial knee reconstruction. Am J Sports Med. 2010;38:339–47.
27. Weimann A, Schatka I, Herbort M, Achtnich A, Zantop T, Raschke M, Petersen W. Reconstruction of the posterior oblique ligament and the posterior cruciate ligament in knees with posteromedial instability. Arthroscopy. 2012;28:1283–9.
28. Liu H, Wang F, Kang H, Chen B, Zhang Y, Ma L. Anatomical reconstruction of the medial collateral ligament and the posterior oblique ligament of the knee. Acta Orthop Belg. 2012;78:400–4.
29. Sherlock MF, Otto D. Antegrade tibial tunnel technique for posterior cruciate ligament reconstruction. Arthroscopy. 2008;24:1301–5.
30. Dong J, Ji G, Zhang Y, Gao S, Wang F, Chen B. Single allograft medial collateral ligament and posterior oblique ligament reconstruction: a technique to improve valgus and rotational stability. Eur J Orthop Surg Traumatol. 2014;24:1025–9.
31. Sims WF, Jacobson KE. The posteromedial corner of the knee: medial-sided injury patterns revisited. Am J Sports Med. 2004;32:337–45.
32. Fujino K, Tajima G, Yan J, Kamei Y, Maruyama M, Takeda S, Kikuchi S, Shimamura T. Morphology of the femoral insertion site of the medial patellofemoral ligament. Knee Surg Sports Traumatol Arthrosc. 2015;23:1–6.

8

Minimally invasive unilateral pedicle screws and a translaminar facet screw fixation and interbody fusion for treatment of single-segment lower lumbar vertebral disease: surgical technique and preliminary clinical results

Peng Huang, Yiguo Wang, Jiao Xu, Bo Xiao, Jianheng Liu, Luyang Che and Keya Mao[*]

Abstract

Background: Conventional open transforaminal lumbar interbody fusion (TLIF) using unilateral pedicle screws and a translaminar facet screw has been performed for many years with good results. The outcomes of minimally invasive TLIF (MIS TLIF) are similar to the good outcomes of open TLIF, with the additional benefits of reducing iatrogenic injury, shortening hospital stays, and reducing the recovery duration. Instead of using small cuts on both sides, we performed MIS TLIF through a single cut using unilateral pedicle screws and a translaminar facet screw. The operative feasibility, efficacy safety, and benefits of single-level MIS TLIF of such techniques require further clarification.

Methods: A total of 60 patients with various single-segment lower lumbar vertebral diseases were treated in our department from January 2010 to March 2013. All the patients were initially performed single-level MIS TLIF using a hybrid construction of unilateral pedicle screws and a translaminar facet screw. Patient demographics and operative data were collected. The clinical outcomes were assessed before surgery and 3, 6, 12, and 24 months after surgery using the visual analog scale (VAS) for back and leg pain and the Oswestry Disability Index (ODI). Radiologic assessment of the lumbar spine with static and dynamic plain radiographs was performed 3, 6, 12, and 24 months after surgery. The fusion rates were assessed by an independent radiologist 2 years after surgery according to the Bridwell interbody fusion grading system.

(Continued on next page)

* Correspondence: maokeya@sina.com
Department of Orthopaedics, Chinese PLA General Hospital, Beijing 100853,
China

(Continued from previous page)

Results: No patients experienced significant postoperative complications. Excepting two cases, 58 cases were followed up for 24–38 months, averaged 29.9 ± 4.1 months. The patients' average age was 46.6 ± 11.5 years, operative time 109.7 ± 17.8 min, intraoperative blood loss 67.3 ± 29.7 ml, length of incision 29.0 ± 3.2 mm, fluoroscopy time 31.1 ± 7.2 s, time to ambulation 20.3 ± 7.0 h, length of hospital stay 5.1 ± 1.1 days, and length of the translaminar facet screw 51.7 ± 3.4 mm. Screw position results: type I, 54 cases with 54 segments; type II, four cases with four segments. There were two (3.4%) translaminar facet screw failures, which were intraoperatively converted to a bilateral pedicle screw fixation procedure and excluded from the research. The postoperative images showed good positioning of the hybrid internal fixation, and all of the translaminar facet screws penetrated the facet joint. Two (3.6%) translaminar facet screws penetrated the lateral lamina and two (3.6%) translaminar facet screws penetrated the medial lamina without any serious neural complications. During the follow-up, there was no screw loosening or pedicle fracture observed. The VAS and ODI scores were significantly improved compared with the preoperative scores (P < 0.05), and the symptoms disappeared gradually. Fifty-one patients (87.9%) achieved grade I fusion radiographically at the final follow-up.

Conclusions: MIS TLIF using a hybrid construction of unilateral pedicle screws and a translaminar facet screw is safe and effective in the treatment of single-segment lower lumbar vertebral disease, and it can be used as an optimal choice for fixation and fusion of some single-segment lower lumbar vertebral diseases.

Keywords: Minimally invasive spinal surgery, Translaminar facet screw fixation, Pedicle screw fixation, Lumbar degenerative disease

Background

Bilateral pedicle screw fixation combined with interbody fusion has been recognized as the "gold standard" treatment for the lumbar vertebral disease, which has a variety of advantages, such as great fixation intensity, excellent stability, and high fusion rate [1–8]. However, with its extensive use in the clinic, many disadvantages of the treatment have been reported, which includes long skin incision, considerable stress of internal fixation by strong fixation, stress shielding in the fixed segment, and the potential accelerated degeneration of adjacent segments [9–11]. Thus, surgeons have searched several modified fixation techniques, such as unilateral pedicle screw (UPS), and UPS plus contralateral translaminar facet screw (UPSFS) which has come into use, and acquired good clinical outcome and satisfied fusion rate [12–14].

Unilateral pedicle screw fixation combined with interbody fusion has been extensively used in the clinic, which has gotten a primarily good clinic result. Significant reductions in operation time, duration of hospitalization, and costs have been cited as the benefits of unilateral pedicle screw fixation (PSF) [12]. And some studies even showed that the unilateral PSF has equivalent fusion rates compared with the bilateral PSF [15]. However, biomedical studies indicated that this method failed to control lateral bending and resist torsional forces, potentially resulting in stress concentration and increasing the risk of internal fixation failure [16–19]. Translaminar facet screw fixation is another important method for lumbar fixation. Many relevant studies confirmed its availability in the clinic application [20, 21]. The translaminar facet screw was first introduced by King in 1948, and this technique involved the insertion of a short screw across the facet joint [22].

Translaminar facet screw fixation (TFSF) was initially described as a form of posterior instrumented fusion for lumbosacral degenerative disease by Magerl in the 1980s [23, 24]. The screw is a long screw that enters through the base of the spinous process on one side, fixes the contralateral facet joint after traversing the lamina, and ends at the base of the transverse process [23]. This procedure has been shown to be a successful technique that offers ease of procedure, smaller incisions, few complications, and reduced implant costs [25–29].

In addition to interbody fusion, TFSF offers a strong alternative to PSF with the same indications. However, the traditional use of TFSF also requires extensive paraspinal muscle retraction for insertion with consequent increased infection rates and muscle injury, and it carries a risk of neural and vascular damage as a result of improperly placed screws [7, 26, 30]. Researchers have attempted to achieve satisfactory lumbar fusion using minimally invasive (MIS) techniques that reduce injury and implant costs.

As a means of providing suitable spine stiffness with minimal injury and implant load, a hybrid construction of unilateral pedicle screws with a contralateral translaminar facet screw has been studied more frequently [14, 18, 31–34]. Biomechanical studies have certified the comparable strengths of bilateral PSF and unilateral pedicle screws and translaminar facet screw combination [18, 31, 33, 34]. Clinical outcomes have shown that open transforaminal lumbar interbody fusion (TLIF) using unilateral pedicle screws and a translaminar facet screw offers good results [14]. However, few studies on MIS TLIF using unilateral pedicle screws and a translaminar facet screw have been reported [32].

Hence, the feasibility, clinical outcomes, and fusion rates of unilateral pedicle screws combined with a translaminar facet screw in single-segment lower lumbar vertebral disease were investigated in this study.

Methods

Ethics statement

This study has been approved by the Ethics Committee of the Chinese PLA General Hospital, and the approval number is K2010-011-02. Written informed consent was obtained from each patient prior to the study.

Inclusion and exclusion criteria

Inclusion criteria were patients with (I) single-segment lower lumbar vertebral disease; (II) chronic low back pain with or without neurological symptoms of lower extremities; and (III) inefficacy after strict conservative treatment for more than 6 months. Imaging findings showed serious single segmental degeneration disease, unilateral intervertebral disc herniation, or lumbar instability, which are consistent with the symptoms and signs. Exclusion criteria were (I) lumbar degenerative spondylolisthesis (II degree or higher); (II) lumbar spondylolysis; (III) serious three-dimensional deformity of lumbar vertebrae; (IV) obvious osteoporosis of lumbar vertebrae; and (V) patients with multi-segment lumbar degenerative disease, revision surgery, spinal tumor, acute spinal trauma, and spinal infections.

General information

This study included 60 patients (34 male, 26 female) aged 22 to 67 years (mean, 46.6 years). All the patients have a history of lumbar degenerative disease and had been treated conservatively for at least 6 months without success. The patients were evaluated with a routine lumbar X-ray, computed tomography (CT), and magnetic resonance imaging at admission, and the signs and symptoms of the patients were consistent with the imaging findings. Fifty-eight patients underwent single-level MIS TLIF by the same experienced surgeon using a hybrid construct fixation with unilateral pedicle screws combined with contralateral translaminar facet screw. It was the first lumbar surgery at that level for all of the patients, and the indication for surgery was chronic low back pain, intermittent claudication, and unilateral radicular complaints. The translaminar facet screw length and the thickness and oblique angle of the laminar were measured according to the preoperative lumbar X-ray and CT. The hybrid construct fixation was used at the L4–L5 level in 23 patients and at the L5–S1 level in 35 patients. Thirty-five patients underwent translaminar fixation on the left side, and 23 patients underwent fixation on the right side. The minimum follow-up was 24 months (range 24 to 38 months).

Surgical technique

The MIS TLIF procedure was performed on the side that appeared symptomatic. Under general anesthesia, the patient was placed in a prone position on a radiolucent operative frame. The surgical procedure consisted of the following steps:

1. Incision and placement of tubular retractor: With the help of a C arm, a longitudinal incision was made in the skin 3–4 cm lateral to the midline on the symptomatic side. The incision was generally 2.5–3 cm long, which was sufficient for the placement of the tubular retractor (METRx system, Medtronic Sofamor Danek, USA).

2. Discectomy, decompression, and fusion: After blunt dissection of the longissimus and multifidus muscles, progressive dilation of the dissected plane was completed. The tubular retractor was then docked over the facet joint at the level of the surgery. After clearance of the reliquus soft tissues under direct vision, the peripheral lamina and the facet joint were exposed. Canals for the pedicle screws were prepared with the help of a C arm. A complete facetectomy was then performed, and the ligamentum flavum was resected. After the traversing and exiting nerve roots were identified, a rigorous discectomy was conducted and the cartilage end plates were removed using curettement. A sufficient local autologous bone graft taken from the removed facet was used to fill the disc space. A single appropriately sized PEEK cage (Concorde, DePuy Spine, USA) packed with locally harvested autologous cancellous bone was inserted obliquely across the disc space. When sufficient decompression was completed, two pedicle screws and a rod (Exp, Depuy Spine, USA) were implanted before the final tightening.

3. Translaminar facet screw fixation: The lateral and laminar angles of the translaminar facet screw to be fused were measured preoperatively using X-ray and CT or MR imaging. After the MIS TLIF and unilateral PSF procedure, the tube was adjusted to provide an oblique view of the base of the superior spinous process. This facilitated the entry of a 2.2-mm-diameter drill. Considering the preoperatively determined lateral and laminar angles, the drill was inserted through the same incision under radiological guidance. During the drill's insertion, care was taken to ensure that it remained within the cortical confines of the lamina. After drilling, a 4.5-mm-diameter cortical screw (AO Spine, USA) of suitable length (usually 45–58 mm) was inserted for fixation, traversing through the lamina and facet joints and terminating at the base of the transverse

process. Accurate placement of the screw was confirmed using the C arm or intraoperative CT prior to wound closure. A representative case is presented in Fig. 1.

Postoperative treatment

Patients received routine postoperative management, including infection prevention, and low-dose hormones and correction of dehydration and gastric mucosal protective measures and bed rest. After waking from anesthesia, the patients were encouraged to actively dorsiflex the ankle and perform straight leg raises with both lower legs. All the patients did not need to have a drainage tube. Patients wore waist support and were encouraged out-of-bed activity 3 to 5 days postoperatively. With the help of a waist girdle, progressive back and abdominal muscle exercises were initiated at the sixth week postoperatively.

Evaluation method

The data recorded for analysis were age, gender, operative time, intraoperative blood loss, length of incision, X-ray exposure time, length of the translaminar facet screw, time to ambulation, length of hospital stay, complications, and the clinical and radiographic results after surgery. After surgery or discharge from the hospital, the patients received regular, close follow-up (at 3 days, 3 months, 6 months, and 1 year postoperation and annually thereafter). Clinical and radiological evaluations were conducted at every follow-up visit. All of the data were collected prospectively after a minimum of 2 years of follow-up. The patients were evaluated using the visual analog scale (VAS) for leg and back pain and the Oswestry Disability Index (ODI), version 2.0. The radiological evaluation included anteroposterior, lateral, oblique, and flexion-extension plain radiography, CT scans, and MRI. Translaminar facet screw and interbody fusion were assessed by imaging. Translaminar facet screw position was classified into three types: type I, the translaminar facet screw is located in the lamina; type II, the translaminar facet screw penetrates the lamina partially; and type III, the translaminar facet screw penetrated the lamina completely [35]. Fusion rates based on the Bridwell interbody fusion grading system were assessed using static and dynamic plain radiography 2 years postoperatively [36]. The Bridwell interbody fusion grading system is provided in Table 1.

Statistical analysis

SPSS 17.0 (SPSS, Chicago, IL) was used for the statistical analyses. Normally distributed continuous variables are shown as the mean ± SD. Analysis of variance (ANOVA) was performed for the VAS and ODI scores. A P value less than 0.05 was considered statistically significant.

Results
General information

A total of 58 patients were followed up in the study. The mean age of the patients was 46.6 ± 11.5 years (range 22–67 years), and the mean follow-up period was 29.9 ± 4.1 months (range 24–38 months).

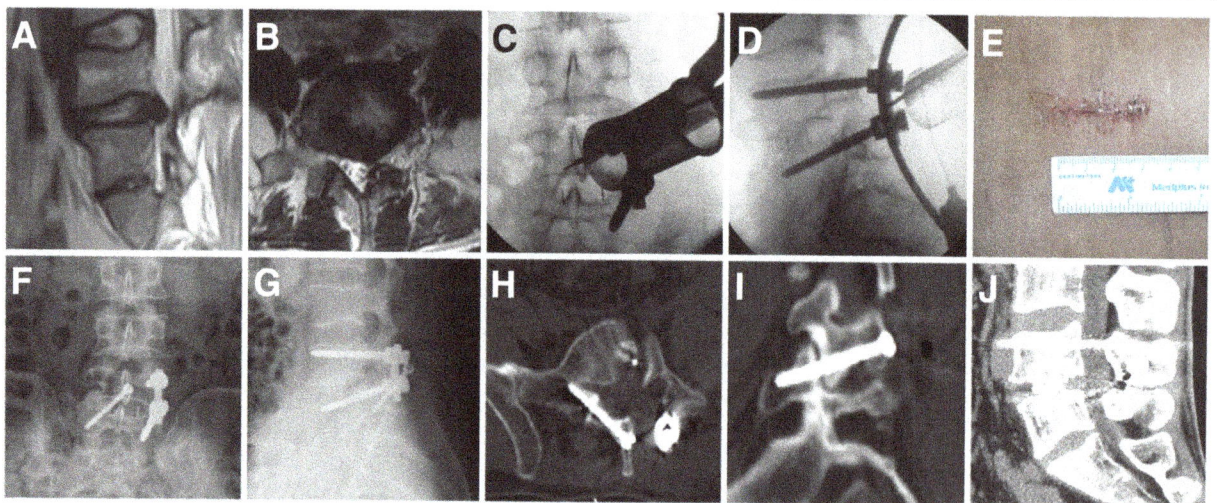

Fig. 1 The preoperative MRI (**a**, **b**) showed a herniated disc. Accurate placement of the translaminar facet screw (**c**, **d**) was accomplished using the C arm intraoperatively. A small skin incision (**e**) was showed. Anteroposterior (**f**) and lateral (**g**) views after MIS TLIF showed good position of the hybrid internal fixation. CT scans (**h–j**) at 2 years after surgery demonstrated solid interbody fusion, and the translaminar facet screw entered through the base of spinous process on one side, fixed the contralateral facet joint after traversing the laminar, and ended at the base of the transverse process

Table 1 Bridwell interbody fusion grading system

Grade	Description
I	Fused with remodeling and trabeculae present
II	Graft intact, not fully remodeled and incorporated, but no lucency present
III	Graft intact, potential lucency present at top and bottom of graft
IV	Fusion absent with collapse/resorption of graft

Operative data

The mean operative time was 109.7 ± 17.8 min (range 73–157 min); the mean intraoperative blood loss was 67.3 ± 29.7 ml (range 26–157 ml); the mean length of incision was 29.0 ± 3.2 mm (range 24–37 mm); the mean fluoroscopy time was 31.1 ± 7.2 s (range 19–53 s); the mean ambulation time was 20.3 ± 7.0 h (range 8–42 h); the mean length of hospital stay was 5.1 ± 1.1 days (range 3–8 days); and the mean translaminar facet screw length was 51.7 ± 3.4 mm (range 45–58 mm). Translaminar facet screw positions were assessed as follows: type I, 54 cases with 54 segments, and type II, four cases with four segments.

Follow-up

During the follow-up, there were significant improvements in both the VAS score for back and leg pain and the ODI scores at all time points compared with the pre-operation scores ($P < 0.05$). The symptoms disappeared gradually. The VAS and ODI scores are listed in Table 2. Fifty-one patients (87.9%) achieved grade I fusion radiographically at the 2-year follow-up. There were no cases of grade III or IV fusions.

Complications

Two (3.4%) cases of small dural tears during decompression were not repaired, and these two patients were kept on bed rest for 10 days with no subsequent postoperative cerebrospinal fluid leakage. One (1.7%) case of fat

Table 2 Results of VAS and ODI score

	VAS back	VAS leg	ODI
Preoperative	6.2 ± 1.8	6.8 ± 1.8	57.7 ± 15.5
Three days after operation	$3.1 \pm 1.5^*$	$1.7 \pm 1.2^*$	-
Three months after operation	$1.8 \pm 1.2^{*\#}$	$1.4 \pm 1.2^*$	$27.6 \pm 11.1^*$
Six months after operation	$1.6 \pm 1.3^{*\#}$	$1.4 \pm 1.3^*$	$25.1 \pm 8.8^*$
One year after operation	$1.4 \pm 1.4^{*\#}$	$1.2 \pm 1.0^{*\#}$	$19.1 \pm 8.6^{*\triangle\triangledown}$
Two years after operation	$1.1 \pm 0.9^{*\#\triangle}$	$0.9 \pm 0.8^{*\#\triangle\triangledown}$	$13.8 \pm 5.8^{*\triangle\triangledown\measuredangle}$
P	0.000	0.000	0.000

Note: "-" stands for no data

*compared with preoperative value, $P < 0.05$; #compared with the value at 3 days after operation, $P < 0.05$; △compared with the value at 3 months after operation, $P < 0.05$; ▽compared with the value at 6 months after operation, $P < 0.05$; ⊿compared with the value at 1 year after operation, $P < 0.05$

liquefaction experienced primary healing after physical therapy and changing of the dressings. There were two translaminar facet screw failures that were intraoperatively converted to pedicle screws (bilateral PSF). The postoperative images showed good positioning of the hybrid internal fixation, and all of the translaminar facet screws penetrated the facet joint. Two (3.6%) translaminar facet screws penetrated the lateral lamina, and two (3.6%) translaminar facet screws penetrated the medial lamina with no serious neural complications. One (1.7%) patient who required temporary new radiculopathy because of translaminar facet screw malpositioning experienced a full recovery within 2 weeks after subsequent corrective surgery.

Discussion

In this study, a tubular retractor was adopted to expose the lamina and articular process. Facetectomy, discectomy, intervertebral clearance, intervertebral bone grafting, and cage placement were then performed. Unilateral pedicle screws combined with a contralateral translaminar facet screw fixation based on preoperative measured data were conducted. Previous studies indicated that translaminar facet screw fixation is a simple, safe, and satisfactory method [29, 37]. Our results revealed that the direction of the drill in the lamina and screw placement were the most important step in this operation. Postoperatively, imaging data indicated that the position of the translaminar facet screws was good (type I, 53 cases with 54 segments; type II, three cases with four segments). In this operation, only a 3–4-cm longitudinal incision was made in the skin lateral to the midline on the symptomatic side, while the muscles, facet joint, and laminar on the contralateral side remained intact, which is important to reduce surgical trauma and blood loss and shorten operative time [38]. The mean operative time was 109.7 ± 17.8 min (range 73–157 min); the mean intraoperative blood loss was 67.3 ± 29.7 ml (range 26–157 ml); the mean length of incision was 29.0 ± 3.2 mm (range 24–37 mm); the mean fluoroscopy time was 31.1 ± 7.2 s (range 19–53 s); the mean ambulation time was 20.3 ± 7.0 h (range 8–42 h); the mean length of hospital stay was 5.1 ± 1.1 days (range 3–8 days); and the mean translaminar facet screw length was 51.7 ± 3.4 mm (range 45–58 mm). The low intraoperative blood loss, small skin incision, reduced trauma, and short operative time all contributed to moderate pain and rapid recovery postoperatively. In addition, all patients wore waist support and were encouraged out-of-bed activity 3 to 5 days postoperatively. With the help of a waist girdle, progressive back and abdominal muscle exercises were initiated at the sixth week postoperatively and no fixation loosening and breakage were observed during the follow-up. Fifty-one patients (87.9%) achieved grade

I fusion radiographically at the 2-year follow-up. There were no cases of grade III or IV fusions. Sethi et al. also achieved bony fusion among 19 patients with low lumbar lesions using unilateral pedicle screws and a translaminar screw fixation technique [14]. The results of Sethi and our study both indicated that unilateral pedicle screw fixation combined with contralateral translaminar facet screw fixation and interbody fusion technique can obtain satisfactory clinical results. Moreover, significant differences in VAS and ODI scores were observed between the final follow-up and preoperation. The leg and back pain, lumbar function, and activities of daily living were obviously improved. Compared with the conventional internal fixation technique [14, 39], our study indicated that unilateral pedicle screw fixation combined with contralateral translaminar facet screw fixation and interbody fusion can obtain the same satisfactory clinical results.

However, several other surgical techniques are available to obtain single segmental lumbar interbody fusion at present. PSF is frequently used to provide temporary spinal stability after spinal surgery until a fusion mass forms [12, 15]. Although it offers the advantage of solid stability, bilateral PSF use is associated with higher implant costs and an increased incidence of neurologic complications [40, 41]. Furthermore, it requires extensive paraspinal muscle retraction for the insertion of the screws, which results in increased rates of infection and muscle injury, and improperly placed screws can lead to neural and vascular damage [7, 26, 30]. With the aim of reducing operative time and implant costs, some researchers have attempted to use unilateral PSF for lumbar spinal fusion [12]. However, unilateral PSF has not been recommended for long fusions despite studies that show comparable fusion rates for unilateral and bilateral PSF [15, 18]. The authors of several biomechanical investigations have demonstrated that unilateral PSF decreases spinal stiffness [18, 19].

Many researchers have shown that translaminar facet screw insertion provides a comparable rate of fusion and satisfactory clinical outcomes provided that the indications are correctly applied [29, 37]. The current study supports the use of TFSF for short-segment fusion in the lumbar spine as a successful technique with the benefits of a relatively simple procedure, smaller incisions, few complications, and reduced implant costs [25–29]. Currently, the hybrid construct of unilateral pedicle screws combined with a contralateral translaminar facet screw is being increasingly investigated because it provides suitable spine stiffness with minimal injury and implant loads [14, 18, 31–34]. Several biomechanical studies have shown that the hybrid construction provides a strength similar to that of bilateral PSF [18, 31, 33, 34]. Sethi and Lee documented the good clinical outcomes of open

TLIF using unilateral pedicle screws and a translaminar facet screw (similar to the system we used in our study), and they suggested that the hybrid construction offered a less expensive and more viable option for single-level lumbar fusion [14]. Jang and Lee published their pilot clinical studies of the unilateral pedicle screw (PS)-based and contralateral facet screw (FS)-based TLIF techniques, and they indicated that TLIF with ipsilateral PS and contralateral FS fixation offered reduced blood loss and soft-tissue injury compared with the conventional TLIF [32].

Researchers have attempted to achieve satisfactory lumbar fusion with MIS techniques while reducing injury and implant costs [42]. The morbidity associated with open TLIF is extensive, and prolonged muscle ischemia occurs as a result of the extensive muscle stripping and retraction that occurs during the surgical approach [43, 44]. The MIS TLIF procedure is used to achieve solid lumbar interbody fusion via a unilateral posterolateral approach, and it has gained recent popularity because it results in smaller wounds, less tissue trauma, and faster recovery [45, 46]. However, wide exposure and expensive implants are required for the insertion of the percutaneous pedicle screws in standard MIS TLIF [14, 32]. In addition, the soft-tissue injuries caused by the insertion of percutaneous pedicle screws include damage to muscles, the adjacent facet, and ligaments. The procedure can cause increased blood loss, infection rate, and postoperative back pain; a longer recovery period; and impaired fusion [30, 44, 47].

For the disadvantages previously mentioned above, we performed MIS TLIF in 58 patients using a hybrid internal fixation system consisting of unilateral pedicle screws and a contralateral translaminar facet screw. The technique of MIS TLIF used in this study was quite different from the standard MIS TLIF [14, 32], and our result revealed that it is characterized by a small incision, reduced trauma, simple operation, high safety, good stability, high fusion rate, and few complications. And we determined that it is feasible and safe to insert a translaminar facet screw under direct vision via a single small incision and that there was no decrease in stiffness or effectiveness compared with the conventional bilateral PSF procedure. Because the anatomical structures surrounding the canal created for the translaminar facet screw include the posterior muscle, the anterior ligamentum flavum, and the superior and inferior pedicle cortical bone, there is a relatively extensive safe area for the insertion of the translaminar facet screw. This safety statement was also justified by the fact that in our study, two (3.6%) translaminar facet screws penetrated the lateral lamina and two (3.6%) translaminar facet screws penetrated the medial lamina with no serious neural complications. Additionally, there was a relatively steep learning curve for this technique.

However, there are several limitations to this current study. Firstly, it is a retrospective investigation, which cannot avoid selection and recall bias completely, despite our trying our best to collect and analyze the data meticulously throughout the study. Secondly, the patients with bilateral radicular symptoms were not included. In fact, our group has already adopted this technique to treat patients with bilateral symptoms and two segment degenerative lumbar disease. Next, we will report the preliminary result of this aspect of the research. Last, but not the least, the sample size in this study was relatively small and the follow-up time of 29.9 months was relatively short to observe the long-term clinical outcome. And it is just a preliminary clinical study about the feasibility of this surgical technique and a clinical result. In the future, well-designed prospective studies with a larger study population and longer follow-up time should be conducted to determine the clinical and radiographic significance of the MIS TLIF technique compared with bilateral PSF technique and other internal fixation methods, providing a convincing evidence-based conclusion.

Conclusion

We have introduced the MIS TLIF technique using a hybrid internal fixation system constructed with unilateral pedicle screws and a contralateral translaminar facet screw which was different from the conventional MIS TLIF. The MIS TLIF technique is safe and effective in the treatment of single-segment lower lumbar vertebral disease, and it can be used as an optimal choice for the fixation and fusion of some single-segment lower lumbar vertebral diseases.

Abbreviations
CT: Computed tomography; ODI: Oswestry Disability Index; PSF: Pedicle screw fixation; TFSF: Translaminar facet screw fixation; TLIF: Transforaminal lumbar interbody fusion; VAS: Visual analog scale

Acknowledgements
This research was performed mainly at the Department of Orthopaedics of the Chinese PLA General Hospital.

Funding
This work was supported by the Project of the National Natural Science Foundation (51372276) and the 12th Five-Year Military Medicine and Health Project (CWS11J110).

Authors' contributions
PH and KM designed the study. YW carried out the study and collected the crucial background information. JX and JL collected the data. BX analyzed the data. JL interpreted the data. PH composed the article. LC did the figure editing. All authors read and approved the final manuscript.

Authors' information
Peng Huang is the first author and Keya Mao is the corresponding author.

Competing interests
The authors declare that they have no competing interests.

References
1. Glaser J, Stanley M, Sayre H, Woody J, Found E, Spratt K. A 10-year follow-up evaluation of lumbar spine fusion with pedicle screw fixation. Spine (Phila Pa 1976). 2003;28(13):1390–5.
2. Brantigan JW, Neidre A, Toohey JS. The Lumbar I/F Cage for posterior lumbar interbody fusion with the variable screw placement system: 10-year results of a Food and Drug Administration clinical trial. Spine J. 2004;4(6):681–8.
3. Cheh G, Bridwell KH, Lenke LG, et al. Adjacent segment disease following lumbar/thoracolumbar fusion with pedicle screw instrumentation: a minimum 5-year follow-up. Spine (Phila Pa 1976). 2007;32(20):2253–7.
4. Oh HS, Kim JS, Lee SH, Liu WC, Hong SW. Comparison between the accuracy of percutaneous and open pedicle screw fixations in lumbosacral fusion. Spine J. 2013;13(12):1751–7.
5. Kim YJ, Lenke LG, Bridwell KH, Cho YS, Riew KD. Free hand pedicle screw placement in the thoracic spine: is it safe. Spine (Phila Pa 1976). 2004;29(3):333–42. discussion 342.
6. Gertzbein SD, Robbins SE. Accuracy of pedicular screw placement in vivo. Spine (Phila Pa 1976). 1990;15(1):11–4.
7. Kim CW, Lee YP, Taylor W, Oygar A, Kim WK. Use of navigation-assisted fluoroscopy to decrease radiation exposure during minimally invasive spine surgery. Spine J. 2008;8(4):584–90.
8. Tuli J, Tuli S, Eichler ME, Woodard EJ. A comparison of long-term outcomes of translaminar facet screw fixation and pedicle screw fixation: a prospective study. J Neurosurg Spine. 2007;7(3):287–92.
9. Zeng ZY, Wu P, Mao KY, et al. Unilateral pedicle screw fixation versus its combination with contralateral translaminar facet screw fixation for the treatment of single segmental lower lumbar vertebra diseases. Zhongguo Gu Shang. 2015;28(4):306–12.
10. Park P, Garton HJ, Gala VC, Hoff JT, Mcgillicuddy JE. Adjacent segment disease after lumbar or lumbosacral fusion: review of the literature. Spine (Phila Pa 1976). 2004;29(17):1938–44.
11. Zencica P, Chaloupka R, Hladíková J, Krbec M. Adjacent segment degeneration after lumbosacral fusion in spondylolisthesis: a retrospective radiological and clinical analysis. Acta Chir Orthop Traumatol Cech. 2010;77(2):124–30.
12. Suk KS, Lee HM, Kim NH, Ha JW. Unilateral versus bilateral pedicle screw fixation in lumbar spinal fusion. Spine (Phila Pa 1976). 2000;25(14):1843–7.
13. Feng ZZ, Cao YW, Jiang C, Jiang XX. Short-term outcome of bilateral decompression via a unilateral paramedian approach for transforaminal lumbar interbody fusion with unilateral pedicle screw fixation. Orthopedics. 2011;34(5):364.
14. Sethi A, Lee S, Vaidya R. Transforaminal lumbar interbody fusion using unilateral pedicle screws and a translaminar screw. Eur Spine J. 2009;18(3):430–4.
15. Kabins MB, Weinstein JN, Spratt KF, et al. Isolated L4-L5 fusions using the variable screw placement system: unilateral versus bilateral. J Spinal Disord. 1992;5(1):39–49.
16. Harris BM, Hilibrand AS, Savas PE, et al. Transforaminal lumbar interbody fusion: the effect of various instrumentation techniques on the flexibility of the lumbar spine. Spine (Phila Pa 1976). 2004;29(4):E65–70.
17. Kasai Y, Inaba T, Kato T, Matsumura Y, Akeda K, Uchida A. Biomechanical study of the lumbar spine using a unilateral pedicle screw fixation system. J Clin Neurosci. 2010;17(3):364–7.
18. Slucky AV, Brodke DS, Bachus KN, Droge JA, Braun JT. Less invasive posterior fixation method following transforaminal lumbar interbody fusion: a biomechanical analysis. Spine J. 2006;6(1):78–85.
19. Goel VK, Lim TH, Gwon J, et al. Effects of rigidity of an internal fixation device. A comprehensive biomechanical investigation. Spine (Phila Pa 1976). 1991;16(3 Suppl):S155–61.
20. Aepli M, Mannion AF, Grob D. Translaminar screw fixation of the lumbar spine: long-term outcome. Spine (Phila Pa 1976). 2009;34(14):1492–8.
21. Pavlov PW, Meijers H, van Limbeek J, et al. Good outcome and restoration of lordosis after anterior lumbar interbody fusion with additional posterior fixation. Spine (Phila Pa 1976). 2004;29(17):1893–9. discussion 1900.
22. King D. Internal fixation for lumbosacral fusion. J Bone Joint Surg Am. 1948;30A(3):560–5.

23. Magerl FP. Stabilization of the lower thoracic and lumbar spine with external skeletal fixation. Clin Orthop Relat Res. 1984;189:125–41.

24. Montesano PX, Magerl F, Jacobs RR, Jackson RP, Rauschning W. Translaminar facet joint screws. Orthopedics. 1988;11(10):1393–7.

25. Reich SM, Kuflik P, Neuwirth M. Translaminar facet screw fixation in lumbar spine fusion. Spine (Phila Pa 1976). 1993;18(4):444–9.

26. Best NM, Sasso RC. Efficacy of translaminar facet screw fixation in circumferential interbody fusions as compared to pedicle screw fixation. J Spinal Disord Tech. 2006;19(2):98–103.

27. Grob D, Bartanusz V, Jeszenszky D, et al. A prospective, cohort study comparing translaminar screw fixation with transforaminal lumbar interbody fusion and pedicle screw fixation for fusion of the degenerative lumbar spine. J Bone Joint Surg Br. 2009;91(10):1347–53.

28. Jang JS, Lee SH, Lim SR. Guide device for percutaneous placement of translaminar facet screws after anterior lumbar interbody fusion. Technical note. J Neurosurg. 2003;98(1 Suppl):100–3.

29. Humke T, Grob D, Dvorak J, Messikommer A. Translaminar screw fixation of the lumbar and lumbosacral spine. A 5-year follow-up. Spine (Phila Pa 1976). 1998;23(10):1180–4.

30. Kawaguchi Y, Matsui H, Tsuji H. Back muscle injury after posterior lumbar spine surgery. A histologic and enzymatic analysis. Spine (Phila Pa 1976). 1996;21(8):941–4.

31. Deguchi M, Cheng BC, Sato K, Matsuyama Y, Zdeblick TA. Biomechanical evaluation of translaminar facet joint fixation. A comparative study of poly-L-lactide pins, screws, and pedicle fixation. Spine (Phila Pa 1976). 1998;23(12):1307–12. Discussion 1313.

32. Jang JS, Lee SH. Minimally invasive transforaminal lumbar interbody fusion with ipsilateral pedicle screw and contralateral facet screw fixation. J Neurosurg Spine. 2005;3(3):218–23.

33. Eskander M, Brooks D, Ordway N, Dale E, Connolly P. Analysis of pedicle and translaminar facet fixation in a multisegment interbody fusion model. Spine (Phila Pa 1976). 2007;32(7):E230–5.

34. Schleicher P, Beth P, Ottenbacher A, et al. Biomechanical evaluation of different asymmetrical posterior stabilization methods for minimally invasive transforaminal lumbar interbody fusion. J Neurosurg Spine. 2008;9(4):363–71.

35. Zeng ZY, Zhang JQ, Song YX, et al. Combination of percutaneous unilateral translaminar facet screw fixation and interbody fusion for treatment of lower lumbar vertebra diseases: a follow-up study. Orthop Surg. 2014;6(2):110–7.

36. Bridwell KH, Lenke LG, McEnery KW, Baldus C, Blanke K. Anterior fresh frozen structural allografts in the thoracic and lumbar spine. Do they work if combined with posterior fusion and instrumentation in adult patients with kyphosis or anterior column defects. Spine (Phila Pa 1976). 1995;20(12):1410–8.

37. Kim KT, Lee SH, Lee YH, Bae SC, Suk KS. Clinical outcomes of 3 fusion methods through the posterior approach in the lumbar spine. Spine (Phila Pa 1976). 2006;31(12):1351–7. discussion 1358.

38. Zeng ZY, Wu P, Yan WF, et al. Mixed fixation and interbody fusion for treatment single-segment lower lumbar vertebral disease: midterm follow-up results. Orthop Surg. 2015;7(4):324–32.

39. Bagan B, Patel N, Deutsch H, Harrop J, Sharan A, Vaccaro AR, et al. Perioperative complications of minimally invasive surgery (MIS): comparison of MIS and open interbody fusion techniques. Surg Technol Int. 2008;17:281–6.

40. Pihlajämaki H, Myllynen P, Böstman O. Complications of transpedicular lumbosacral fixation for non-traumatic disorders. J Bone Joint Surg Br. 1997;79(2):183–9.

41. Castro WH, Halm H, Jerosch J, Malms J, Steinbeck J, Blasius S. Accuracy of pedicle screw placement in lumbar vertebrae. Spine (Phila Pa 1976). 1996;21(11):1320–4.

42. Cao Y, Chen Z, Jiang C, Wan S, Jiang X, Feng Z. The combined use of unilateral pedicle screw and contralateral facet joint screw fixation in transforaminal lumbar interbody fusion. Eur Spine J. 2015;24:2607–13.

43. Rosenberg WS, Mummaneni PV. Transforaminal lumbar interbody fusion: technique, complications, and early results. Neurosurgery. 2001;48(3):569–74. discussion 574–5.

44. Gejo R, Matsui H, Kawaguchi Y, Ishihara H, Tsuji H. Serial changes in trunk muscle performance after posterior lumbar surgery. Spine (Phila Pa 1976). 1999;24(10):1023–8.

45. Foley KT, Holly LT, Schwender JD. Minimally invasive lumbar fusion. Spine (Phila Pa 1976). 2003;28:S26–35.

46. Humphreys SC, Hodges SD, Patwardhan AG, Eck JC, Murphy RB, Covington LA. Comparison of posterior and transforaminal approaches to lumbar interbody fusion. Spine (Phila Pa 1976). 2001;26(5):567–71.

47. Rantanen J, Hurme M, Falck B, et al. The lumbar multifidus muscle five years after surgery for a lumbar intervertebral disc herniation. Spine (Phila Pa 1976). 1993;18(5):568–74.

9

Gallie technique versus atlantoaxial screw-rod constructs in the treatment of atlantoaxial sagittal instability

Bo Yuan, Shengyuan Zhou, Xiongsheng Chen*, Zhiwei Wang, Weicong Liu and Lianshun Jia

Abstract

Background: The objectives of this study are to investigate the clinical curative effect of Gallie technique and atlantoaxial screw-rod constructs (SRC) on atlantoaxial sagittal instability and determine the indication of Gallie technique.

Methods: Data of 49 patients with atlantoaxial sagittal instability from February 2008 to May 2015 were analyzed retrospectively. The visual analog scale (VAS) score and the neck disability index (NDI) were used to evaluate the curative effect. Postoperative radiological outcomes were used to evaluate the stability of atlantoaxial joint and bone fusion. Perioperative parameters such as blood loss, operation time, radiographic exposure times, and hospital expense were also recorded and analyzed.

Results: Forty-nine patients (36 men and 13 women) were included in this study. The mean age was 41.4 ± 8.9 (range from 19 to 64). All patients were followed up for 24–67 months. Among these patients, 25 of these patients underwent Gallie surgery and 24 underwent SRC surgery. The pain in the occipitocervical area of all the patients has been relieved. NDI scores and VAS scores were lower in Gallie group than in SRC group in early postoperative period. The proportion of the patients who achieved good bone fusion within 3 months after operation was 88.0% (22/25) in the Gallie group and 100% (24/24) in the SRC group. The Gallie group is lower than the SRC group in blood loss, operation time, radiographic exposure times, and hospital expense. Statistical difference was observed between the two groups.

Conclusions: For patients with atlantoaxial instability who has (1) the atlantodental interval (ADI) which is bigger than 5 mm on lateral flexion-extension X-ray, or Anderson-D'Alonzo type II odontoid fracture, (2) no asymmetry between odontoid process and lateral mass on open-mouth anterior-posterior X-ray, and (3) no dislocation of lateral mass joint on the CT 3D reconstruction, Gallie technique can be chosen as a safe and effective method if atlantoaxial reduction can be achieved preoperatively. Compared with SRC, Gallie technique can relieve the pain in the occipitocervical area earlier and it can shorten operation time and reduce intraoperative bleeding, radiographic exposure times, and hospital expense effectively. However, for patients with irreducible atlantoaxial dislocation, the Gallie technique should be used with caution.

Keywords: Atlantoaxial, Instability, Titanium cable, Screw-rod constructs

* Correspondence: chenxiongsheng@vip.sohu.com
Department of Orthopedic Surgery, Shanghai Changzheng Hospital, Second
Military Medical University, Shanghai 200003, People's Republic of China

Background

As a special part of the cervical spine in human body, atlantoaxial complex bears approximately 50% of rotary motion and 12% of flexion and extension movement of the cervical spine [1]. Without intervertebral disc between the atlas and the axis, the stability of atlantoaxial complex relies solely on the atlantoaxial joint and the transverse ligament [2, 3]. Any injury of structure above may cause atlantoaxial instability [4]. Due to its specificity in structure and position, atlantoaxial instability may cause neck pain and stiffness, activity limitation, and progressive compression of the spinal cord. Therefore, recovering normal anatomical position within a short period of time and maintaining its stability are needed for the treatment of atlantoaxial instability to prevent further spinal cord injury.

The original operation method presented by Mixter [5] and Gallie [6] was the posterior cervical wiring of lamina of C1 and C2 (Gallie technique). This technique limits the anterior displacement of atlas effectively with the principle of tension band. However, many empirical studies [7, 8] have shown that the Gallie system allowed more rotation in any direction than the atlantoaxial pedicle screw technique. Screw-rod constructs (SRC) have been the mainstream in the treatment of atlantoaxial instability. Compared with Gallie technique, the SRC technique has higher operative difficulty and incidence of vascular injury. However, not all atlantoaxial instability is accompanied by rotational instability. There are merits of Gallie technique for treatment of patients with atlantoaxial sagittal instability caused by simple transverse ligament injury or odontoid fractures.

There are few reports on the classification of atlantoaxial instability and the comparison of the wiring technique and the screw-rod technique for the treatment of atlantoaxial sagittal instability. Therefore, a comparison was conducted to investigate the clinical curative effect of the Gallie technique and the SRC technique on atlantoaxial sagittal instability to determine the indication of Gallie technique.

Methods

Clinical data

Data of patients with atlantoaxial sagittal instability from February 2008 to May 2015 in the Department of Spine Surgery, Shanghai Changzheng Hopital, were analyzed retrospectively.

We defined a subtype of atlantoaxial instability, which had the following radiologic features: (1) the atlantodental interval (ADI) which is bigger than 5 mm on lateral flexion-extension X-ray, or Anderson-D'Alonzo type II odontoid fracture, (2) no asymmetry between odontoid process and lateral mass on open-mouth anterior-posterior X-ray, and (3) no dislocation of lateral mass joint on the CT 3D reconstruction. The patients with these features can be diagnosed as atlantoaxial sagittal instability.

The inclusion criteria included (1) the patients who were diagnosed as atlantoaxial sagittal instability and (2) the patients who showed no symptom of spinal cord compression.

The exclusion criteria were (1) atlantoaxial rotatory dislocation; (2) arch fracture, infection, or tumor of atlas; (3) incomplete, short, absence of posterior arch of atlas, or spinal process of axis; (4) patients with severe osteoporosis; and (5) patients unable to tolerate surgery or external fixation.

Treatment protocols

All patients underwent continuous skull traction for 3 to 14 days before operation. Atlantoaxial reduction was examined during traction with cervical lateral X-ray.

After general anesthesia with endotracheal intubation, patients were placed in the prone position on a plaster bed. Atlantoaxial reduction was confirmed with C-arm X-ray. In the Gallie group, from posterior tubercle of C1 to 15 mm on both sides and lamina and spinous process of C2 were freed by subperiosteal exposure through a standard posterior midline approach. Posterior arch of C1 was separated from dural sac. Double titanium cables passed through the front of posterior arch of C1 closely and crossed through the lower edge of spinous process of C2. Autologous iliac crest bone harvested from posterior superior iliac spine was refined to fishtail bone and grafted between decorticated lamina of C2 and posterior arch of C1. All patients were routinely immobilized with neck and chest brace for 12 weeks. In the SRC group, from posterior tubercle of C1 to isthmus on both sides and C2 and spinous process of C3 were freed by subperiosteal exposure through a standard posterior midline approach. Pedicle screws or lateral mass screws were inserted into C1, and pedicle screws or par screws were inserted into C2. After connecting the rods between the C1 and C2 screws, bone graft fusion and postoperative external fixation were taken in the same way as the Gallie group. Anterior cervical release and reduction were needed for patients who were unable to achieve reduction under traction preoperatively. Patients were placed in the prone position after general anesthesia. Scar tissue was exposed and removed between the anterior arch of C1 and dens, and around lateral mass of C1 through right anterior cervical transverse incision. Gallie or SRC surgery was undertaken after the atlantoaxial reduction through X-ray. All the operations were completed by the same treatment group.

Clinical and radiological assessment

Clinical and radiographic data were obtained before surgery, at 1 week and 3, 6, and 12 months after surgery, and annually thereafter. Visual analog scale (VAS) and neck disability index (NDI) were used to evaluate the neck pain of the patients. Cervical spine X-ray and CT were used to evaluate the bone fusion. Delayed union was defined as fusion time longer than 3 months. If delayed union occurred, patients will need to do radiographic evaluations every month until fusion. Non-union was defined as failure to achieve fusion at 9 months or failure of fixation [9].

Perioperative parameters such as blood loss, operation time, radiographic exposure times, and hospital expense were recorded and analyzed.

Statistical analysis

The SPSS for Window (version 16.0) was used for the analysis. For continuous variables, data were expressed as mean ± standard deviation. t test was used to compare continuous variables (age, follow-up duration, blood loss, operation time, total cost). Chi-square test of Fisher's exact test was used to compare categorical variables (gender, type of instability, bone fusion rate). VAS and NDI scores at different time points within the group were compared using one-way ANONA, and pairwise comparison was conducted with LSD t test. VAS and NDI scores were compared using unpaired t test between groups. Significance was defined as $P < 0.05$.

Result

A total of 49 patients met the inclusion criteria. Twenty-five of these patients underwent Gallie surgery and 24 underwent SRC surgery. The mean followed-up duration was 40.4 ± 13.4 months for the Gallie group and 33.3 ± 6.5 months for the SRC group. The baseline data are shown in Table 1. There was no significant difference between the two groups in terms of age, sex, type of instability, and time from injury to surgery. The patients were divided into two historical groups. In the early years of this period, most of patients underwent Gallie surgery, and in the following years, most of patients underwent SRC surgery. For this reason, the follow-up duration was significantly different between the two groups.

Intraoperative findings showed that the posterior arch of C1 of all the patients were complete. The procedures were successful, and there was no nerve damage and cerebrospinal fluid leakage. There was no infection of donor site of iliac bone after operation.

Clinical follow-up results are shown in Table 2 and Figs. 1 and 2. The pain levels in the occipitocervical areas of all the patients have been relieved 3 months after operation. At that time, the NDI scores for the Gallie group and the SRC group were reduced to 8.1 and 11.1 respectively. The VAS scores for the Gallie group and the SRC group were reduced to 2.9 and 3.6 respectively. The difference of NDI and VAS scores 3 months after operation was statistically significant between two groups.

Perioperative parameters are shown in Table 3. Blood loss in the Gallie group was significantly lower than that

Table 1 Demographic data of the patients

Characteristic	Gallie group (n = 25)	SRC group (n = 24)	P value
Age (year)	40.2 ± 9.5	42.6 ± 8.2	ND
Sex (male/female)	17:8	19:5	ND
Type of instability			ND
Odontoid fracture	10	11	
Atlantoaxial dislocation	13	13	
Reoperation	2	0	
Time from injury to surgery			ND
Less than 3 weeks	6	5	
More than 3 weeks	19	19	
Follow-up duration (month)	40.4 ± 13.4	33.3 ± 6.5	<0.05

Data are expressed as mean ± standard deviation unless otherwise indicated

in the SRC group ($P < 0.05$). Operation time in the Gallie group was also significantly lower than that in the SRC group ($P < 0.001$). Radiographic exposure times in the Gallie group were significantly lower than that in the SRC group ($P < 0.001$). The cost of patients in the Gallie group was significantly lower than that of patients in SRC group ($P < 0.001$).

Radiological evaluation is shown in Table 3. Typical cases are shown in Figs. 3 and 4. Delayed union was observed in one case in the Gallie group who was asked to continue using external fixation and take radiographic evaluations on a monthly basis. He did not achieve good bone fusion until the 6th month after operation. Non-union occurred in two

Table 2 Clinical outcomes

Characteristic	Gallie group (n = 23)	SRC group (n = 20)	P value
NDI score			
Pre-op	17.4 ± 5.1	16.7 ± 4.9	ND
Post-op 3 months	8.1 + 1.6	11.1 + 4.0	<0.05
Post-op 6 months	3.8 + 1.7	5.1 + 1.8	<0.05
Post-op 12 months	2.4 + 1.0	2.9 + 1.3	ND
Post-op 24 months	1.7 + 1.2	1.9 + 1.1	ND
Last follow-up	0.8 ± 0.8	0.9 ± 0.9	ND
VAS score			
Preo-op	5.4 ± 1.0	5.2 ± 1.5	ND
Post-op 3 months	2.9 + 0.7	3.6 + 0.9	<0.01
Post-op 6 months	1.6 + 0.6	1.8 + 0.7	ND
Post-op 12 months	0.7 + 0.7	0.8 + 0.6	ND
Post-op 24 months	0.4 + 0.5	0.4 + 0.5	ND
Last follow-up	0.4 ± 0.5	0.3 ± 0.5	ND

Data are expressed as mean ± standard deviation unless otherwise indicated
Pre-op preoperative, *Post-op* postoperative, *NDI* neck disability index, *VAS* visual analog scale

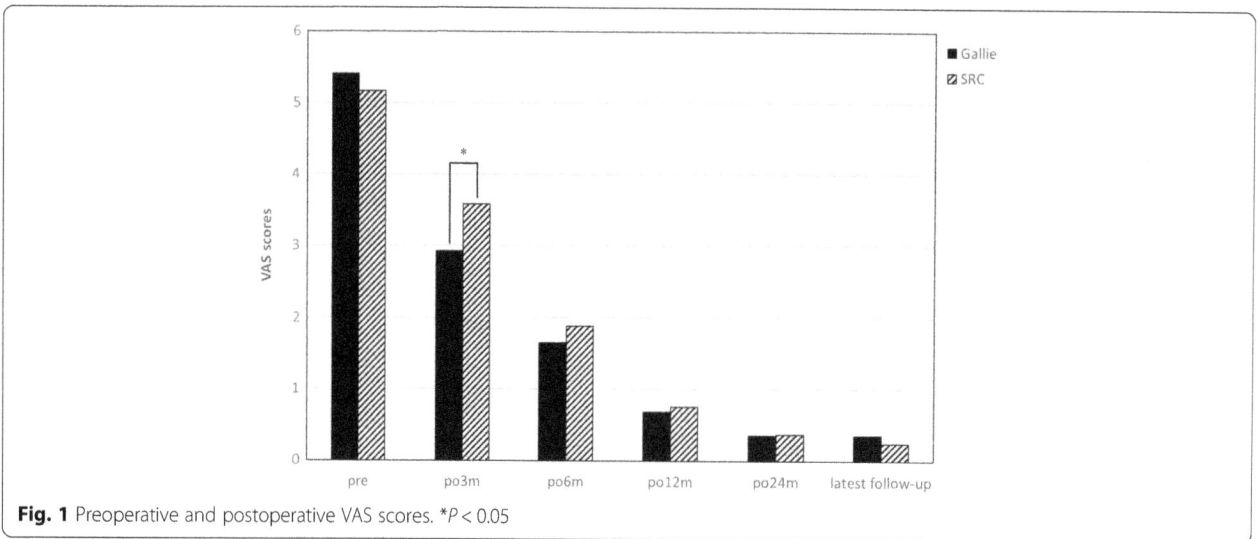

Fig. 1 Preoperative and postoperative VAS scores. *P < 0.05

cases with irreducible atlantoaxial dislocation in the Gallie group who underwent anterior cervical release and reduction before the Gallie surgery. Then, they converted to the SRC surgery (Fig. 5). No deformation, displacement, or breakage of titanium cables or screws was observed in the remaining patients in the radiological evaluation. Two patients underwent the Gallie surgery due to the failure of anterior odontoid screw fixation (Fig. 6). Good internal fixation position and bone fusion were shown after the Gallie surgery.

Discussion

The key to the surgical treatment of atlantoaxial instability is to reconstruct the stable atlantoaxial structures. Wiring fixation and bone graft fusion method like traditional Gallie and Brooks techniques [6, 10] has the advantage of being easy to perform and less traumatic to soft tissues. The Gallie technique can limit the anterior

displacement of atlas effectively and enhance the sagittal stability of C1–C2. In recent years, the posterior screw and the rod system, including the transarticular screw, the pedicle screw, the lateral mass screw, the pars screw, and the laminar screw, have taken an increasingly dominant role. The atlantoaxial pedicle screw, pioneered by Goel et al. [11] and modified by Harms et al. [12], was one of the most commonly applied techniques. Moreover, the biomechanical stability of atlantoaxial pedicle screw is significantly higher than that of the wiring technique [7, 8], as well as that of the transarticular screw technique [2, 13]. In terms of the bone fusion rates, there is no distinction between the atlantoaxial pedicle screw and the transarticular screw technique [14, 15].

In the previous literatures [1, 9, 16–18], the Gallie technique was reported to have low bone fusion rate and poor clinical efficacy. According to the biomechanical studies of Papagelopoulos et al. [7] and Grob et al. [19],

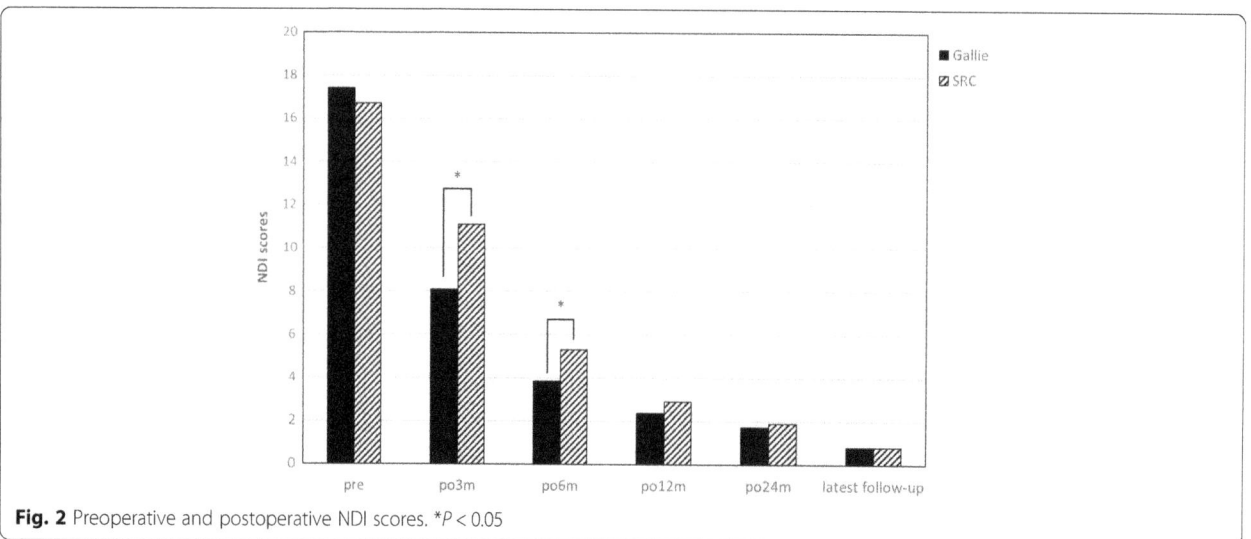

Fig. 2 Preoperative and postoperative NDI scores. *P < 0.05

Table 3 Radiological evaluation of patients and perioperative parameters of patients

Characteristic	Gallie group (n = 23)	SRC group (n = 20)	P value
Bone fusion rate	22/25	24/24	ND
Blood loss (ml)	134.4 ± 67.4	216.3 ± 136.3	<0.05
Operation time (min)	96.6 ± 17.1	122.5 ± 17.3	<0.001
Radiation exposure times	2.2 ± 0.4	3.5 ± 0.7	<0.001
Total cost (¥ᵃ)	35795.3 ± 6254.0	53361.9 ± 6356.7	<0.001

Data are expressed as mean ± standard deviation unless otherwise indicated
ᵃSeven Chinese Yuan equals one US dollar

the Gallie technique had low resistance to rotation motion. However, the classification of atlantoaxial instability was not taken into consideration in their studies. The atlantoaxial instability can be divided into three types: anterior dislocation, posterior dislocation, and rotational instability. Simple atlantoaxial sagittal instability is defined as excessive flexion and extension movement between atlas and axis caused by odontoid fracture or transverse ligament injury etc., with or without atlantoaxial dislocation. The anatomical and biomechanical studies [7, 20–22] have shown that alar ligament and capsular ligament are primarily responsible for limiting excessive rotatory motion. When the injury of above the ligaments occurs, the range of motion in rotation of the atlantoaxial complex increases obviously. However, the atlantoaxial complex tends to increase the range of motion in the flexion and the extension when simple odontoid fracture or transverse ligament injury occurs. In addition, the atlas fracture may cause displaced lateral mass and loss of C0–C2 height, known as "buoy phenomenon" [23, 24], which may induce ligament laxity and instability of atlantoaxial complex. That was why we excluded the patients with atlantoaxial rotatory subluxation and atlas fracture.

The VAS scores and the NDI scores of 49 patients with atlantoaxial sagittal instability complex in this study were significantly lower than that in the past. The proportion of patients achieved good bone fusion within 3 months after the operation was 88.0% (22/25) in the Gallie group and 100% (24/24) in the SRC group. Good bone fusion rate in the two groups showed no significant statistical difference. Delayed union was observed in one

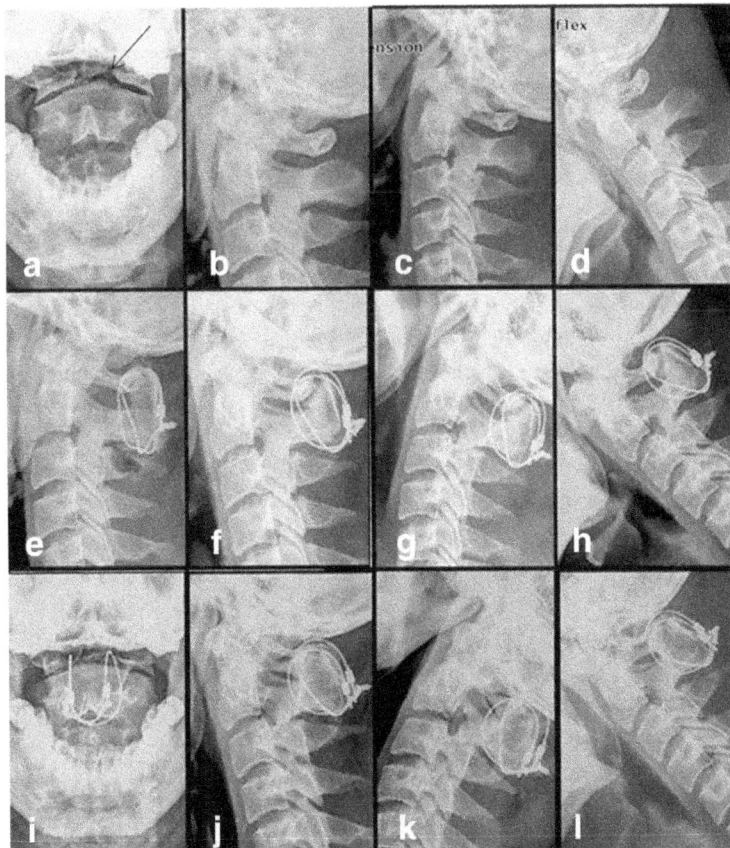

Fig. 3 A 27-year-old man had old odontoid fracture caused by accident. **a–d** Preoperative X-ray showed fracture line was located at the bottom of odontoid (*arrow*), revealing an atlantoaxial instability. **e–l** X-ray obtained on the 1st day, the 3rd month, the 6th month, the 1st year, and the 2nd year postoperatively showed bone fusion

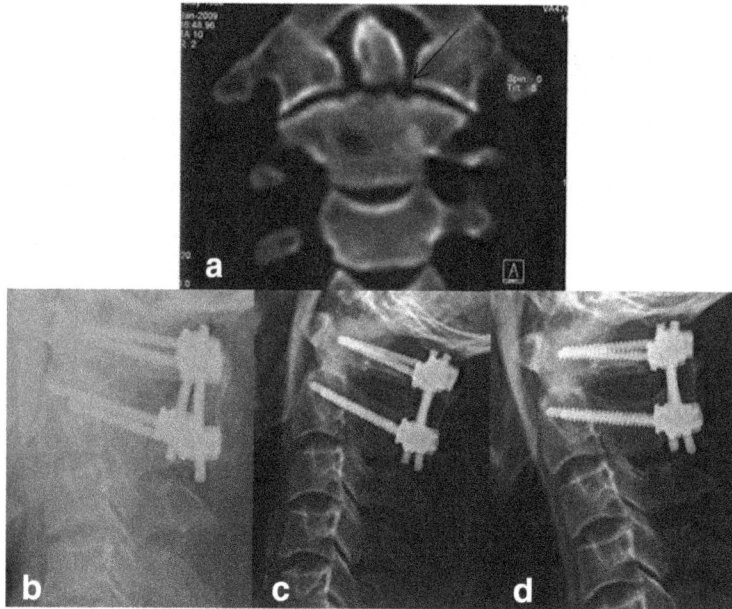

Fig. 4 A 46-year-old man had type II odontoid fracture caused by traffic accident. **a** Preoperative computed tomography (CT) showed fracture line was located at the bottom of odontoid (*arrow*). **b** Lateral radiograph obtained on the 1st day after the surgery showed the position of C1 lateral mass–C2 pedicle screws and the autogenous bone block. **c, d** Dynamic lateral radiographs showed bone fusion in the 3rd month postoperatively

case in the Gallie group, who achieved good bone fusion in the 6th month after the operation. This coincides closely with study of Lin et al. [9]. Non-union occurred in two cases with irreducible atlantoaxial dislocation in the Gallie group. Old dislocation resulted in a lot of scar tissues and contracture of ligament, even bony fusion. Even though reduction can be achieved after the anterior cervical release surgery, the cables tended to deform due to huge long-term sagittal stress [25]. Therefore, the Gallie technique should be used with caution for patients with irreducible atlantoaxial dislocation. The Gallie technique is able to establish stable atlantoaxial complex for patients with atlantoaxial sagittal instability caused by simple odontoid fracture or transverse ligament injury. On the contrary, in terms of blood loss, operation time, radiographic exposure times, and hospital expense, the Gallie

technique is significantly better than the SRC technique. This is associated with small exposure, less damage to attachment of atlantoaxial muscle, and low cost of titanium cable. Compared with the SRC technique, the Gallie technique can relieve the pain in the occipitocervical area earlier.

In addition, the complication rates of the Gallie technique is also lower than that of the SRC technique. The insertion of C1 lateral mass screw may cause irritation of nerve root of C2. Lee et al. [26] investigated the feasibility of C1 pedicle screw fixation in patients whose atlas vertebral artery groove height is less than 4 mm. Huang et al. [27] attempted to choose a higher entry point to prevent occipital neuralgia.

Four C1 lateral mass screws were inserted in the patients in the SRC group. Although no irritation of nerve root of C2 occurred, the average amount of bleeding during

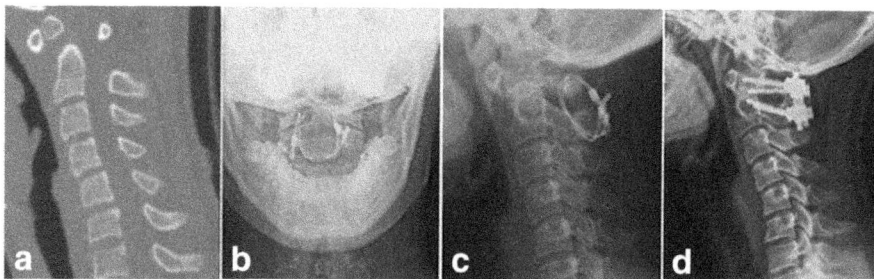

Fig. 5 A 17-year-old woman had Os odontoideum. **a** Preoperative CT showed uncombined odontoid process. **b, c** Postoperative X-ray obtained at the 6th month after the Gallie fixation showed that there was no bridging bone around the iliac bone graft. **d** Lateral radiographs obtained in the 24th month after the Gallie fixation showing bone fusion

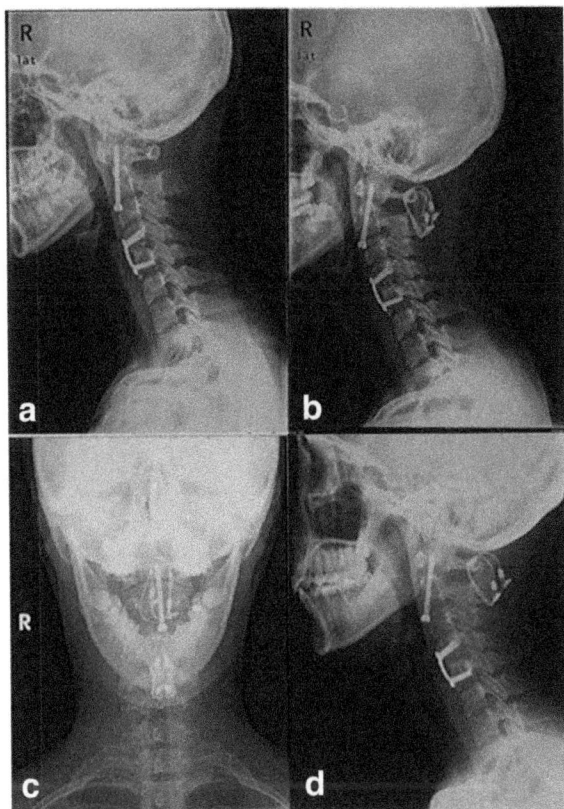

Fig. 6 A 19-year-old woman had type II odontoid fracture caused by traffic accident. **a** Lateral radiograph showed atlantoaxial dislocation was still present. **b** Lateral radiograph obtained at 1 day after the Gallie fixation showed good reduction of atlas. **c, d** Open-mouth and lateral radiographs obtained at 18 months after the Gallie fixation, showing bone fusion

have (1) the atlantodental interval (ADI) which is bigger than 5 mm on lateral flexion-extension X-ray, or Anderson-D'Alonzo type II odontoid fracture, (2) no asymmetry between odontoid process and lateral mass on open-mouth anterior-posterior X-ray, and (3) no dislocation of lateral mass joint on the CT 3D reconstruction. Compared with the SRC technique, the Gallie technique can relieve the pain in occipitocervical area in a shorter period of time. It can also reduce intraoperative bleeding, radiographic exposure times, and hospital expense effectively. However, for patients with irreducible atlantoaxial dislocation, the Gallie technique should be used with caution. Although aided by external fixation brace after Gallie surgery, these patients may occur non-fusion.

Abbreviations
ADI: Atlantodental interval; NDI: Neck disability index; SRC: Screw-rod constructs; VAS: Visual analog scale

Acknowledgements
Not applicable.

Funding
Not applicable.

Authors' contributions
BY and SYZ contributed equally to this work. XSC, BY, and SYZ designed the study. BY, ZWW, and WCL collected and analyzed the data. BY and SYZ were major contributors in writing the manuscript. XSC and LSJ supervised the study. All authors read and approved the final manuscript.

Competing interests
The authors declare that they have no competing interests.

operation was 216.3 ± 136.3 ml, of which the standard deviation was much larger than that of the Gallie group. Injury of the venous plexus was seen in two patients during operation, and the bleeding volume was more than 500 ml. The SRC technique may cause uncontrollable bleeding of the venous plexus.

Besides, though biomechanical strength of the Gallie technique was not ideal compared with the SRC technique [7, 13], aided by external fixation brace and excellent health guidance, no breakage of titanium cables was observed in our study. Both the Gallie technique and the SRC technique could establish stable atlantoaxial complex for patients with atlantoaxial sagittal instability. The Gallie technique distinguishes from the SRC because it can shorten the operation time, reduce intraoperative bleeding, and accelerate recovery period.

Conclusion
Gallie technique can be chosen as a safe and effective method if atlantoaxial reduction can be achieved preoperatively for patients with atlantoaxial instability who

References
1. Hood B, Hamilton DK, Smith JS, Dididze M, Shaffrey C, Levi AD. The use of allograft and recombinant human bone morphogenetic protein for instrumented atlantoaxial fusions. World Neurosurg. 2014;82:1369–73. doi:10.1016/j.wneu.2013.01.083*10.1016/j.wneu.2013.01.083.
2. Du JY, Aichmair A, Kueper J, Wright T, Lebl DR. Biomechanical analysis of screw constructs for atlantoaxial fixation in cadavers: a systematic review and meta-analysis. J Neurosurg Spine. 2015;22:151–61. doi:10.3171/2014.10.SPINE13805*10.3171/2014.10.SPINE13805.
3. Kalantar SB. Fractures of the C1 and C2 vertebrae. Semin Spine Surg. 2013;25:23–35. doi:10.1053/j.semss.2012.07.002*10. doi: 1053/j.semss.2012.07.002.
4. Nightingale RW, Winkelstein BA, Knaub KE, Richardson WJ, Luck JF, Myers BS. Comparative strengths and structural properties of the upper and lower cervical spine in flexion and extension. J Biomech. 2002;35:725–32.
5. Mixter SJ, Osgood RB. IV. Traumatic lesions of the atlas and axis. Ann Surg. 1910;51:193–207.
6. Gallie WE. Fractures and dislocations of the cervical spine. Am J Surg. 1939;46:495–9.
7. Papagelopoulos PJ, Currier BL, Hokari Y, Neale PG, Zhao C, Berglund LJ, Larson DR, An KN. Biomechanical comparison of C1-C2 posterior arthrodesis techniques. Spine (Phila Pa 1976). 2007;32:E363–70. doi:10.1097/BRS.0b013e318060cc65.
8. Sim HB, Lee JW, Park JT, Mindea SA, Lim J, Park J. Biomechanical evaluations of various C1-C2 posterior fixation techniques. Spine. 2011;36:E401–7. doi:10.1097/BRS.0b013e31820611ba.

9. Lin Q, Wang X, Zhou X, Chen H, Shen X, Yuan W, Tsai N. A comparison of the Gallie technique and casting versus the harms technique for the treatment of odontoid fractures. J Orthop Trauma. 2011;25:670–3. doi:10.1097/BOT. 0b013e318214b59e.

10. Brooks AL, Jenkins EB. Atlanto-axial arthrodesis by the wedge compression method. J Bone Joint Surg Am. 1978;60:279–84.

11. Goel A, Laheri V. Plate and screw fixation for atlanto-axial subluxation. Acta Neurochir (Wien). 1994;129:47–53.

12. Harms J, Melcher RP. Posterior C1-C2 fusion with polyaxial screw and rod fixation. Spine (Phila Pa 1976). 2001;26:2467–71.

13. Melcher RP, Puttlitz CM, Kleinstueck FS, Lotz JC, Harms J, Bradford DS. Biomechanical testing of posterior atlantoaxial fixation techniques. Spine (Phila Pa 1976). 2002;27:2435–40. doi:10.1097/01.BRS.0000031262.05676.E0.

14. Kim JY, Oh CH, Yoon SH, Park H, Seo HS. Comparison of outcomes after atlantoaxial fusion with transarticular screws and screw-rod constructs. J Korean Neurosurg S. 2014;55:255. doi:10.3340/jkns.2014.55.5.255.

15. Elliott RE, Tanweer O, Boah A, Morsi A, Ma T, Frempong-Boadu A, Smith ML. Comparison of screw malposition and vertebral artery injury of C2 pedicle and transarticular screws: meta-analysis and review of the literature. J Spinal Disord Tech. 2014;27:305–15. doi:10.1097/BSD.0b013e31825d5daa.

16. Stulik J, Vyskocil T, Sebesta P, Kryl J. Atlantoaxial fixation using the polyaxial screw–rod system. Eur Spine J. 2007;16:479–84. doi:10.1007/s00586-006-0241-6.

17. Jin G, Wang H, Li L, Cui S, Duan J. C1 posterior arch crossing screw fixation for atlantoaxial joint instability. Spine. 2013;38:E1397–404. doi:10.1097/BRS. 0b013e3182a40869.

18. El Masry MA, El Assuity WI, Sadek FZ, Salah H. Two methods of atlantoaxial stabilisation for atlantoaxial instability. Acta Orthop Belg. 2007;73:741.

19. Grob D, Crisco JR, Panjabi MM, Wang P, Dvorak J. Biomechanical evaluation of four different posterior atlantoaxial fixation techniques. Spine (Phila Pa 1976). 1992;17:480–90.

20. Li S, Ni B, Xie N, Wang M, Guo X, Zhang F, Wang J, Zhao W. Biomechanical evaluation of an atlantoaxial lateral mass fusion cage with C1-C2 pedicle fixation. Spine (Phila Pa 1976). 2010;35:E624–32. doi:10.1097/BRS.0b013e3181cf412b.

21. Wong ST, Ernest K, Fan G, Zovickian J, Pang D. Isolated unilateral rupture of the alar ligament. J Neurosurg Pediatr. 2014;13:541–7. doi:10.3171/2014.2. PEDS13527.

22. Debernardi A, D'Aliberti G, Talamonti G, Villa F, Piparo M, Collice M. The craniovertebral junction area and the role of the ligaments and membranes. Neurosurgery. 2015;76 Suppl 1:S22–32. doi:10.1227/01.neu.0000462075.73701.d2.

23. Li-Jun L, Ying-Chao H, Ming-Jie Y, Jie P, Jun T, Dong-Sheng Z. Biomechanical analysis of the longitudinal ligament of upper cervical spine in maintaining atlantoaxial stability. Spinal Cord. 2014;52:342–7. doi:10.1038/sc.2014.8.

24. Li L, Teng H, Pan J, Qian L, Zeng C, Sun G, Yang M, Tan J. Direct posterior C1 lateral mass screws compression reduction and osteosynthesis in the treatment of unstable Jefferson fractures. Spine. 2011;36:E1046–51. doi:10. 1097/BRS.0b013e3181fef78c.

25. Wang S, WCYM. Novel surgical classification and treatment strategy for atlantoaxial dislocations. Spine. 2013. doi: 10.1097/BRS.0b013e3182a1e5e4

26. Lee SH, Kim ES, Eoh W. Modified C1 lateral mass screw insertion using a high entry point to avoid postoperative occipital neuralgia. J Clin Neurosci. 2013;20: 162–7. doi:10.1016/j.jocn.2012.01.045.

27. Huang D, He S, Pan J, Hui H, Hu H, He B, Li H, Zhang X, Hao D. Is the 4 mm height of the vertebral artery groove really a limitation of C1 pedicle screw insertion? Eur Spine J. 2014;23:1109–14. doi:10.1007/s00586-014-3217-y.

10

Risk factors for acute surgical site infections after lumbar surgery

Qi Lai[1,2], Quanwei Song[1,2], Runsheng Guo[1,2], Haidi Bi[1,2], Xuqiang Liu[1,2], Xiaolong Yu[1,2], Jianghao Zhu[1,2], Min Dai[1,2] and Bin Zhang[1,2]*

Abstract

Background: Currently, many scholars are concerned about the treatment of postoperative infection; however, few have completed multivariate analyses to determine factors that contribute to the risk of infection. Therefore, we conducted a multivariate analysis of a retrospectively collected database to analyze the risk factors for acute surgical site infection following lumbar surgery, including fracture fixation, lumbar fusion, and minimally invasive lumbar surgery.

Methods: We retrospectively reviewed data from patients who underwent lumbar surgery between 2014 and 2016, including lumbar fusion, internal fracture fixation, and minimally invasive surgery in our hospital's spinal surgery unit. Patient demographics, procedures, and wound infection rates were analyzed using descriptive statistics, and risk factors were analyzed using logistic regression analyses.

Results: Twenty-six patients (2.81%) experienced acute surgical site infection following lumbar surgery in our study. The patients' mean body mass index, smoking history, operative time, blood loss, draining time, and drainage volume in the acute surgical site infection group were significantly different from those in the non-acute surgical site infection group ($p < 0.05$). Additionally, diabetes mellitus, chronic obstructive pulmonary disease, osteoporosis, preoperative antibiotics, type of disease, and operative type in the acute surgical site infection group were significantly different than those in the non-acute surgical site infection group ($p < 0.05$). Using binary logistic regression analyses, body mass index, smoking, diabetes mellitus, osteoporosis, preoperative antibiotics, fracture, operative type, operative time, blood loss, and drainage time were independent predictors of acute surgical site infection following lumbar surgery.

Conclusions: In order to reduce the risk of infection following lumbar surgery, patients should be evaluated for the risk factors noted above.

Keywords: Postoperative infection, Lumbar surgery, Risk factor, Prevention, Strategy

Background

Acute surgical site infection (ASSI) following lumbar surgery is a serious complication with significant morbidity and economic burden. Despite the use of prophylactic antibiotics and improvements in surgical techniques and postoperative care, acute wound infections continue to affect patients after lumbar surgery [1–3]. Patients with ASSI have longer hospital stays, higher reoperation rates, and serious back pain [4]. Although China's financial

* Correspondence: acker11.@126.com
[1]Department of Orthopedics, Artificial Joints Engineering and Technology Research Center of Jiangxi Province, The First Affiliated Hospital of Nanchang University, 17 Yongwai Street, Nanchang, Jiangxi 330006, People's Republic of China
[2]Department of Orthopedics, Multidisciplinary Therapy Center of Musculoskeletal Tumor, The First Affiliated Hospital of Nanchang University, Nangchang 330006, Jiangxi, China

investment in healthcare is growing along with a corresponding increase in medical insurance, the medical costs for a patient with an ASSI after lumbar surgery have increased to be within the range of $ 0.5–2 million.

ASSI after lumbar surgery is a commonly reported complication. Studies from European populations report infection rates ranging from 9.3 to 20% [5, 6]. Although techniques for spinal surgery have improved with regard to postoperative infections and wound complications, the infection rates are still high. Additionally, although many scholars have published findings related to surgical wound infections, they did not perform a systematic assessment of the risk factors for ASSI following lumbar surgery. Unlike previous studies, our study had a large sample size, and we performed a comprehensive assessment of the risk factors of ASSI. Moreover, we focused on ASSI, which is significantly different from the SSI that was reported in other studies. The aim of our study was to analyze the risk factors for ASSI following lumbar surgery, including fracture fixation, lumbar fusion, and minimally invasive lumbar surgery in order to provide clinicians with a theoretical basis for preventing ASSI after lumbar surgery. Our goal was to help reduce the infection rate and the patients' physical, mental, and economic burdens.

Methods

After approval by our hospital's ethics committee, we performed a review of all lumbar surgeries performed at the orthopedic department of The First Affiliated Hospital of Nanchang University to identify patients who developed an ASSI. All surgeries were performed by the director of spine surgery. Patients who underwent lumbar fusion, internal fracture fixation, and minimally invasive surgery between January 2014 and December 2016 were identified by searching the hospital's medical record database. During this period, 1367 patients underwent lumbar surgery. Cases of lumbar vertebra fracture, lumbar intervertebral disc herniation, lumbar canal stenosis, degenerative lumbar spondylolisthesis, and scoliosis were considered in this analysis.

Identification of acute surgical site infection

ASSIs as classified according to the criteria of the Centers for Disease Control and Prevention in China were studied. An infection was considered to be an ASSI when it occurred at the surgical site within 2 weeks after surgery. ASSI was defined as an infection involving the deep soft tissue muscle and fascia, in contrast to a superficial infection with only infected skin and subcutaneous tissue. Additional criteria for ASSI were the presence of at least one classical sign of inflammation (pain, swelling, redness, increased local temperature) and drainage of purulent fluid from the operative incision, spontaneous wound dehiscence, or an abscess or other signs of infection on observation, reoperation, or histopathological or radiological investigation [7, 8].

Data collection

Patients were selected according to the following criteria: (1) a preoperative diagnosis of lumbar vertebra fracture, lumbar intervertebral disc herniation, lumbar canal stenosis, degenerative lumbar spondylolisthesis, or scoliosis and (2) patients with complete data who underwent lumbar fusion surgery. Patients were excluded if they had a primary lumbar infection, such as lumbar spine tuberculosis, or non-lumbar surgery; were less than 18 years old; were dependent on pain or psychotropic medications; or had cognitive or mental disorders. Each procedure was performed by board-certified spinal surgeons at a dedicated tertiary general hospital. Data review was then performed, and missing data of 444 patients were excluded.

Risk factors were analyzed, including patient-related risk factors such as sex, age, body mass index (BMI), educational level, type of disease, smoking, alcohol consumption, long-term hormone use, hypertension, chronic obstructive pulmonary disease (COPD), osteoporosis, diabetes, nutritional status, and procedure-related risk factors such as preoperative antibiotics, operative time, intraoperative blood loss, intraoperative blood transfusion, number of internal fixation metals, postoperative drainage time, and drainage volume.

Statistical analysis

Twenty-six patients were found to have ASSI after lumbar surgery and were defined as the infection group; the other 897 patients were defined as the control group. The count data were analyzed by the chi-square test, and the measurement data were analyzed by an independent sample t test. Binary logistic regression controlled for confounding characteristics and identified independent predictors of postoperative surgical site infections. All the data were processed by SPSS 23.0 statistical software (IBM Corp., Armonk, NY). $p < 0.05$ was considered to be statistically significant.

Results

Overall, 1367 patients were identified who met our inclusion criteria. A total of 368 patients with incomplete information because of transfer to another hospital and 76 patients who declined the operation on the day of surgery were excluded. Thus, 923 patients were included in this analysis. Twenty-six patients were diagnosed with lumbar ASSI. The incidence of ASSI was 2.81%.

Age, BMI, smoking history, number of internal fixation metals, operative time, blood loss, operative incision, drainage tube, drainage time, and drainage volume were the measurement data analyzed by the t test. The mean BMI, smoking history, operative time, blood loss, drainage time, and drainage volume in the ASSI group were significantly different from those in the non-ASSI group ($p < 0.05$, Table 1). Additionally, sex, alcohol intake, educational level, diabetes mellitus, COPD, osteoporosis, preoperative antibiotics, long-term hormone use, intraoperative blood transfusion, nutritional status, hypertension, type of disease, and operative type were analyzed as count data by the chi-square test. Diabetes mellitus, COPD, osteoporosis, preoperative antibiotics, type of disease, and operative type in the ASSI group were found to have statistically significant differences compared to the non-ASSI group ($p < 0.05$, Table 2). Finally, the risk factors for the statistical differences were analyzed by binary logistic regression. BMI,

Table 1 The differences of risk factors in the infection and non-infection groups were analyzed by *t* test (measurement data)

Risk factors	ASSI (mean ± SEM, *n* = 26)	Non-ASSI (mean ± SEM, *n* = 897)	*t*	*p*
Age (year)	54.58 ± 2.710	54.93 ± 0.5503	0.1090	0.9132
BMI (kg/m^2)	24.85 ± 0.9210	22.76 ± 0.1179	2.935	*0.0034*
Smoking (year)	21.27 ± 2.765	10.18 ± 0.3913	4.770	*<0.0001*
Number of internal fixation metals (piece)	5.423 ± 0.4374	5.252 ± 0.07764	0.3703	0.7112
Operative time (min)	208.5 ± 7.439	170.7 ± 2.776	2.307	*0.0212*
Blood loss (ml)	916.2 ± 72.66	696.5 ± 12.79	2.886	*0.0040*
Operative incision (cm)	13.38 ± 0.8340	11.93 ± 0.2319	1.061	0.2889
drainage tube (root)	1.538 ± 0.1385	1.394 ± 0.0306	0.7985	0.4248
Time of draining (day)	3.808 ± 0.3283	2.146 ± 0.05885	4.745	*<0.0001*
Capacity draining (ml)	440.0 ± 45.92	236.7 ± 8.072	4.230	*<0.0001*

Italicized value is statistically different

Table 2 The differences of risk factors in the infection and non-infection groups were analyzed by Chi-square test (count data)

Risk factors		ASSI (*n* = 26)	Non-ASSI (*n* = 897)	x^2	*p*
Sex	Male	20	550	2.606	0.106
	Female	6	347		
Drink wine	Yes	19	550	1.478	0.224
	No	7	347		
Academic career	≤High school	24	770	0.897	0.349
	>High school	2	127		
Diabetes mellitus	Yes	17	382	5.351	*0.021*
	No	9	515		
COPD	Yes	10	563	6.340	*0.012*
	No	16	334		
Osteoporosis	Yes	19	476	4.069	*0.044*
	No	7	421		
Preopreative antibiotics	Yes	19	456	5.004	*0.025*
	No	7	441		
Type of disease	Fracture	15	308	6.059	*0.014*
	Others	11	589		
Operative type	Open	23	621	4.431	*0.035*
	Others	3	276		
Long-term use of hormone	Yes	6	98	3.732	0.053
	No	20	799		
Intraoperative blood transfusion	Yes	5	206	0.614	0.433
	No	21	567		
Nutritional status	Good	19	687	0.173	0.667
	Poor	7	210		
Hypertension	Yes	4	245	1.825	0.177
	No	22	652		

Italicized value is statistically different

Table 3 Binary logistic regression model for the development of ASSI after lumbar surgery

Risk factors		Exp (B) (95% C.I. of Exp (B))	p
Patient-related risk factors	Age (year)	0.729(0.544–0.976)	0.34
	Sex	0.000(0.000–2.294)	0.074
	BMI (kg/m²)	2.888(1.059–7.875)	0.038
	Smoking (year)	1.684(1.008–2.813)	0.047
	Drink wine	2.180(0.241–9.771)	0.121
	Academic career	3.337(0.012–9.383)	0.265
	Diabetes mellitus	2.200(0.046–1.102)	0.020
	COPD	0.000	0.987
	Osteoporosis	1.842(0.151–4.836)	0.044
	Nutritional status	0.000(0.000–162.412)	0.220
	Fracture	2.916(0.156–5.308)	0.001
	Hypertension	0.011(0.00–13.221)	0.213
	Long-term use of hormone	0.551(0.151–4.836)	0.105
Procedure-related risk factors	Preoperative antibiotics	2.030(0.005–5.216)	0.025
	Operative type	1.374(0.010–4.445)	0.035
	Operative incision (cm)	1.027(0.555–1.899)	0.993
	Operative time (min)	1.014(0.987–1.042)	0.030
	Blood loss (ml)	1.022(0.999–1.045)	0.024
	Number of internal fixation metals (piece)	22.589(0.891–572.990)	0.059
	Intraoperative blood transfusion	0.000(0.000–0.417)	0.413
	Drainage tube (root)	0.019(0.000–11.327)	0.225
	Time of draining (day)	4.983(1.641–15.140)	0.033
	Capacity draining (ml)	1.008(0.990–1.025)	0.392

DM, osteoporosis, COPD, preoperative antibiotics, fracture and operative type are classification variables; BMI, smoking, operative time, blood loss, operative incision, capacity draining, and time of draining are continuous variables (Sig./$p < 0.05$ was considered to be statistically significant. Exp (B) >1 were risk factors and <1 were protective factors). Italicized value is statistically different

smoking, diabetes mellitus, osteoporosis, preoperative antibiotics, fracture, operative type, operative time, blood loss, and drainage time were independent predictors of ASSI following lumbar surgery ($p < 0.05$ and Exp (B) > 1, Table 3).

Discussion

This study analyzed 923 patients who underwent lumbar surgery and assessed 23 possible risk factors. Importantly, we identified new risk factors of osteoporosis and traumatic fracture. Next, we analyzed the results of our research.

Rates of acute surgical site infections after lumbar surgery

Surgical site infections are the most common hospital-acquired infections that occur in the postoperative period [9]. However, the reported incidence of postoperative spinal infections varies widely, from 0.7 to 16% [10–13]. The reason for this wide range may be that different factors evaluated during the preoperative period have different rates of postoperative infection. Overall, however, there are relatively few reports on lumbar

ASSIs. The incidence of ASSI following lumbar surgery has been shown to be lower without the use of internal fixation of the posterior spine, such as in minimally invasive surgery [14]. The rate of ASSI following lumbar surgery has been reported to be 2.6 to 3.8% [15] following internal fixation lumbar surgery. In our study, 26 of 923 patients were diagnosed with acute surgical site infection following lumbar surgery, an infection rate of 2.81%. Therefore, it is one of the key problems encountered by orthopedists and patients.

Analysis of risk factors

Numerous factors influence the development of ASSI after lumbar surgery, and they may be divided into two categories: (1) unchangeable and strictly patient-related and (2) changeable or procedure-related.

Patient-related risk factors

BMI When performing surgery on obese patients with a thick layer of subcutaneous fat, it is necessary to cut through a large amount of oily liquid. The sterile gauze often becomes saturated with liquefied fat from the surgical incision in obese patients, and bacteria can become embedded in the incision, increasing the risk of infection. It has been reported in the literature [14, 15] that BMI is a risk factor for postoperative complications; a 5-kg/m^2 increase in BMI is associated with a 10% increase in the risk of postoperative complications, especially surgical site infection. In our study, we also found that a higher BMI was associated with a greater risk of ASSI. Therefore, orthopedic surgeons should assess patients' BMI preoperatively and should be especially vigilant in caring for the surgical incisions of obese patients in the postoperative period.

Smoking Tar, nicotine, and other toxic substances are absorbed into the bodies of patients with a long history of smoking. Many scholars have described the physical effects of smoking. Lin AH et al. [16] reported that reactive oxygen species in smokers will attack polyunsaturated fatty acids in the biological membranes, leading to lipid peroxidation and the formation of a large number of small-molecule lipid peroxidation products, such as malondialdehyde, acetone, and pentanaldehyde, which reflect the degree of lipid oxidative damage. Therefore, the products of lipid peroxidation can be directly or indirectly caused by injury and functional changes of cells. Finally, the surgical sites in smokers heal more slowly, and the risk of infection is increased. In our study, we found that the longer the smoking history, the greater the risk of ASSI. Therefore, orthopedic surgeons should assess patients' smoking history preoperatively and should carefully monitor for ASSI in patients with a long smoking history.

Diabetes mellitus Surgical site infections are related to the presence of diabetes mellitus. Thus, ASSI following lumbar surgery may be associated with diabetes mellitus. Patients with diabetes mellitus may have lesions in the blood vessels, including in the small vessels and the microvasculature [17]. Therefore, when the vessels are cut, large vessels and microvessels may be occluded, leading to ischemia and hypoxia in the incision tissue and, finally, to infection or a lack of healing at the lumbar surgical site. The immune function of patients with diabetes mellitus is inhibited because of serious functional damage to the cell and a decrease in platelet growth factors [18]. Therefore, the probability of acquired infection is significantly increased. Using logistic regression analysis, we also found that diabetes mellitus was associated with ASSI following lumbar surgery. Therefore, orthopedic surgeons should monitor blood glucose levels in patients preoperatively and should not perform lumbar surgery until the glucose levels return to normal with insulin or hypoglycemic agents.

Osteoporosis On logistic regression analysis of 923 patients who underwent lumbar surgery, we discovered that osteoporosis was related to ASSI following lumbar surgery; no previous study has reported a relationship between osteoporosis and SSI or ASSI. Thus, the specific mechanism to explain how osteoporosis affects ASSI following lumbar surgery is unclear. Our results could be explained in two ways. There were relatively few infections in this study, which could have affected the statistical analysis results. However, we think that osteoporosis may indeed be associated with ASSI following lumbar surgery, and this is a newly discovered factor. We suppose that a vertebral body with osteoporosis cannot be firmly fixed using internal fixation, resulting in loosening of the pedicle screws. Additionally, the operation time and bleeding in patients with osteoporosis were significantly higher than in those without osteoporosis. In the future, further study is needed regarding the mechanism of osteoporosis and ASSI.

Traumatic fracture Similar to osteoporosis, we found that traumatic fracture was a risk factor for ASSI following lumbar surgery in our logistic regression analysis. Few studies have reported that lumbar fracture can increase the risk of ASSI following lumbar surgery. Thus, as for osteoporosis, the specific mechanism of how traumatic fractures affect ASSI following lumbar surgery is unclear. We suppose that traumatic fractures can damage blood vessels and tissues and stimulate a bodily or local inflammatory response, leading to a large number of inflammatory factors into the blood.

Procedure-related risk factors

Use of antibiotics According to our clinical experience and literature review, the postoperative use of antibiotics is an important measure for preventing infection. However, it is very controversial whether the use of preoperative antibiotics can reduce ASSIs following lumbar surgery. Scholars [19] hold that cleaning surgical incisions with a first- or second-generation cephalosporin can prevent bacterial infection, and surgical incision of pollution available third-generation cephalosporins. The judicial use of preoperative antibiotics may be a very useful prophylactic measure. However, some scholars believe that antibiotics should not be used before surgery, as they may produce drug resistance. Therefore, this is a very controversial issue. In our logistic regression analysis of 923 patients who underwent lumbar surgery, we discovered that the lacking of preoperative antibiotics was related to lumbar ASSI. We believe that administering a second-generation cephalosporin 30 min prior to the surgery is essential for preventing infection.

Type of operation In our retrospective analysis, we discovered that the rate of infection for patients undergoing open surgery was significantly higher than that for minimally invasive surgery. Our logistic regression analysis showed open surgery to be a significant factor. Additionally, Koutsoumbelis et al. [20] stated that open surgery was not only traumatic with respect to bleeding, but there are also risks from tissue exposure to air, perhaps resulting in an increased risk of surgical site infections. We, therefore, believe that open surgery is more likely to cause ASSI than is minimally invasive surgery and that patients indicated for minimally invasive surgery should choose it when possible.

Operative time Lumbar surgery requires a very meticulous and careful surgery because it involves sites around the spinal cord, so the operation time is significantly longer than that for other sites. The lengthy surgery may lead to tissue ischemia and hypoxia, with slow postoperative incision healing, resulting in an increased infection risk. Additionally, some studies [8, 21] have reported that a lumbar operation time of >3 h is associated with a significantly increased risk of postoperative infection. Moreover, many scholars believe that operative time is a risk factor for postoperative infection. Similarly, we found that operative time was related to ASSI following lumbar surgery. Therefore, surgeons should try to decrease the operation time during lumbar surgery.

Blood loss during the operation Continuous bleeding during surgery not only affects the operation but also increases the operation time, while bacteria in the blood can circulate deep into the incision and increase the risk of postoperative infection. Relevant studies [22, 23] report that when the amount of blood loss is >800 ml, the risk of postoperative infection increased. In our analysis, we also showed that blood loss was a risk factor for lumbar ASSI. Increased intraoperative bleeding is primarily due to injury to the spinal canal venous plexus from fusion decompression, so the venous plexus should be carefully operated and blocked with bipolar coagulation.

Postoperative drainage time Two drainage tubes are usually placed after lumbar surgery in our hospital. Therefore, we analyzed the association between drainage (duration, number of drains, and capacity) and ASSI following lumbar surgery. We found that drainage time was a risk factor for ASSI. In addition, Ando and Tamaki [24] reported that non-standardized drainage following lumbar surgery can easily lead to a deep incision infection. Ahmed et al. [25] considered that a postoperative drainage time of >72 h significantly increased the risk of ASSI. A drainage tube placed too shallow may cause deep congestion and hematoma, and one placed too

deep is likely to cause infection. Therefore, we suggest that the optimal drainage tube placement time is 48 h.

Study limitations
The limitation of this study was an insufficient case of infection, which could have led to inadequate analysis of some factors and to other risk factors not being identified. Thus, a larger sample should be used in future studies to validate these results.

Conclusions
We discovered that BMI, smoking, diabetes mellitus, osteoporosis, traumatic fracture, open operation, operative time, operative blood loss, drainage time, and no preoperative use of antibiotics were associated with ASSIs following lumbar surgery. Despite measures intended to reduce the incidence of ASSI following lumbar surgery, they remain a common and potentially dangerous complication. Therefore, prevention is ideal, and an improved understanding of the risk factors will allow preventive measures to be improved. Surgeons should adequately analyze and evaluate risk factors in patients and then develop a prevention program. Once an infection is diagnosed, the authors recommend surgery to remove the lesion of infection, retention of the internal fixation material, and catheter drainage with a 3000-ml NaCl rinse daily for 7–12 days. Additionally, antibiotics should be used according to bacterial culture results.

Abbreviations
ASSI: Acute surgical site infections; BMI: Body mass index; COPD: Chronic obstructive pulmonary disease

Acknowledgements
We greatly appreciate the assistance of Dr. Sheng Huang and Editage who provided English language editing, and we greatly appreciate the assistance of Huiqiang Yu, Professor of Statistics, who revised the statistical methods of this study.

Funding
All research costs were covered by three projects, the Gan-Po Talents Project 555 of Jiangxi Province, the Jiangxi Province Health Department of Science and Technology Plan (700639004), and the Jiangxi Science and Technology Support Plan.

Authors' contributions
QL, BZ, and MD conceived and designed the study. QL, QS, and RG performed the experiments. HB and XL analyzed the data. QL and BZ wrote the paper. JZ, XY, BZ, and MD reviewed and edited the manuscript. All authors read and approved the manuscript.

Authors' information
QL, QS, RG, HB, XY, and JZ are masters' graduate students.

Competing interests
The authors declare that they have no competing interests.

References

1. Pullter Gunne A, Mohamed A, Skolasky R, et al. The presentation, incidence, etiology, and treatment of surgical site infections after spinal surgery. Spine. 2010;35:1323–8.
2. Wang TY, Back AG, Hompe E, Wall K, Gottfried ON. Impact of surgical site infection and surgical debridement on lumbar arthrodesis: a single-institution analysis of incidence and risk factors. J Clin Neurosci. 2017;39:164–9.
3. Lim S, Edelstein AI, Patel AA, Kim BD, Kim JY. Risk Factors for Postoperative Infections Following Single Level Lumbar Fusion Surgery. Spine (Phila Pa 1976). 2014. [Epub ahead of print].
4. Veeravagu A, Patil CG, Lad SP, et al. Risk factors for postoperative spinal wound infections after spinal decompression and fusion surgeries. Spine (Phila Pa 1976). 2009;34:1869–72.
5. Meredith DS, Kepler CK, Huang RC, Brause BD, Boachie-Adjei O. Postoperative infections of the lumbar spine: presentation and management. Int Orthop. 2012;36(2):439–44.
6. Sansur CA, Smith JS, Coe JD, et al. Scoliosis research society morbidity and mortality of adult scoliosis surgery. Spine (Phila Pa 1976). 2011;36:E593–7.
7. Nolan MB, Martin DP, Thompson R, Schroeder DR, Hanson AC, Warner DO. Association between smoking status, preoperative exhaled carbon monoxide levels, and postoperative surgical site infection in patients undergoing elective surgery. JAMA Surg. 2017;152(5):476–83.
8. Fei Q, Li J, Lin J, et al. Risk factors for surgical site infection after spinal surgery: a meta-analysis. World Neurosurg. 2016;95:507–15.
9. Asomugha EU, Miller JA, McLain RF. Surgical site infections in posterior lumbar surgery: a controlled-cohort study of epidural steroid paste. Spine (Phila Pa 1976). 2017;42(1):63–9.
10. Schimmel JJ, Horsting PP, de Kleuver M, et al. Risk factors for deep surgical site infections after spinal fusion. Eur Spine J. 2010;19(10):1711–9.
11. Smith JS, Shaffrey CI, Sansur CA, et al. Rates of infection after spine surgery based on 108,419 procedures: a report from the Scoliosis Research Society Morbidity and Mortality Committee. Spine (Phila Pa 1976). 2011;36:556–63.
12. Gelalis ID, Arnaoutoglou CM, Politis AN, et al. Bacterial wound contamination during simple and complex spinal procedures. A prospective clinical study. Spine J. 2011;11:1042–8.
13. Memtsoudis SG, Vougioukas VI, Ma Y, et al. Perioperative morbidity and mortality after anterior, posterior, and anterior/posterior spine fusion surgery. Spine (Phila Pa 1976). 2011;36:1867–77.
14. Olsen MA, Nepple JJ, Riew KD. Risk factors for surgical site infection following orthopeadic spinal operations. J Bone Joint SurgAm. 2008;90(1):62–9.
15. Iona C, James W-MD, et al. The diagnosis and management of infection following instrumented spinal fusion. Eur Spine J. 2008;17:445–50.
16. Lin AH, Liu MH, Ko HB, Perng DW, Lee TS, Kou YR. Inflammatory effects of menthol vs. non-menthol cigarette smoke extract on human lung epithelial cells: a double-hit on TRPM8 by reactive oxygen species and menthol. Front Physiol. 2017;8:263.
17. Umemura T, Kawamura T, Hotta N. Pathogenesis and neuroimaging of cerebral large and small vessel disease in type 2 diabetes: a possible link between cerebral and retinal microvascular abnormalities. J Diabetes Investig. 2017;8(2):134–48.
18. Zou D, Chen Y. Pathogenesis and treatment of diabetic microvascular complications [J]. Chinese J Diabetes. 2005;05:26–27.
19. Trampuz A, Zimmerli W. Antimicrobial agents in orthopaedic surgery: prophylaxis and treatment. J Drugs. 2006;66(8):1089–105.
20. Koutsoumbelis S, Hughes AP, Girardi FP, et al. Risk factors for postoperative infection following posterior lumbar instrumented arthrodesis. J Bone Jt Surg. 2011;93-A:1627–33.
21. Parchi PD, Evangelisti G, Andreani L, et al. Postoperative spine infections. Orthop Rev (Pavia). 2015;7(3):5900.
22. Fang A, Hu SS, Endres N, Bradford DS. Risk factors for infection after spinal surgery. Spine. 2005;30:1460–5.
23. Demura S, Kawahara N, Murakami H, et al. Surgical site infection in spinal metastasis: risk factors and countermeasures. Spine. 2009;34:635–9.
24. Ando M, Tamaki T, et al. Surgical site infection in spinal surgery: a comparative study between 2-octyl-cyanoacrylate and staples for wound closure. Eur Spine J. 2014;23(4):854–62.
25. Ahmed R, Greenlee JD, Traynelis VC. Preservation of spinal instrumentation after development of postoperative bacterial infection in patients undergoing spinal arthrodesis. J Spinal Disord Tech. 2012;25(6):299–302.

11

High-grade bursal-side partial rotator cuff tears: comparison of mid- and long-term results following arthroscopic repair after conversion to a full-thickness tear

Nuri Aydin and Bedri Karaismailoglu*

Abstract

Background: Partial-thickness rotator cuff tears (PTRCTs) are one of the leading causes of shoulder dysfunction. Successful results have been reported with different treatment techniques, but the long-term consequences of these procedures are not yet clearly known. The purposes of this study were to evaluate and compare the mid- and long-term clinical outcomes of arthroscopically repaired bursal-side PTRCTs after conversion to full-thickness tears and identify the possible effects of age, gender, and hand dominance on clinical outcomes.

Methods: Twenty-nine patients who had undergone arthroscopic repair of a significant bursal-side PTRCT were functionally evaluated. The repair was made after conversion to a full-thickness tear. The average patient age was 55. 2 years (range 35–69 years, SD ±7.6 years). Clinical outcomes were evaluated at 2 and 5 years after surgery. Constant Shoulder Score (CSS) and Visual Analogue Scale for Pain (VAS pain) were used as outcome measures.

Results: The average CSS improved from 38.9 preoperatively to 89.2 and 87.8 at 2 and 5 years after surgery, respectively ($p < 0.001$). The average VAS pain score decreased from 7.90 preoperatively to 1.17 and 1.31 at 2 and 5 years after surgery, respectively ($p < 0.001$). A significant improvement was detected in patient functional outcomes and VAS pain scores at 2 and 5 years after surgery compared with the preoperative period. The patients who underwent surgery from their non-dominant extremity showed a significantly higher CSS increase relative to those who underwent surgery on the dominant extremity ($p = 0.022$).

Conclusions: Arthroscopic repair of high-grade bursal-side PTRCTs after conversion to full-thickness tears is a reliable surgical technique with good functional outcomes and pain relief both at mid- and long-term follow-ups. Surgery on the non-dominant side may be related to better functional outcomes.

Keywords: Partial rotator cuff tears, Bursal side, Shoulder arthroscopy, Arthroscopic repair, Surgical outcome

Background

Arthroscopic repair of full-thickness rotator cuff tears has been reported to improve functional scores and promote healing [1–3]. Partial-thickness rotator cuff tears (PTRCTs) are characterized by a partial disruption in the tendon fibres. Ellman [4] classified PTRCTs arthroscopically according to the location (articular, bursal, or interstitial) and depth of the tear. Ellman grade III tears, which involve more than 6 mm or 50% of the tendon

thickness, are also known as high-grade PTRCTs. Bursal-side tears typically occur in middle/older-aged patients (>40 years of age) as a result of intraarticular pathology or impingement and are less common than articular-side tears [5].

PTRCT management usually starts with conservative treatment, particularly when concomitant tendon and bursal inflammation are present. If the tear is deep and the symptoms are related to the tear rather than the inflammation, conservative treatment is rarely helpful, and early surgery is recommended by some authors [6]. Even if some factors such as age, activity level, tendon quality, and

* Correspondence: bedrikio@hotmail.com
Orthopaedics and Traumatology Department, Istanbul University Cerrahpasa Medical Faculty, Kocamustafapasa Cad. No:53, Fatih, Istanbul, Turkey

surgeon experience may affect the decision, debridement is generally preferred for Ellman grade I–II tears, whereas repair is indicated for high-grade (>50% depth) PTRCTs due to the limited healing capacity of the rotator cuff and the risk of tear progression [7]. Arthroscopic PTRCT repair is accomplished using the transtendinous technique or repair after conversion to a full-thickness tear [7, 8].

The main objective of this study was to evaluate and compare the mid- and long-term clinical outcomes of patients who underwent arthroscopic repair of bursal-side PTRCTs after conversion to full-thickness tears. The effects of patient age, gender, and hand dominance on the clinical outcome were investigated.

Methods

After obtaining approval from the local Ethics Committee (06-01-2015/A-38), we retrospectively reviewed 42 patients (42 consecutive shoulders) who had bursal-side PTRCTs and underwent surgery between May 2009 and January 2012. All tears were treated arthroscopically using a single-row repair technique after conversion to a full-thickness tear.

Patient selection

The inclusion criteria of this study were as follows: (1) pain and disability during daily living activities for at least 6 months, (2) no benefit from shoulder physiotherapy, (3) bursal-side partial supraspinatus tear evident on magnetic resonance imaging (MRI), and (4) high-grade (>50%) bursal-side partial supraspinatus tear diagnosed by intraoperative examination. The exclusion criteria were as follows: (1) previous surgery of the affected shoulder or cervical spine, (2) concomitant shoulder instability, (3) concomitant rheumatologic disease, or (4) concurrent shoulder procedures (repair of subscapularis, infraspinatus or teres minor tears, biceps tenotomy or tenodesis, distal clavicular resection, or labral repair). Twenty-nine patients met the inclusion criteria for the study and returned for postoperative clinical evaluations. Nine patients were lost to follow-up, and four patients did not meet the inclusion and exclusion criteria.

Clinical evaluation

The patients were evaluated preoperatively and postoperatively at 2 and 5 years after surgery using the Constant Shoulder Score (CSS) and Visual Analogue Scale for Pain (VAS pain) and [9]. All of the pre- and postoperative evaluations were performed by the same surgeon. The data were collected prospectively during routine patient follow-ups, and the functional outcomes were investigated retrospectively according to patient age, gender, and hand dominance.

Preoperative imaging

Preoperative radiographs of the shoulder were obtained in all patients to determine if any bony lesions or arthritic pathology were present. All patients were preoperatively evaluated by MRI to identify PTRCTs and diagnose concomitant abnormalities. The grade of rotator cuff tear was determined by intraoperative examination, and patients with tears larger than half (>50%) of the cuff thickness were included in this study [10].

Surgical technique

The operations were performed under general anaesthesia with intravenous cefuroxime antibiotic prophylaxis in beach chair position by the first author. After inserting the arthroscope through a standard posterior portal, an anterior portal was established lateral to the coracoid process with the help of a spinal needle. This portal was used to assess any intraarticular pathologies. The lateral portal was established inferior to the lateral border of the acromion. After assessment of the glenohumeral joint, the arthroscope was redirected to the subacromial space. Subacromial decompression was performed using a radiofrequency device (Dyonics RF-S Whirlwind 90 Prob, Smith & Nephew, Memphis, USA). Acromioplasty was performed starting anteriorly and progressing posterolaterally in all patients using a 4.5-mm burr (Smith & Nephew, Memphis, USA) from the lateral portal. In the case of a curved or hooked acromion, a flat acromion was created. Degenerative tissue was debrided. The bursal-side PTRCT, which was determined preoperatively by MRI, was confirmed with intraoperative examination, and the grade of the tear was measured using a 6-mm arthroscopic probe. Bursal-side PTRCTs were converted to full-thickness tears with a 4.5-mm shaver. After preparing the footprint of the supraspinatus tendon over the bony tuberosity, an absorbable anchor (Twinfix AB 5.0 mm, Smith & Nephew, Memphis, USA) was placed at a 45° angle. The single-row suture anchor fixation technique was used in all tears. The sutures were passed through the tendons in a horizontal mattress fashion using arthroscopic suture passers (Elite Pass Suture Shuttle, Smith & Nephew, Memphis, USA) and tied with a sliding knot. The operations were completed at the closure of the portals with absorbable sutures.

Postoperative rehabilitation

The patients were discharged on the same day or the day after the surgery. A standard postoperative rehabilitation protocol for full-thickness rotator cuff repair was followed. The arm was maintained in a simple arm sling for 6 weeks. Pendulum and self-assisted circumduction exercises were started immediately after the surgery. Passive range of motion exercises including abduction, external rotation, and forward elevation were initiated during the second postoperative week. Self-assisted active exercises were started at 6 weeks after surgery. Six months after surgery, patients were allowed to engage in heavy manual work and over-head activities.

Statistical analyses

A paired t test was used to assess differences in pre- and postoperative CSSs. The analyses of variance (ANOVA) test was used to compare the results according to age, gender, and hand dominance. Statistical analyses were performed using SPSS program, version 22.0 (SPSS Inc.). Standard deviation (SD) was used as a measure of variability. The results are presented with two decimal places.

Results

The mean patient age was 55.2 years (range 35–69 years, SD ±7.6 years), and the patient cohort included 20 females and 9 males. Five patients underwent surgery on their non-dominant sides, whereas the others underwent surgery on their dominant sides. No intra- or perioperative complications occurred, and none of the patients underwent revision surgery. Before surgery, the average CSS was 38.9 (range 20–68, SD ±11.6), and the average VAS pain score was 7.90 (range 6–10, SD ±0.81). The patients were re-evaluated at 2 and 5 years after surgery. At 2 years after the surgery, the average CSS was 89.2 (range 61–100, SD ±12.2), and the average VAS pain score was 1.17 (range 0–3, SD ±0.92). At 5 years after surgery, the average CSS was 87.8 (range 65–100, SD ±12.38), and the average VAS pain score was 1.31 (range 0–4, SD ±0.96). The CSS increases between the preoperative period and the 2nd postoperative year and between the preoperative period and the 5th postoperative year were both statistically significant ($p < 0.001$) (Table 1) (Fig. 1). Between the 2nd and 5th postoperative years, a slight decrease (1.4 points) in average CSSs was observed, but this change was not statistically significant (Fig. 1). The VAS pain score decrease was also

Table 1 Significance of CSS and VAS pain score change over time by paired t test

	Mean difference	SD	p value
Constant Shoulder Score			
Preop–Postop 2nd year	−50.34	17.65	<0.001*
Preop–Postop 5th year	−48.93	19.29	<0.001*
Postop 2nd year–5th year	1.41	17.36	0.66
VAS Pain Score			
Preop–Postop 2nd year	6.72	1.16	<0.001*
Preop–Postop 5th year	6.58	1.18	<0.001*
Postop 2nd year–5th year	−0.13	0.99	0.46

CSS and VAS pain score improvements were statistically significant between the preoperative period and the 2nd postoperative year and between the preoperative period and the 5th postoperative year (both $p < 0.001$) *$p < 0.05$
Preop preoperative, *Postop* postoperative

statistically significant between the preoperative period and the 2nd postoperative year and between the preoperative period and the 5th postoperative year (both $p < 0.001$) (Table 1). The slight increase in average VAS pain score (0.14 points) between the 2nd and 5th postoperative years was not statistically significant.

When the hand dominance was considered, the patients who underwent surgery on their non-dominant sides showed significantly higher CSS increases between the preoperative period and the 2nd postoperative year ($p = 0.022$) and between the preoperative period and the 5th postoperative year ($p = 0.017$) compared with the patients who underwent surgery on their dominant sides (Table 2) (Fig. 1). Between the 2nd and 5th postoperative years, the patients who underwent surgery on their non-dominant sides showed a slight average CSS increase (1.80 points), whereas the patients who underwent surgery on their dominant sides showed a slight decrease (2.08 points), but these changes were not statistically significant (Fig. 1). Even though it was not statistically significant, the VAS pain score decrease in the patients who underwent surgery on their non-dominant sides continued between the 2nd and 5th postoperative years, whereas a slight increase was observed in the patients who underwent surgery on their dominant sides (Table 3).

When patient age was considered, the differences in CSSs between the preoperative period and the 2nd postoperative year were not statistically significant. However, older patients (>55 years of age) maintained their clinical outcomes through the 5th postoperative year, whereas younger patients (≤55 years of age) showed a slight clinical deterioration. As a result, older patients showed significantly greater improvements in CSSs between the preoperative period and the 5th postoperative year compared with younger patients ($p = 0.042$) (Table 2). Males showed greater CSS improvements compared with females between the preoperative period and the 2nd postoperative year, although this difference was not statistically significant. Males showed a decrease in average CSSs between the 2nd and 5th postoperative years, whereas females showed a slight increase. However, these differences were not statistically significant (Table 2). VAS pain score change differences between groups regarding age and gender were also not statistically significant (Table 3).

Discussion

In this study, statistically significant improvements in function and pain relief were detected in patients with bursal-side PTRCTs repaired arthroscopically after conversion to full-thickness tears, even 5 years after surgery. The change in functional outcome between the mid- and long-term follow-ups was not statistically significant. Undergoing surgery on the non-dominant side was found to be a possible factor that would positively affect

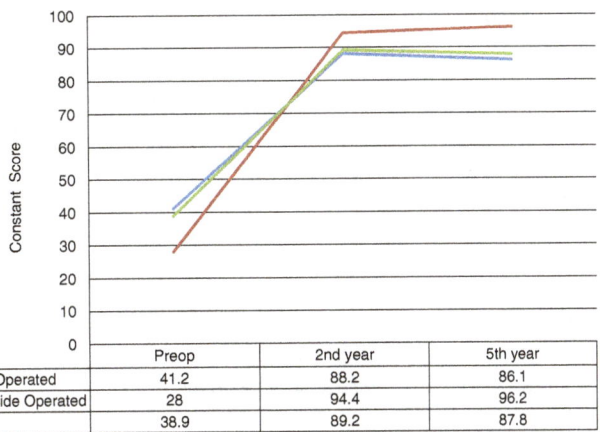

Fig. 1 Graph comparing the mean CSSs calculated preoperatively and at 2 and 5 years after surgery and the difference regarding hand dominance

	Preop	2nd year	5th year
Dominant Side Operated	41.2	88.2	86.1
Non-dominant Side Operated	28	94.4	96.2
Overall	38.9	89.2	87.8

the clinical outcome, although no statistically significant differences were observed regarding age and gender.

PTRCT repair may be performed either as a transtendon repair [11] or after conversion to a full-thickness tear [12]. No consensus in the literature exists regarding the best treatment choice. Some authors claim that conversion to a full-thickness tear and debridement of the degenerative tissue creates an environment with better healing capacity, similar to that observed for acute tears [13]. Some other authors prefer transtendon repair to preserve the remaining healthy fibres and restore the original rotator cuff footprint. In several studies comparing the two techniques, no significant differences in the functional outcomes and pain relief have been detected [8, 14]. In a recent meta-analysis of clinical results from articular-side PTRCTs treated with these two techniques, the authors reported no difference between clinical outcomes, but they did determine a higher re-tear rate in the group treated after conversion to full-thickness tears [15]. However, no similar results or meta-analysis exist for bursal-side PTRCTs in the literature.

Most of the previous studies have investigated articular-side PTRCTs, and fewer studies have reported functional outcomes following bursal-side tears. Bursal- and articular-side PTRCTs differ in their mechanisms of injury. It is believed that bursal-side tears are more related to an abnormal acromion causing extrinsic pressure over the tendon, whereas articular-side tears are more associated with intrinsic degeneration of the tendon itself [16]. Thus, the healing capacities between these two conditions may differ, and the outcomes of articular-side tears may not correlate with those of bursal-side tears. Upon closer inspection of the studies involving bursal-side tears, a controversy remains regarding which surgical technique yields the best clinical outcome. Koh et al. and Xiao and Cui achieved good clinical outcomes at 2-year follow-ups in their studies that included 38 and 48 patients, respectively, with high-grade bursal-side PTRCTs repaired arthroscopically by transtendon repair [11, 17]. Donohue et al. reported

Table 2 Average CSSs according to hand dominance, age, and gender (values; mean ± SD) with comparison of follow-up scores by ANOVA and the associated p values

Patient information		Average Constant Shoulder Score (±SD)					
		Preoperative	Postoperative		p value*		
			2 years	5 years	Pre–Po2	Pre–Po5	Po2–Po5
Operated extremity	Dominant side (n = 24)	41.16 (±2.17)	88.16 (±2.49)	86.08 (±2.49)	0.022*	0.017*	0.724
	Non-dominant side (n = 5)	28.0 (±4.75)	94.40 (±5.46)	96.20 (±5.46)			
Age	>55 years (n = 17)	36.70 (±9.99)	91.35 (±9.73)	91.33 (±2.04)	0.137	0.042*	0.673
	≤55 years (n = 12)	42.0 (±13.40)	86.25 (±15.05)	82.83 (±15.45)			
Gender	Female (n = 20)	38.60 (±10.15)	87.05 (±11.67)	89.00 (±11.77)	0.298	0.183	0.356
	Male (n = 9)	39.55 (±15.02)	94.11 (±12.71)	85.22 (±14.67)			

Patients who underwent surgery on their non-dominant extremities showed statistically significant CSS improvements between the preoperative period and the 2nd postoperative year and between the preoperative period and the 5th postoperative year (p < 0.05). Older patients (>55 years of age) showed greater CSS increases between the preoperative period and the 5th postoperative year relative to younger patients (p = 0.042) *p < 0.05
Pre preoperative, Po2 2nd postoperative year, Po5 5th postoperative year

Table 3 Average VAS pain scores according to hand dominance, age, and gender (values; mean ± SD) with comparison of scores according to follow-up years by ANOVA and the associated *p* values

Patient information		VAS pain score (±SD)					
		Preoperative	Postoperative		*p* value*		
			2 years	5 years	Pre–Po2	Pre–Po5	Po2–Po5
Operated extremity	Dominant side (*n* = 24)	8.04 (±0.75)	1.29 (±0.95)	1.50 (±0.93)	0.661	0.824	0.423
	Non-dominant side (*n* = 5)	7.20 (±0.83)	0.60 (±0.45)	0.40 (±0.63)			
Age	>55 (*n* = 17)	8.12 (±0.85)	1.29 (±0.84)	1.47 (±0.94)	0.541	0.341	0.609
	≤55 (*n* = 12)	7.58 (±0.66)	1.00 (±1.04)	1.08 (±0.99)			
Gender	Female (*n* = 20)	7.90 (±0.85)	1.15 (±0.93)	1.40 (±1.04)	0.580	0.605	0.973
	Male (*n* = 9)	7.89 (±0.78)	1.22 (±0.97)	1.11 (±0.78)			

The VAS pain score change differences between groups were not statistically significant *$p < 0.05$
Pre preoperative, *Po2* 2nd postoperative year, *Po5* 5th postoperative year

similar good results with articular, intratendinous, and bursal high-grade partial tears repaired arthroscopically after conversion to full-thickness tears in a study including 20 patients in each group [18]. In several studies, the authors compared the clinical results of bursal- and articular-side PTRCTs. Kim et al. did not determine any differences in re-tear rates between these two injuries but found superior clinical results at 2 years of follow-up for high-grade bursal-side tears compared with articular tears, which were treated after conversion to full-thickness tears [19]. Considering our results, this study has concluded that arthroscopic repair of bursal-side PTRCTs after conversion to full-thickness tears yields good clinical outcomes at both the mid- and long-term follow-ups.

Aleem et al. reviewed 55 patients who were operated bilaterally for full-thickness rotator cuff tears. Even though the clinical outcomes were better in the patients who underwent surgery on their non-dominant sides, the difference was not statistically significant [20]. In our study, the patients who underwent surgery on their non-dominant extremities showed a greater and statistically significant average CSS increase, revealing that hand dominance is an important factor for clinical outcome. Our results may be related to low patient adherence to postoperative activity limitations in those who underwent surgery on their dominant extremities. Although it was not statistically significant, the continuing decrease in VAS pain scores between the 2nd and 5th postoperative years in patients who underwent surgery on their non-dominant extremities, in contrast to the slight increase in the patients who underwent surgery on their dominant extremities, also supports this finding.

In our study, the average CSS improvement was statistically higher in older patients compared with younger patients not at the 2nd year but at the 5th year of follow-up. This is in contrast to the current literature, which claims that older patients have more persistent tears and younger patients have better clinical results

[21, 22]. Our finding of a greater average CSS at long-term follow-up in older patients might be related to activity restrictions due to ageing, which allows for better healing in the repaired tendon.

In our study, males and young patients showed a decrease in average CSS between the 2nd and 5th postoperative years, but this difference was not statistically significant. This situation might be explained by the overuse of the operated extremity by young and male patients to a greater extent than old and female patients during their occupational, daily, and recreational activities.

Even though we observed significant clinical improvement in high-grade bursal-side PTRCTs treated arthroscopically after conversion to full-thickness tears, our study also had several limitations. First, no postoperative MRI or ultrasonography was obtained to investigate tendon integrity and possible re-ruptures. Second, there was no control group of patients treated with a different surgical technique to which we can compare our results. Therefore, it is not possible to conclude that the technique we used is superior to any others. Finally, the number of patients was small, and nine patients were lost to follow-up, which negatively affected the strength of our study.

Despite these limitations, this study has several strengths. First, all surgeries were performed by the same shoulder surgeon with the same surgical technique in the same group of patients with no additional lesions or interventions, which reduced the possible variability in clinical outcomes due to the surgeon, repair technique, or concomitant pathologies. Second, prospective data collection makes the results of this study reliable. Finally, to our knowledge, our study is the first to report the long-term results of high-grade bursal-side PTRCTs repaired arthroscopically after conversion to full-thickness tears and compare long-term results with mid-term results. Additionally, the effect of the relationship between hand dominance and operated side on clinical outcomes of high-grade bursal-side PTRCTs has not been reported in previous studies.

Conclusion

Arthroscopic repair of bursal-side PTRCTs after conversion to full-thickness tears showed good functional outcomes and pain relief in long-term follow-up. The patients who underwent surgery on their non-dominant sides achieved better clinical outcomes than did the patients who underwent surgery on their dominant sides, and the difference was statistically significant. This situation might be related to lower patient compliance with activity limitations and extremity protection in those who underwent surgery on their dominant sides.

Acknowledgements
Not applicable.

Funding
None.

Authors' contributions
NA performed the surgeries and participated in the preparation of the manuscript. BK completed the clinical evaluations of the patients and the statistical analysis and participated in the preparation of the manuscript. Both authors read and approved the final manuscript.

Authors' information
NA is the Associate Professor at the Department of Orthopaedics, Istanbul University Cerrahpasa Medical Faculty, SECEC (European Society for Surgery of the Shoulder and Elbow) Committee Member.

Competing interests
The authors declare that they have no competing interests.

References

1. Boileau P, Brassart N, Watkinson DJ, Carles M, Hatzidakis AM, Krishnan SG. Arthroscopic repair of full-thickness tears of the supraspinatus: does the tendon really heal? J Bone Joint Surg Am. 2005;87:1229–40.
2. Lafosse L, Brozska R, Toussaint B, Gobezie R. The outcome and structural integrity of arthroscopic rotator cuff repair with use of the double-row suture anchor technique. J Bone Joint Surg Am. 2007;89:1533–41.
3. Park JY, Siti HT, Keum JS, Moon SG, Oh KS. Does an arthroscopic suture bridge technique maintain repair integrity?: a serial evaluation by ultrasonography. Clin Orthop Relat Res. 2010;468:1578–87.
4. Ellman H. Diagnosis and treatment of incomplete rotator cuff tears. Clin Orthop Relat Res. 1990;254:64–74.
5. Neer CS. Impingement lesions. Clin Orthop Relat Res. 1983;173:70–7.
6. Fukuda H, Mikasa M, Yamanaka K. Incomplete thickness rotator cuff tears diagnosed by subacromial bursography. Clin Orthop Relat Res. 1987;223:51–8.
7. Weber SC. Arthroscopic debridement and acromioplasty versus mini-open repair in the treatment of significant partial-thickness rotator cuff tears. Arthroscopy. 1999;15:126–31.
8. Shin SJ. A comparison of 2 repair techniques for partial-thickness articular-sided rotator cuff tears. Arthrosc - J Arthrosc Relat Surg. 2012;28:25–33.
9. Constant CR, Murley AH. A clinical method of functional assessment of the shoulder. Clin Orthop Relat Res. 1987;214:160–4.
10. Spencer EE Jr, Dunn WR, Wright RW, Wolf BR, Spindler KP, McCarty E, et al. Interobserver agreement in the classification of rotator cuff tears using magnetic resonance imaging. Am J Sport Med. 2008;36:99–103.
11. Xiao J, Cui G. Clinical and structural results of arthroscopic repair of bursal-side partial-thickness rotator cuff tears. J Shoulder Elb Surg. 2015;24:e41–6.
12. Deutsch A. Arthroscopic repair of partial-thickness tears of the rotator cuff. J Shoulder Elb Surg. 2007;16:193–201.
13. Brockmeier SF, Dodson CC, Gamradt SC, Coleman SH, Altchek DW. Arthroscopic intratendinous repair of the delaminated partial-thickness rotator cuff tear in overhead athletes. Arthrosc - J Arthrosc Relat Surg. 2008;24:961–5.
14. Franceschi F, Papalia R, Del Buono A, Vasta S, Costa V, Maffulli N, et al. Articular-sided rotator cuff tears: which is the best repair? A three-year prospective randomized controlled trial. Int Orthop. 2013;37:1487–93.
15. Sun L, Zhang Q, Ge H, Sun Y, Cheng B. Which is the best repair of articular-sided rotator cuff tears: a meta-analysis. J Orthop Surg Res. 2015;10:84.
16. Nakajima T, Rokuuma N, Hamada K, Tomatsu T, Fukuda H. Histologic and biomechanical characteristics of the supraspinatus tendon: reference to rotator cuff tearing. J Shoulder Elb Surg. 1994;3:79–87.
17. Koh KH, Shon MS, Lim TK, Yoo JC. Clinical and magnetic resonance imaging results of arthroscopic full-layer repair of bursal-side partial-thickness rotator cuff tears. Am J Sports Med. 2011;39:1660–7.
18. Donohue NK, Nickel BT, Grindel SI. High-grade articular, bursal, and intratendinous partial-thickness rotator cuff tears: a retrospective study comparing functional outcomes after completion and repair. Am J Orthop. 2016;45:e254–60.
19. Kim KC, Shin HD, Cha SM, Park JY. Repair integrity and functional outcome after arthroscopic conversion to a full-thickness rotator cuff tear: articular-versus bursal-side partial tears. Am J Sports Med. 2014;42:451–6.
20. Aleem AW, Syed UAM, Wascher J, Zoga AC, Close K, Abboud JA, et al. Functional outcomes after bilateral arthroscopic rotator cuff repair. J Shoulder Elb Surg. 2016;25:1668–73.
21. Grasso A, Milano G, Salvatore M, Falcone G, Deriu L, Fabbriciani C. Single-row versus double-row arthroscopic rotator cuff repair: a prospective randomized clinical study. Arthrosc J Arthrosc Relat Surg. 2009;25:4–12.
22. Kamath G, Galatz LM, Keener JD, Teefey S, Middleton W, Yamaguchi K. Tendon integrity and functional outcome after arthroscopic repair of high-grade partial-thickness supraspinatus tears. J Bone Joint Surg Am. 2009;91:1055–62.

12

Biomechanical analysis of the posterior bony column of the lumbar spine

Jiukun Li[1†], Shuai Huang[2†], Yubo Tang[3], Xi Wang[1] and Tao Pan[1*]

Abstract

Background: Each part of the rear bone structure can become an anchor point for an attachment device. The objective of this study was to evaluate the stiffness and strength of different parts of the rear lumbar bone structure by axial compression damage experiments.

Methods: Five adult male lumbar bone structures from L2 to L5 were exposed. The superior and inferior articular processes, upper and lower edges of the lamina, and upper and lower edges of the spinous process were observed and isolated and then divided into six groups ($n = 10$). The specimens were placed between the compaction disc and the load platform in a universal testing machine, which was first preloaded to 5.0 N tension to eliminate water on the surface and then loaded to the specimen curve decline at a constant tension loading rate of 0.01 mm/s, until the specimens had been destroyed.

Results: Significant differences in mechanical properties were found among different parts of the rear lumbar bone structure. Compared with other parts, the lower edge of the lamina has good mechanical properties, which have a high modulus of elasticity; the superior and inferior articular processes have greater ultimate strength, which can withstand greater compressive loads; and the mechanical properties of the spinous process are poor, and it is significantly stiffer and weaker than the lamina and articular processes.

Conclusion: These data can be useful in future spinal biomechanics research leading to better biomechanical compatibility and provide theoretical references for spinal implant materials.

Keywords: Mechanical properties, Compression test, Lamina, Articular process, Spinous process

Background

Transforaminal interbody fusion (TLIF) was developed as an alternative method for mitigating the risks and limitations associated with posterior lumbar interbody fusion (PLIF). TLIF involves attachment of adjacent vertebral bodies with implants to achieve a fusion effect. Pedicle screw fixation and rod attachment are popular, and bilateral pedicle screw–rod attachment has been widely used. Meanwhile, unilateral pedicle screw procedures have been conducted in PLIF and are a safe and cost-effective method to perform the PLIF procedure [1]. Recent reports show that the minimally invasive posterior lumbar interbody fusion (MI-PLIF) technique is a safe procedure with fewer complications and a high fusion rate [2, 3].

Pedicle screw fixation and rod attachment are popular, but their application has been limited by postoperative complications and high costs [4, 5]. Both unilateral and bilateral pedicle screw–rod attachments in one- or two-segment lumbar spinal fusion have comparable complication rates [6, 7]. Furthermore, if the primary operation with pedicle screw fixation and rod attachment fails, a damaged posterior bony structure makes subsequent rebuilding and stabilization of the spine more challenging [6, 7].

On the basis of the three-column spine theory [8], the spine is divided into three columns: the anterior column, column, and posterior column. When the anterior column is in a pathological state as a result of spondylolisthesis and/or degenerative disc disease, the original spine biomechanical properties change significantly, resulting in spinal load redistribution after attachment. In a

* Correspondence: pantaozs6y@163.com
†Equal contributors
[1]Department of Orthopaedic Surgery, The Sixth Affiliated Hospital of Sun Yat-sen University, 26 Yuancun Er Heng Road, Guangzhou, Guangdong 510655, China
Full list of author information is available at the end of the article

pathological state or a fixed state, the function of the anterior column completely diminishes. Thus, the posterior column bears all the pressure, indicating that the posterior structure of the lumbar spine plays a non-negligible role in the reconstruction of the lumbar spine for stability, which provides the theoretical foundation for posterior lumbar fusion [9].

With the advances in biomechanics and material science research, new posterior fixation devices are emerging. Each bone structure of the rear lumbar column can become an anchor point for an attachment device. We have also designed a newly developed shape-memory alloy hook in a TLIF, which can achieve immediate stability [10].

Previous biomechanical studies have shown that the stiffness of the vertebral pedicle is the hardest part, but it just conveys directly the stress of the rear structure to the front vertebral body as a pedicle screw channel and then effectively completes the three-column spine attachment, which has become the gold standard posterior lumbar fusion [11]. However, the pedicle screw placement damages the pedicle structure or the attachment fastness decreased because of osteoporosis and the screw can cause a fatigue fracture, loosening, or even detaching. If the patient does not appear to have lumbar spondylolisthesis or instability, performing the three-column fixation is not necessary. The main role of the facet joints of the spine is anti-rotation and anti-shear, although it is not a major structural function to resist spine compression. However, biomechanical studies show that translaminar facet joint screws [12] can also provide good fixed effect through a facet anchor point. The spinous process, the rearmost bone structure, can achieve spinal canal decompression by interspinous separation or attachment of devices to maintain its height. These devices can reduce disc pressure through their elastic means and thus provide flexible mounting pressure to reduce adjacent segment degeneration [13]. However, the strength and stiffness of the spinous process will decrease and result in spinous process fracture and cause fracture attachment failure in patients with osteoporosis. In addition, these devices damage the interspinous ligament between the spinous process. Studies have shown that complete rear spine ligament complex plays an important role in lumbar stability [8]. There are also studies of a design called Ni-Ti "U" shape-memory alloy devices [10], which anchor to the lamina–lamina, lamina–facet, and transverse process–transverse process, avoiding damaging the posterior lumbar bone structure and protecting the intact spinal motion unit, more in line with the biomechanical characteristics of the spine. In addition, the Harrington's system unit commonly used in scoliosis also anchors to the lamina–facet. These posterior attachment devices can be designed to anchor to the pedicle, articular process, lamina, transverse, or spinous process; however, whether these different bony structures of the anchor point have different mechanical properties, no relevant literature has been reported.

Previous research has focused on biomechanical performance testing and stress–strain analyses of the spine and intervertebral discs; however, mechanical testing for rear lumbar bone structure is rarely reported. The purpose of this study was to evaluate the differences in the stiffness and strength of each rear lumbar bone anchor point by studying axial compression damage. This information can provide the basic mechanics for a clinical spinal attachment device by determining the optimal implant location, and it can probably be used to develop a trauma model using finite element analysis.

Methods

Specimen preparations

Five adult male lumbar structures were obtained from the Department of Anatomy of Guilin Medical College, and the experiment followed an institutional medical ethics procedure. Individual vertebra, with the paraspinal muscles, interspinous ligament, spinal cord, and other soft tissues removed, were isolated. The L2 to L5 posterior column bone structures were exposed and observed, and the superior and inferior articular processes, upper and lower edges of the lamina, and upper and lower edges of the spinous processes were isolated (Fig. 1a). Using the appropriate anatomical site, these samples were divided into six groups (n = 10): the superior articular process (group 1), inferior articular process (group 2), upper edge of the lamina (group 3), lower edge of the lamina (group 4), upper edge of the spinous process (group 5), and lower edge of the spinous process (group 6). Before mechanical testing, all specimens were tested using contact and imaging studies to rule out deformities, degenerative changes, fractures, cancer, osteoporosis, and other pathological abnormalities (Fig. 1b, c). With their upright positions, the cortical axis of all specimens coincided with the central axis of the specimen, and both ends were embedded and fixed with denture powder and denture resin to make compressed samples [14]. The mean length of the exposed bone in the denture powder block was considered as the original length L_0, which was measured thrice using a vernier caliper, with the mean value accuracy of 0.01 mm (Fig. 1d). Due to the irregular geometry of the embedded specimens, these compressed samples could not be processed into standard test pieces. In accordance with engineering mechanics "worst" principle, the smallest cross section of the specimen was surrounded with a small wire (Fig. 1e) and copied to a 1-mm grid paper as the load plane (Fig. 1f) and then measured thrice to derive the mean as the force face S_0. All the specimens were wrapped and sealed with saline-infiltrated gauze and frozen properly at –20 °C for further compression testing.

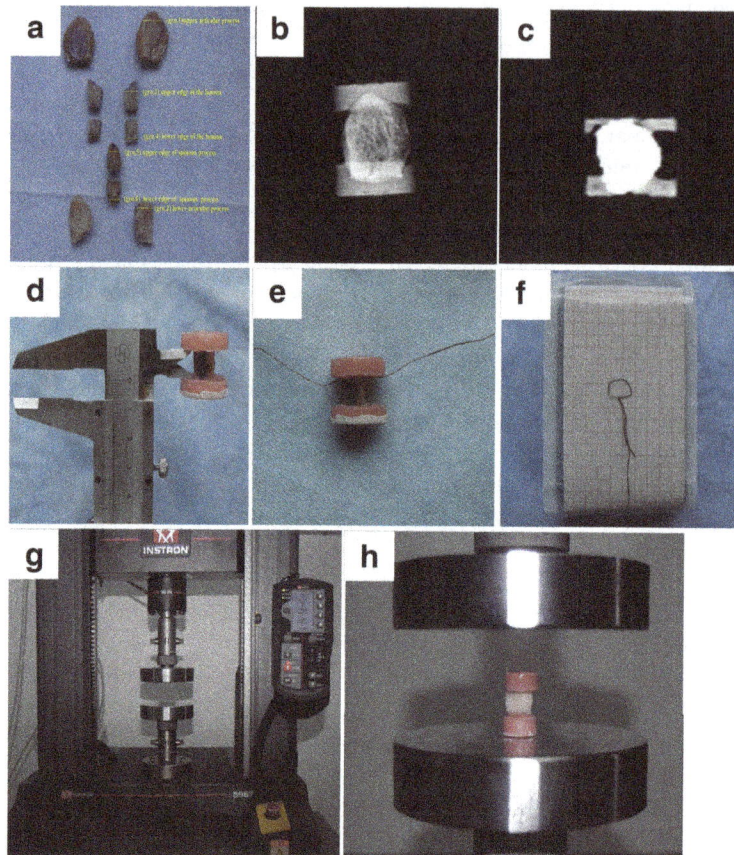

Fig. 1 Preparation and measurement of bone specimens. The samples were divided into six groups (**a**). All specimens were tested using imaging studies to rule out pathological abnormalities (**b**, **c**). Measurement of the original length L_0 (**d**). Measurement of force face S_0 (**e**, **f**). Universal testing machine (**g**). The central axis of the specimen coincided with two platen center connections to achieve the shaft load (**h**)

Compression testing

Before compression testing, all bone specimens from the −20 °C freezer were naturally thawed at room temperature. Subsequently, the specimens were placed between the compact disc and the load platform (Fig. 1h) in a universal testing machine (Fig. 1g), and the central axis of the specimens was coincided with two platen center connections to achieve a shaft load. All specimens were first preloaded to 5.0 N tension to eliminate water on their surfaces and then loaded to the specimen curve [15] at a constant 0.01 mm/s loading rate [16] until the specimen was destroyed. The loading data were transferred by a mechanical load sensor, and the material testing software program automatically recorded the elastic modulus, stress–strain, and other original data [16]. Typical specimen stress–strain curves were pretreated (Fig. 2a), and the fitting curves of each group are presented in Fig. 2b. Stress was calculated by dividing the applied force for specimens by the measurement of the cross-sectional area. Strain was calculated by dividing the actual deformation of specimens by individual original length. The elastic

modulus was determined as the slope of the linear section of stress–strain curve within a strain range of 0.02. The maximum strain, ultimate strength, and maximum load of each specimen were determined when the curve declined, at which the bone specimen began to develop fractures.

Statistical analysis

Statistical analyses were performed using SPSS 19.0 software. The Kruskal–Wallis test was used between groups; hence, the one-way analysis of variance (ANOVA) was feasibly performed in each group after the normality test with normal distribution was completed. The Levin test showed heterogeneity of variance without assuming homogeneity of the case, and Dunnett-T3 method was used in each group for multiple comparison procedures. $P < 0.05$ was considered as statistically different.

Results

The descriptive statistics of the mechanical parameters for each group are shown in Table 1. The normal distribution and homogeneity of variance test results are shown in Table 2. Table 3 shows that all groups were

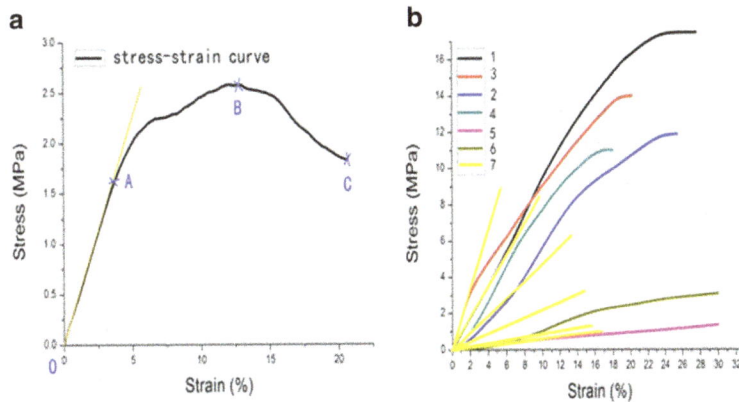

Fig. 2 Typical stress–strain curve (**a**). Each group fitting curve (**b**). **a** A typical stress–strain plot is divided into three parts: the elastic, plastic, and breaking phases; the horizontal and vertical axes represent the strain and stress diagrams, respectively. The OA segment is the elastic stage, representing the slope of the curve; the AB segment is the plastic stage, where B is the maximum load corresponding with ultimate strength; and the BC segment is the fracture stage, where C is the point for the specimen to completely fracture. The curve has a good linear relationship (OA), then increased before B and decreased to C. Each group fitting curve is represented in **b**. All curves are stopped at the maximum compressive stress, each set of the curves in the initial stage gradually separated, and no overlap is observed. The slope of the curve in each group set up on the edge of the lamina group, curve peaks corresponding to the maximum pressure on the facet group

analyzed using ANOVA, and a pairwise comparison of each group was made.

Our results demonstrated that, for elastic modulus, the upper edge of lamina had the largest elastic modulus (117.20 ± 5.95 Mpa, Table 1) (Fig. 3a), significantly different among all six groups ($P < 0.05$, Table 3) while there is no significant difference between the inferior articular process and the lower edge of lamina ($P > 0.05$, Table 3). When compared with othe group, the upper and lower edge of the spinous process had smallest elastic modulus vaule, significantly lower than othe groups ($P < 0.05$, Table 3).

The inferior articular process had the ultimate strength maximum value (15.56 ± 2.76 MPa, Table 1) (Fig. 3c), and no significant difference was found in the upper edge of the lamina ($P > 0.05$, Table 3). However, the edge of the lamina ultimate strength (15.56 ± 2.76 MPa, Table 1) was greater than the inferior articular process (10.99 ± 2.68 MPa, Table 1). The inferior articular process had a higher ultimate strength value than the upper edge of the lamina ($P < 0.05$, Table 3). The maximum load of the upper and

lower edges of the spinous process was significantly lower than that of each group ($P < 0.05$, Table 3).

For maximum load, no significant difference between the superior and inferior articular processes ($P > 0.05$, Table 3), among which the inferior articular process carried the maximum capacity (1170.79 ± 247.59 N, Table 1) (Fig. 3d), and the three carrying capacities were significantly higher than those of the lower edge of the lamina ($P < 0.05$, Table 3). The maximum load of the upper and lower edges of the spinous process was significantly lower than that of each group ($P < 0.05$, Table 3), but the upper edge of the spinous process was greater than its lower edge ($P < 0.05$).

For the ultimate strain, the inferior articular process had the maximum strain (Fig. 3b), and no significant difference was found between the superior and inferior articular processes ($P > 0.05$, Table 3) but was significantly higher than the upper and lower edge of lamina ($P < 0.05$, Table 3); there was no significant difference between the superior articular process and upper edge of the lamina group ($P > 0.05$), but greater than the

Table 1 Descriptive statistics of the mechanical parameters of the six groups ($x ± s$, $n = 10$)

Group numbers	Elastic modulus (MPa)	Maximum strain (%)	Ultimate strength (MPa)	Maximum load (N)
1	62.58 ± 11.07	26.35 ± 3.00	10.99 ± 2.68	1039.14 ± 419.97
2	82.32 ± 16.46	30.82 ± 4.00	15.56 ± 2.76	1170.79 ± 247.59
3	117.20 ± 5.95	22.16 ± 6.09	14.71 ± 3.89	914.48 ± 242.13
4	79.95 ± 13.57	18.39 ± 3.25	11.54 ± 2.62	489.02 ± 77.88
5	47.35 ± 5.80	14.64 ± 2.48	3.47 ± 0.315	196.76 ± 14.27
6	14.86 ± 2.43	14.56 ± 2.23	0.76 ± 0.04	59.52 ± 6.00

1 superior articular process group, *2* inferior articular process group, *3* upper edge of the lamina group, *4* lower edge of the lamina group, *5* upper edge of the spinous process group, *6* lower edge of the spinous process group

Table 2 Results of normal distribution and homogeneity of the variance test of mechanical parameters

Mechanical parameters	Nonparametric	Normality test	ANOVA	Homogeneity test
Elastic modulus (MPa)	$\chi^2 = 51.919$	$P = 0.000 < 0.05$	$F = 111.195$	$P = 0.000$
Maximum deformation (%)	$\chi^2 = 42.519$	$P = 0.000 < 0.05$	$F = 42.528$	$P = 0.000$
Ultimate strength (MPa)	$\chi^2 = 46.820$	$P = 0.000 < 0.05$	$F = 59.557$	$P = 0.000$
Maximum load (N)	$\chi^2 = 50.075$	$P = 0.000 < 0.05$	$F = 30.787$	$P = 0.000$

The Kruskal–Wallis test prompted significant differences between groups; one-way analysis of variance (ANOVA) was feasibly performed in each group; the normality test conformed to normal distribution ($P = 0.000$); and the Levin test showed heterogeneity of variance ($P = 0.000$)

lower edge of the lamina ($P < 0.05$, Table 3). No significant difference was found between the upper and lower edges of the lamina ($P > 0.05$, Table 3). The spinous minimum limit strain was significantly lower than that in each group ($P < 0.05$, Table 3).

Discussion

Each point of the rear lumbar bone structure may become an anchor point for a posterior attachment device. However, the difference in stiffness and strength of these anchor points is still poorly understood. No previous report was found regarding the mechanical properties of these anchor points measured with compression testing. In this study, we used the traditional and conventional compression platen methods [17] with a universal testing machine to perform uniaxial compression testing directly on specimens. This method is simple, and data

Table 3 Pairwise comparison table of the mechanical parameters of the six groups (Dunnett-T3)

Elastic modulus (MPa)	Ultimate strain (%)	Maximum load (N)	Ultimate strength (MPa)
P1–2 > 0.05	P1–2 > 0.05	P1–2 > 0.05	P1–2 < 0.05
P1–3 < 0.05	P1–3 > 0.05	P1–3 > 0.05	P1–3 > 0.05
P1–4 > 0.05	P1–4 < 0.05	P1–4 < 0.05	P1–4 > 0.05
P1–5 < 0.05	P1–5 < 0.05	P1–5 < 0.05	P1–5 < 0.05
P1–6 < 0.05	P1–6 < 0.05	P1–6 < 0.05	P1–6 < 0.05
P2–3 < 0.05	P2–3 < 0.05	P2–3 > 0.05	P2–3 > 0.05
P2–4 > 0.05	P2–4 < 0.05	P2–4 < 0.05	P2–4 < 0.05
P2–5 < 0.05	P2–5 < 0.05	P2–5 < 0.05	P2–5 < 0.05
P2–6 < 0.05	P2–6 < 0.05	P2–6 < 0.05	P2–6 < 0.05
P3–4 < 0.05	P3–4 > 0.05	P3–4 < 0.05	P3–4 > 0.05
P3–5 < 0.05	P3–5 < 0.05	P3–5 < 0.05	P3–5 < 0.05
P3–6 < 0.05	P3–6 < 0.05	P3–6 < 0.05	P3–6 < 0.05
P4–5 < 0.05	P4–5 > 0.05	P4–5 < 0.05	P4–5 < 0.05
P4–6 < 0.05	P4–6 > 0.05	P4–6 < 0.05	P4–6 < 0.05
P5–6 < 0.05	P5–6 > 0.05	P5–6 < 0.05	P5–6 < 0.05

$P < 0.05$ was considered statistically significant

1 superior articular process group, 2 inferior articular process group, 3 upper edge of the lamina group, 4 lower edge of the lamina group, 5 upper edge of the spinous process group, 6 lower edge of the spinous process group

are reliable. Our results indicated that different parts of the rear lumbar spine bone structure exhibited significant differences in mechanical properties, which could provide useful reference data regarding the best lumbar rear mooring points.

The most important information for evaluating the merits of a material is whether the material has high rigidity (stiffness) and compressive strength (strength). Our results showed that the axial pressure of the upper and inferior articular process group was 1170.79 ± 247.59 N and 1039.14 ± 419.97 N, respectively, suggesting that stress values of the articular process were significantly higher than those of the lamina and spinous processes, which strongly confirmed that the facet joints have an important bearing function on the spine mechanics.

In the lumbar motion segment, the three-joint complex consisted of the adjacent upper and lower vertebrae, front disc, and upper and lower facet joints that are located on both sides of the rear column [18]. The complex plays an important role in the spine mechanics transfer and guides the limited free movement of the lumbar spine, where the facet joints (lumbar facet joint) were second only to the front lumbar intervertebral joints for bearing stress and serving a stabilizing role. However, the facet joint determines its specific mechanical properties due to its large variation [19]. Our results theoretically and directly proved that the facet joint has an important bearing function on the mechanical properties, and this is consistent with conclusions from many previous studies [20].

In the comparative analysis of mechanical properties, we compared the upper edge of the lamina with the upper articular process and the lower edge of the lamina with the lower articular process. With a comprehensive comparison, the upper and lower articular processes had greater intensity with a strong ability to withstand compression loads, whereas the upper and lower edges of the lamina had high hardness with a strong ability to resist external deformation, which can be used as an ideal anchor point for rear lumbar attachment device.

An intriguing finding of this study is that the strength and stiffness of the spinous process, as the

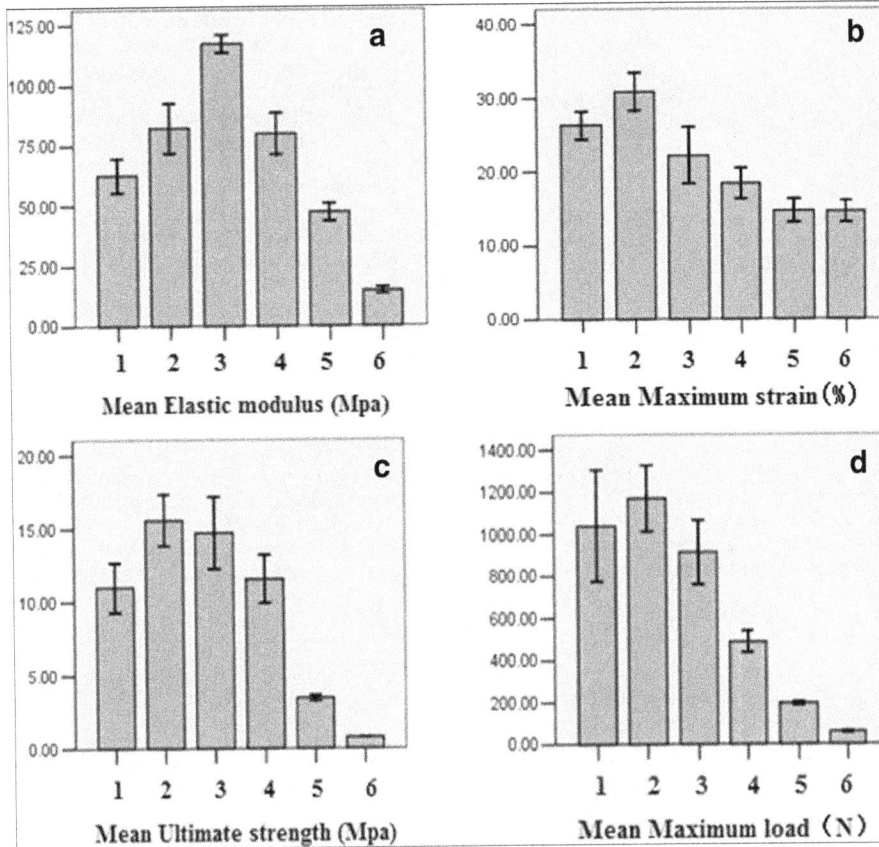

Fig. 3 Six groups of histogram specimen mechanical parameters. **a** For each set of elastic modulus, the elastic modulus at maximum is the upper edge of lamina. **b** For each set of elastic strain, ultimate strain at maximum is the inferior articular process. **c** The ultimate strength at maximum is the inferior articular process. **d** The maximum load at maximum is the inferior articular process

rearmost bone structure of lumbar column, were significantly lower than other bone parts by the comparative statistical analysis. In the design of the tension band interspinous device, Golish et al. [21] measured the carrying capacity of the L4 spinous process as 453 ± 16 N when the center line was not reduced, and after depressing, the carrying capacity decreased to 264 ± 99 N; the carrying capacity of the L5 spinous process was 517 ± 190 N. When the midline was not reduced, the carrying capacity decreased to 269 ± 184 N after depressing. When the spinous process of the lumbar spine was loaded with clamps and hooks, Shepherd et al. [22] found that the carrying capacity of L3 and L4 spinous processes was 339 N. The N values of the spinous process measured in our test were smaller than those in other reports, which may be caused by bone loss with time during storage because the bone strength was significantly and positively correlated to the bone mineral density. However, in our study, specimens of each group were collected from the same conditions, and the experimental results by statistical analysis indicated that the stiffness

and strength of the upper and lower edges of the spinous process were significantly weaker than those of the lamina and articular processes. This strongly confirmed that the spinous process was not the best anchor point for an attachment device and that the interspinous attachment device used for posterior lumbar non-fusion could not effectively achieve spinal decompression on other rear bone parts.

Conclusions

Compared with other bone anchor points, the upper and lower edges of the lamina have good mechanical properties, and the upper and lower articular processes have greater strength than the other parts. The mechanical properties of the spinous process were not relevant among those bone anchor points. Our data can be used for future biomechanics research on the spine and can provide a theoretical reference for improving biomechanical compatibility of the implant material.

Abbreviations
MI-PLIF: Minimally invasive posterior lumbar interbody fusion; PLIF: Posterior lumbar interbody fusion; TLIF: Transforaminal interbody fusion

Acknowledgements
None.

Funding
This work was supported by the "Key Science and Technology Planning Project of Guangzhou, China" Grant (2009A1-E031-3).

Authors' contributions
TP and JL conceived and designed the study. SH and YT performed the experiments. XW wrote the paper. JL and SH contributed equally to this work. All authors read and approved the manuscript.

Competing interests
The authors declare that they have no competing interests.

Author details
[1]Department of Orthopaedic Surgery, The Sixth Affiliated Hospital of Sun Yat-sen University, 26 Yuancun Er Heng Road, Guangzhou, Guangdong 510655, China. [2]Department of Orthopaedic Surgery, The Second Affiliated Hospital of Guangzhou Medical University, Guangzhou 510260, China. [3]Department of Pharmacy, The First Affiliated Hospital of Sun Yat-sen University, Guangzhou 510080, China.

References
1. Bingqian C, Feng X, Xiaowen S, et al. Modified posterior lumbar interbody fusion using a single cage with unilateral pedicle screws: a retrospective clinical study. J Orthop Surg Res. 2015;10:98.
2. Hentenaar B, Spoor AB, de Waal MJ, Diekerhof CH, den Oudsten BL. Clinical and radiological outcome of minimally invasive posterior lumbar interbody fusion in primary versus revision surgery. J Orthop Surg Res. 2016;11:2.
3. Chen C, Cao X, Zou L, Hao G, Zhou Z, Zhang G. Minimally invasive unilateral versus bilateral technique in performing single-segment pedicle screw fixation and lumbar interbody fusion. J Orthop Surg Res. 2015;10:112.
4. Lau D, Lee JG, Han SJ, Lu DC, Chou D. Complications and perioperative factors associated with learning the technique of minimally invasive transforaminal lumbar interbody fusion (TLIF). J Clin Neurosci. 2011; 18(5):624–7.
5. Chrastil J, Patel AA. Complications associated with posterior and transforaminal lumbar interbody fusion. J Am Acad Orthop Surg. 2012; 20(5):283–91.
6. Tormenti MJ, Maserati MB, Bonfield CM, et al. Perioperative surgical complications of transforaminal lumbar interbody fusion: a single-center experience. J Neurosurg Spine. 2012;16(1):44–50.
7. Fu L, Chang MS, Crandall DG, Revella J. Comparative analysis of clinical outcomes and complications in patients with degenerative scoliosis undergoing primary versus revision surgery. Spine (Phila Pa 1976). 2014; 39(10):805–11.
8. Denis F. The three column spine and its significance in the classification of acute thoracolumbar spinal injuries. Spine (Phila Pa 1976). 1983;8(8):817–31.
9. Hernandez-Labrado GR, Polo JL, Lopez-Dolado E, Collazos-Castro JE. Spinal cord direct current stimulation: finite element analysis of the electric field and current density. Med Biol Eng Comput. 2011;49(4):417–29.
10. Wang X, Xu J, Zhu Y, et al. Biomechanical analysis of a newly developed shape memory alloy hook in a transforaminal lumbar interbody fusion (TLIF) in vitro model. PLoS One. 2014;9(12):e114326.
11. Shin HC, Yi S, Kim KN, Kim SH, Yoon DH. Posterior lumbar interbody fusion via a unilateral approach. Yonsei Med J. 2006;47(3):319–25.
12. Magerl FP. Stabilization of the lower thoracic and lumbar spine with external skeletal fixation. Clin Orthop Relat Res. 1984;189:125–41.
13. Kong DS, Kim ES, Eoh W. One-year outcome evaluation after interspinous implantation for degenerative spinal stenosis with segmental instability. J Korean Med Sci. 2007;22(2):330–5.
14. Keaveny TM, Morgan EF, Niebur GL, Yeh OC. Biomechanics of trabecular bone. Annu Rev Biomed Eng. 2001;3:307–33.
15. Hou Y, Yuan W, Kang J, Liu Y. Influences of endplate removal and bone mineral density on the biomechanical properties of lumbar spine. PLoS One. 2013;8(11):e76843.
16. Snyder SM, Schneider E. Estimation of mechanical properties of cortical bone by computed tomography. J Orthop Res. 1991;9(3):422–31.
17. Linde F, Gothgen CB, Hvid I, Pongsoipetch B. Mechanical properties of trabecular bone by a non-destructive compression testing approach. Eng Med. 1988;17(1):23–9.
18. Jaumard NV, Welch WC, Winkelstein BA. Spinal facet joint biomechanics and mechanotransduction in normal, injury and degenerative conditions. J Biomech Eng. 2011;133(7):071010.
19. Adams MA, Hutton WC. The effect of posture on the role of the apophysial joints in resisting intervertebral compressive forces. J Bone Joint Surg Br. 1980;62(3):358–62.
20. Goto K, Tajima N, Chosa E, et al. Mechanical analysis of the lumbar vertebrae in a three-dimensional finite element method model in which intradiscal pressure in the nucleus pulposus was used to establish the model. J Orthop Sci. 2002;7(2):243–6.
21. Golish SR, Fielding L, Agarwal V, Buckley J, Alamin TF. Failure strength of lumbar spinous processes loaded in a tension band model. J Neurosurg Spine. 2012;17(1):69–73.
22. Shepherd DE, Leahy JC, Mathias KJ, Wilkinson SJ, Hukins DW. Spinous process strength. Spine (Phila Pa 1976). 2000;25(3):319–23.

Risk factors for retear of large/massive rotator cuff tears after arthroscopic surgery: an analysis of tearing patterns

Hisao Shimokobe[1], Masafumi Gotoh[3*], Hirokazu Honda[3], Hidehiro Nakamura[1], Yasuhiro Mitsui[3], Tatsuyuki Kakuma[2], Takahiro Okawa[3] and Naoto Shiba[1]

Abstract

Background: Previous studies have evaluated the risk factors for retear of large/massive rotator cuff tears (RCTs) that were treated arthroscopically; however, most studies did not evaluate tear patterns. The present study hypothesized that postoperative risk factors are affected by the tearing patterns in large/massive cuff tears in patients undergoing arthroscopic rotator cuff repair (ARCR).

Methods: One hundred fifty patients with large/massive cuff tears underwent ARCR at our institution. Of these, 102 patients were enrolled in this study, with an average symptom duration of 36.3 ± 43.9 months and average age of 63.9 $\pm$ 9.4 years. According to the arthroscopic findings and magnetic resonance imaging (MRI), the 102 patients were divided into three groups based on the tendon location: anterosuperior tears ($N = 59$, group AS), posteosuperior tears ($N = 21$, group PS), and anteroposterior-extending tears ($N = 22$, group APE). Functional outcome was evaluated preoperatively and postoperatively using the Japanese Orthopedic Association (JOA) score and the University of California, Los Angeles (UCLA) score. Retear was evaluated with MRI at a minimum of 1 year after surgery, using Sugaya's classification; Types IV and V were considered postoperative retears. Factors affecting postoperative retear were examined with univariate and multivariate analyses.

Results: JOA/UCLA scores significantly improved postoperatively in the three groups ($P < 0.01$ for all). Postoperative retear was noted in 26 of 102 patients (25.5%) in this series: 10 patients in group AS (16.9%), 9 in group PS (42.9%), and 7 in group APE (31.8%). The retear rate was significantly higher in group PS than in the other two groups ($P = 0.02$). Multivariate analysis showed that decreased preoperative active external rotation range was a unique risk factor for postoperative retear in the PS and APE groups (95% confidence interval: 0.02–0.18, cut-off value: 25°, with an area under the curve of 0.90, $P = 0.0025$).

Conclusions: Although multivariate analysis failed to detect significant risk factor for retear in patients with anterosuperior large/massive cuff tears who undergo ARCR, it demonstrated that active external rotation less than 25° before surgery is a significant risk factor in those with posterosuperior large/massive tears. This study may help surgeons understand the results of arthroscopic surgery in patients with large/massive tears.

Keywords: Tearing pattern, Arthroscopic rotator cuff repair, Postoperative retear

* Correspondence: gomasa@med.kurume-u.ac.jp
[3]Department of Orthopaedic Surgery, Kurume University Medical Center,
155-1 Kokubu-machi Kurume, Fukuoka 839-0863, Japan
Full list of author information is available at the end of the article

Background

Arthroscopic rotator cuff repair (ARCR) produces good clinical results, although retear is a significant concern after surgery. Compared with small- and middle-sized rotator cuff tears (RCTs), the retear rate is relatively high in large and massive tears, even if the tear is completely covered during surgery [1–4]; some authors reported that the retear rate was 40–94% in these tears [3–6].

A number of studies have consistently sought to determine the risk factors for postoperative retear in large and massive cuff tears. For example, a recent systematic review reported that the risk factors for retear after ARCR in RCTs included age, tear size, fatty degeneration (FD), the number of tendons involved, acromiohumeral interval, surgical technique, and bone mineral density [7]. One study used a multivariate regression analysis to demonstrate that preoperative FD of the infraspinatus was the most independent predictor of retear in large and massive RCTs in patients who underwent ARCR [8]. Kim et al. [9] reported that the extent of retraction was importantly associated with retear after surgery.

Based on the tendon location involved, large and massive RCTs are classified into three types: anterosuperior tears, posteosuperior tears, and anteroposterior-extending tears. However, previous studies collectively examined large and massive RCTs without sub-dividing the tear pattern as described above. Therefore, the purposes of the present study were to evaluate risk factors affecting postoperative retear in each group. We hypothesized that in large and massive tears, the risk factors for postoperative retear differ among the groups, when sub-divided by the tear pattern.

Methods

The patients provided informed consent, and this retrospective study was approved by the authorized institutional review board at the Ethical Committee of Kurume University (#12333).

Patients

Between April 2005 and August 2013, 150 patients with cuff tears defined as large or massive [6] underwent ARCR in our institution. The inclusion criteria were (1) individuals who had large or massive rotator cuff tears that repaired completely during surgery, (2) those who were available for evaluation of function and magnetic resonance imaging (MRI) preoperatively and at a minimum of 1 year after surgery, and (3) those who underwent an appointed postoperative rehabilitation program. The exclusion criteria were (1) individuals with advanced glenohumeral arthritis or fractures around the shoulder, (2) those who underwent open repair, partial repair, revision surgeries, or any previous shoulder surgery, (3) those who had MRI film without the "Scapula - Y" view on the sagittal-oblique plane, (4) those who refused to undergo

postoperative clinical assessment and MRI, and (5) those who had preoperative stiffness that showed less than 100° in passive elevation or 10° in external rotation [10]. Consequently, 102 patients were enrolled in this study.

According to the arthroscopic and MRI findings, the 102 patients were divided into three groups based on the tendon location: anterosuperior tears [11] in the subscapularis and the supraspinatus, in which the tear extended from the lesser tuberosity to the superior facet (N = 59, group AS); posteosuperior tears in the supraspinatus and the infraspinatus/teres minor, in which the tear extended from the superior facet to the middle or inferior facet (N = 21, group PS); and anteroposterior-extending tears, in which the tear extended from the lesser tuberosity to the middle or inferior facet (N = 22, group APE). When large or massive tears were evaluated according to the classification of DeOrio and Cofield [12], there were 56 patients with a large tear (94.9%) and 3 patients with a massive tear (5.1%) in Group AS, 19 patients with a large tear (90.5%) and 3 patients with a massive tear (9.5%) in group PS, and 15 patients with a large tear (58.2%) and 7 patients with massive tears (31.8%) in group APE. There was no statistical difference in demographic data among the three groups, except for the incidence of hypertension and distribution of massive tears. Details of the patients' characteristics are shown in Table 1.

Surgical procedure

Arthroscopic surgery was indicated when successful non-operative treatment, such as anti-inflammatory medications, physical therapy, subacromial or glenohumeral injections of corticosteroids or hyaluronic acid, or activity modification, was not achieved within 3 months of the first visit.

ARCR was conducted with the patient in the beach chair position under general anesthesia. At first, a glenohumeral examination was performed through a posterior portal and then transferred to the subacromial bursa. After making a lateral portal, we identified the ruptured tendon edge and evaluated its flexibility by grasping the tendon and reducing the edge to the original footprint. Capsular release was conducted from the anterior, anterolateral, or posterolateral portal; if needed, tenotomy of the long head biceps was performed. The method of cuff repair was selected based on the operative findings, tendon mobility, and tear condition with a single-row, double-row, or suture bridge technique (Table 1).

Rehabilitation protocol

Postoperatively, the patient's arm was fixed into a sling with an abduction pillow. Passive range of motion (ROM) exercises of the shoulder were conducted 4 days after surgery. Active ROM exercises and isometric exercise were

Table 1 Patient demographic data

	Group AS (N = 59)	Group PS (N = 21)	Group APE (N = 22)
Age (years)	62.8 ± 10.6 (39–82)	64.9 ± 8.8 (43–78)	66.4 ± 5.8 (54–76)
Sex: male (%)/female (%)	30 (50.1%)/29 (49.1%)	13 (62%)/8 (38%)	13 (59%)/9 (41%)
Side: right (%)/left (%)	43 (72.9%)/16 (27.1%)	11 (52.4%)/10 (47.6%)	19 (86.4%)/3 (13.6%)
Symptom duration (week)	30.8 ± 30.3 (4–156)	53.9 ± 69.9 (4–275)	34.1 ± 40.9 (2–150)
Trauma (%)	34 (57.6%)	16 (76.2%)	12 (54.5%)
Complication			
Diabetes Mellitus (%)	7(11.9%)	16 (76.2%)	2 (9.0%)
Hypertension (%)	16(27.1%)	* 3 (14.3%)	10(45.5%)
De Orio and Cofield's classification			
Large (%)	56 (94.9%)	19 (90.5%)	15 (58.2%)
Massive (%)	3 (5.1%)	2 (9.5%)	*7 (31.8%)
Surgical procedure			
Suture bridge (%)	40 (67.8%)	14 (66.7%)	17 (77.3%)
Simgle row (%)	14 (23.7%)	4(19.0%)	2 (9.0%)
Double row (%)	5 (8.5%)	3 (14.3%)	3 (13.7%)
LHB tenotomy (%)	29 (49.2%)	6 (28.6%)*	13 (59.0%)

Data are presented as mean ± standard deviation unless otherwise indicated LHB, long head biceps
*Statistically significant (P < .05) among the three groups

started 6 weeks after surgery, and isotonic muscle strengthening exercises began 12 weeks after surgery.

Evaluation of functional outcome

Functional outcome was evaluated preoperatively and postoperatively. The visual analog scale was used to measure pain (rest, night, and motion), the range of active motion was measured with a goniometer, muscle strength was measured with a handheld dynamometer (Micro FET2, Hoggan Health Industry, West Jordan, UT, USA), Japanese Orthopedic Association (JOA) score, and the University of California, Los Angeles (UCLA) score. An independent physiotherapist who was blinded to this study performed physical tests.

Evaluation of structural outcome

Acromiohumeral distance was evaluated, using the Oizumi classification [13], on plain radiographs that were taken with the patients standing and their arm held in a neutral position.

Tear length and width were measured on MRI using the protocol of Davidson et al. [14] FD of the supraspinatus, the infraspinatus/teres minor, and the subscapularis were evaluated on the most lateral oblique sagittal T2-weighted MRI with the scapular body (the "Y-view") [15, 16], using both Goutallier classification system and ImageJ [14]. The infraspinatus and teres minor were combined into a single measurement, because their borderline was not always clearly confirmed [17]. Muscle atrophy (MA) was evaluated using the relative ratio of the cross-sectional area of the subscapularis, supraspinatus, and infraspinatus/teres minor muscle belly to that of the supraspinatus fossa. For this measurement, we used ImageJ using the protocol of Nakamura et al. [18]

Retear of the rotator cuff was evaluated using Sugaya's classification [19]: type I, sufficient thickness and evenly low intensity; type II, sufficient thickness and heterogeneous high intensity; type III, repaired cuff tear that kept its continuity but had insufficient thickness; type IV, minor discontinuity and the torn area was minimal in the sagittal plane; and type V, major discontinuity and torn area spread in the sagittal plane. Patients with types IV and V were admitted with postoperative retear [20]. An experienced, orthopedics-trained radiologist who was blinded to the study reviewed these images.

Statistical analysis

The statistical analysis was performed with JMP11 software (SAS, Cary, NC, USA). The Kruskal-Wallis test or χ^2 test was used to compare the continuous or nominal variables in demographics and functional and structural outcomes among the three groups. A Wilcoxon test was used for comparing the preoperative and postoperative functional outcomes in each group. Spearman's ρ was calculated to observe the nonparametric correlation of structural outcomes and clinical outcomes. The correlation between the data evaluated with Goutallier's classification and ImageJ was examined with Spearman's correlation coefficient. For identifying the risk factors for retear after surgery, univariate analysis was first performed in each group; then, multivariate logistic regression was performed using a step wise manner. A receiver-operating curve was calculated to detect the cut-off value when significance was noted in the multivariate analysis. The level of significance was defined for all calculations as $P < .05$. Data are expressed as a mean value with standard deviation.

Results
Preoperative and postoperative functional outcome
Preoperative JOA scores significantly improved from 57.9 ± 19.9 points preoperatively to 87.4 ± 10.0 points postoperatively in group AS, from 56.9 ± 15.4 points to 89.9 ± 6.6 points in group PS, and from 61.7 ± 7.5 points to 83.0 ± 11.4 points in group APE. Consistently, UCLA scores significantly improved from 18.2 ± 5.0 points preoperatively to 28.3 ± 7.2 points postoperatively in Group AS, from 17 ± 4.7 points to 29.4 ± 3.8 points in group PS, and from 15.9 ± 4.0 points to 28.3 ± 5.9 points in group APE. There were no significant differences of postoperative JOA/UCLA scores among the groups. The clinical outcomes scores are shown in Table 2.

Rest, motion, and night pain levels in the three groups were significantly improved postoperatively, except for rest pain in group APE, but it tended to have significance ($P = 0.06$). Most of the parameters in ROM and muscle strength in the three groups significantly improved or tended to have statistical significance after surgery.

Preoperative structural outcome
In the Oizumi classification, Class 0 was observed in 19, 6, and 3 patients; Class I in 30, 7, and 8 patients; Class II in 8, 7, and 4 patients, and Class III in 2, 1, and 5 patients in Group AS, PS, and APE, respectively. Only two patients in group APE had Class IV.

The average retraction of the torn tendon was 29.1 ± 6.2 mm in group AS, 31.2 ± 10.4 mm in group PS, and 37.1 ± 8.7 mm in group APE. The extent of the retraction was significantly larger in group PS and APE than group AS ($P = 0.02$). The average width of the torn tendon was 34.7 ± 66.0 mm in group AS, 37.2 ± 10.4 mm in group PS, and 45.7 ± 89.8 mm in group APE. The extent

of the width was significantly larger in group PS and APE than in group AS ($P = 0.002$).

The average MA in group AS was 246.5 ± 83.5% in the subscapularis, 76.2 ± 19.8% in the supraspinatus, and 220 ± 51.9% in the infraspinatus/teres minor. For group PS, MA was 220.3 ± 67.4% in the subscapularis, 78.9 ± 18.6% in the supraspinatus, and 183.4 ± 38.5% in the infraspinatus/teres minor; for group APE, MA was 252.1 ± 82.4% in the subscapularis, 71.3 ± 16% in the supraspinatus, and 187.4 ± 54.8% in the infraspinatus/teres minor.

The average FD, measured with Image J, for group AS was 5.35 ± 8.25% in the subscapularis, 7.84 ± 10.24% in the supraspinatus, and 3.35 ± 4.92% in the infraspinatus/teres minor; for group PS, FD was 3.5 ± 5.2% in the subscapularis, 11.42 ± 10.15% in the supraspinatus, and 8.52 ± 9.23% in the infraspinatus/teres minor; and for group APE, FD was 6.0 ± 7.23% in the subscapularis, 12.2 ± 9.7% in the supraspinatus, and 6.05 ± 5.2% in the infraspinatus/teres minor.

A low-grade Goutallier stage (stages 0 to 2) was seen in over 80% patients in all three groups. A high-grade Goutallier stage (stages 3 and 4) in group AS was seen in the subscapularis of two patients, supraspinatus of nine patients, and infraspinatus/teres minor of two patients; in Group PS, in the subscapularis of no patients, supraspinatus of three patients, and infraspinatus/teres minor of three patients. In Group APE, a high-grade Goutallier stage was seen in the subscapularis of two patients, supraspinatus of five patients, and infraspinatus/teres minor of three patients. The global fatty degeneration index (GFDI) was 1.02 ± 0.62 in Group AS, 1.36 ± 0.5 in group PS, and 1.29 ± 0.5 in group APE. There was no significant difference among the three groups in GFDI (Table 3).

Postoperative structural outcome
Postoperative retear (Sugaya types IV and V) was noted in 26 of 102 patients (25.5%) in this series: 10 patients in group AS (16.9%), 9 patients in group PS (42.9%), and 7 patients in group APE (31.8%). The retear rate was

Table 2 Preoperative and postoperative clinical outcome in three groups

	Group AS ($N = 59$)	Group PS ($N = 21$)	Group APE ($N = 22$)
JOA score			
Preoperative	57.9 ± 19.9(0–89.5)	56.9 ± 15.4(12–82)	61.7 ± 7.5 (46–78.5)
Postoperative	87.4 ± 10.0(65–100)	89.9 ± 6.6 (80.5–99.5)	83.0 ± 11.4 (60–96)
P value	< 0.001	< 0.001	< 0.001
UCLA score			
Preoperative	18.2 ± 5.0 (7–31)	17 ± 4.7 (9–26)	15.9 ± 4.0 (8–23)
Postoperative	28.3 ± 7.2 (20–35)	29.4 ± 3.8 (22–35)	28.3 ± 5.9 (17–35)
P value	< 0.001	< 0.001	< 0.001

JOA Japanese Orthopedic Association, UCLA University of California, Los Angeles

Table 3 Preoperative structural outcome in three groups

	Group AS (N = 59)	Group PS (N = 21)	Group API: (N = 22)
Oizumi classification			
Grade O	19 (32.2%)	6(28.6%)	3 (13.6%)
Grade I	30 (50.8%)	7 (33.3%)	8 (36.4%)
Grade II	8 (13.6%)	7 (33.3%)	4(18.2%)
Grade III	2 (3.4%)	1 (4.8%)	5 (22.7%)
Grade IV	0 (0%)	0 (0%)	2 (9.1%)
Retraction (mm)	29.1 ± 6.2	31.2 ± 10.4	37.1 ± 8.7
Width (mm)	34.7 ± 6.0	37.2 ± 10.4	45.0 + 9.8
Muscle atrophy (%)			
SSC	246.5 ± 83.5	220.3 ± 67.4	252.1 ± 82.4
SSP	76.2 ± 19.8	78.9 ± 18.6	71.3 ± 16
ISP/TM	220.4 ± 51.9	183.4 ± 38.5	187.4 ± 54.8
Fatty degeneration (%)			
SSC	5.35 ± 8.25	3.5 ± 5 20	6.0 ± 7.23
SSP	7.84 ± 10.24	11.42 ± 10.15	12.2 ± 9.7
ISP/IM	3.35 ± 4.92	8.52 ± 9.23	6.05 ± 5.2
Goutallier classification SSC			
Stage 0	24 (40.7%)	9 (42.9%)	6 (27.3%)
Stage 1	26 (44.1%)	8 (38.1%)	5 (22.7%)
Stage 2	7 (11.9%)	4 (19.0%)	9 (40.9%)
Stage 3	2 (3.4%)	0 (0%)	1 (4.5%)
Stage 4	0 (0%)	0 (0%)	1 (4.5%)
Goutallier classification SSP			
Stage 0	13 (22%)	2 (9.5%)	2 (9.0%)
Stage 1	16 (27.1%)	5 (23.8%)	5 (22.7%)
Stage 2	21 (35.6%)	11 (52.4%)	10 (45.5%)
Stage 3	7 (11.9%)	2 (9.5%)	1 (4.5%)
Stage 4	2 (3.4%)	1 (4.8%)	4 (18.2%)
Goutallier classification ISP/TM			
Stage 0	28 (47.5%)	5 (22.7%)	5 (22.7%)
Stage 1	26 (44.1%)	6 (27.3)	9 (40.9%)
Stage 2	3 (5.0%)	7 (31.8%)	5 (22.7%)
Stage 3	2 (3.4%)	3 (13.6%)	1 (4.5%)
Stage 4	0 (0%)	0 (0%)	2 (9.0%)
GFDI	1.02 ± 0.62	1.36 + 0.5	1.29 ± 0.5

SSC subscapularis, SSP supraspinatus, ISP/TM infraspinatus/teres minor, GFDI global fatty degeneration index

significantly higher in group PS than in groups AS and APE (P = 0.02) (Table 4).

Surgical technique and postoperative retear

Suture bridge technique was performed in 71 patients: 40 in group AS;14 in group PS; 17 in group APE. Postoperative retear occurred in 16 patients (22.5%): 6 in group AS (15.0%); 4 in group PS (28.6%); 6 in group APE (35.3%).

Single-row technique was performed in 20 patients: 14 in group AS; 4 in group PS; 2 in group APE. Postoperative retear occurred in 8 patients (40.0%): 4 in group AS (28.6%); 3 in group PS (75.0%); 1 in group APE (50.0%).

Double-row technique was performed in 11 patients: 5 in group AS; 3 in group PS; 3 in group APE. Postoperative retear occurred in 2 patients (18.2%): none in group AS (0.0%); 2 in group PS (66.7%); none in group APE (0.0%). Details are shown in Table 5.

Table 4 Postoperative retear (SUGAYA's classification)

SUGAYA	Group AS (N = 59)	Group PS (N = 21)	Group APE (N = 22)	Total
Type I	28 (45.8%)	8 (38%)	6 (27.3%)	
Type II	13 (22%)	2 (9.5%)	3 (13.6%)	
Type III	8 (13.6%)	2 (9.5%)	6 (27.3%)	
Type IV	8 (13.6%)	4 (19%)	3 (13.6%)	15
Type V	2 (3.4%)	5 (23.8%)	4 (18.2%)	11
Retear	10 (16.9%)	9 (42.9%)	7 (31.8%)	26 (25.5%)

Risk factors affecting postoperative retear

First, various parameters were evaluated to determine the risk factors for retear after surgery, using univariate analysis. Retraction ($P = 0.039$), width ($P = 0.0023$), FD of the supraspinatus ($P = 0.0043$), the Goutallier classification of the supraspinatus ($P = 0.001$), and GFDI ($P = 0.008$) were significant risk factors in group AS: Preoperative active external rotation range ($P = 0.001$), preoperative muscle strength of flexion ($P = 0.02$), and FD of the infraspinatus/teres minor ($P = 0.048$) were evaluated using ImageJ in group PS. FD of the supraspinatus ($P = 0.002$) and the infraspinatus/teres minor ($P = 0.0074$) were evaluated using ImageJ and GFDI ($P = 0.0123$) in group APE. The Goutallier stage of the infraspinatus in group PS and APE was not a significant risk factor, but it tended to have statistical significance (Table 6).

Next, multivariate analysis using stepwise methods was performed. Preoperative external rotation range was the only risk factor for postoperative retear in groups PS and APE ($P = 0.014$ and $P = 0.016$, respectively). For the prediction of postoperative retear, receiver operating characteristic (ROC) curve analysis demonstrated that the cut-off value in the preoperative external rotation range was 25°, showing that the retear risk increased 2.12-fold as the preoperative external rotation range decreased by 5° (Fig. 1).

Table 5 Univariate analysis in three groups

	Healed (N = 76)	Retear (N = 26)	Total (N = 102)
Suture bridge	55 (77.5%)	16 (22.5%)	71
Group AS	34 (85.0%)	6 (15.0%)	40
Group PS	10 (71.4%)	4 (28.6%)	14
Group APE	11 (64.7%)	6 (35.3%)	17
Single row	12 (60.0%)	8 (40.0%)	20
Group AS	10 (71.4%)	4 (28.6%)	14
Group PS	1 (25.0%)	3 (75.0%)	4
Group APE	1 (50.0%)	1 (50.0%)	2
Double row	9 (81.8%)	2 (18.2%)	11
Group AS	5 (100%)	0 (0%)	5
Group PS	1 (33.3%)	2 (66.7%)	3
Group APE	3 (100%)	0 (0%)	3

Correlation between active external rotation range and its related variables

Since multivariate analysis showed that active external rotation range (AERR) is a unique risk factor for postoperative retear in groups PS and APE, we further evaluated the correlation between AERR and its related variables in these groups. There was statistical significance between AERR and FD, using ImageJ ($r = -0.36$, $P = 0.04$). External rotation strength (ERS) was not significant, but it showed a trend ($P = 0.06$). For FD of the infraspinatus, statistical significance was seen between the evaluation methods, using the Goutallier classification and ImageJ ($r = 0.82$, $P < 0.0001$) (Table 7).

Discussion

The present study investigated the risk factors for retear after ARCR in large and massive cuff tears, dividing these tears into three groups (i.e., group AS, PS, and APE). Although univariate analysis revealed that the groups had different characteristics, step-wise multivariate analysis showed that preoperative, decreased active external rotation in group PS and APE was a unique risk factor for retear after surgery, with a cut-off value of 25°. To our knowledge, such data have not been reported.

Previous studies that used multivariate analysis demonstrated that the Goutallier stage of the infraspinatus is a risk factor for postoperative retear in large and massive tears [8, 21]. In the present study, the Goutallier stage of the infraspinatus in Group PS and APE was a significant factor for postoperative retear in univariate analysis, but not in multivariate analysis. The average Goutallier stage of the infraspinatus was relatively low (0.9) in the present study, compared with 1.2 in a study by Oh et al. [8] and 2.1 in a study by Chung et al. [21] Thus, this may partly explain why the Goutallier stage of the infraspinatus did not reach statistical significance in the present study.

FD of the infraspinatus caused postoperative retear and led to limitations of external rotation [22]. Loss of active external rotation is related to tears in the infraspinatus and teres minor [23]. In the present study, there was a significant correlation between the decrease of active external rotation range and FD, evaluated with ImageJ. Taken together, these results supported our data that decreased

Table 6 Correlation between active external rotation range (AERR) and its related variables

Group AS (N = 59)	P value	Group PS (N = 21)	P value	Group APE (N = 22)	P value
Retraction	0.039	Preoperative ER	0.001	SSP FD	0.002
Width	0.0023	Preoperative FLEX MS	0.02	ISP/TM FD	0.0074
SSP FD	0.0043	ISP/TM FD	0.048	GFDI	0.012
Goutallier SSP	0.001				
GFDI	0.0084	*Goutallier ISP	0.08	*Goutallier ISP	0.068

ER external rotation, MS muscle strength, FD fatty degeneration, GFDI global fatty degeneration index
*There were no significant differences or trends

active external range is significantly associated with postoperative retear in patients who undergo ARCR for treatment of large or massive tears.

In the present study, multivariate analysis showed that decreased active external range before surgery was a risk factor for retear in group PS and APE. The preoperative characteristics in these two groups revealed a similar tendency, except for distribution of large or massive tears. Thus, less fatty involvement of the subscapularis in the two groups may have contributed to the similar data.

In AS cuff tears, the retear rate after surgery was reported to be 6–18% [24–26]. Consistent with these studies, our study found 10 postoperative retear cases (16.9%, N = 59 cases) in group AS. A previous study found that the Goutallier stage of the subscapularis was associated with postoperative retear in AS cuff tears [25], while the Goutallier stage of the supraspinatus was responsible for retear after ARCR in the present study. A high-grade Goutallier stage was found in the supraspinatus in nine cases (15.3%) and in the subscapularis in two cases (3.4%) in group AS. Thus, this might have

affected our data. Although univariate analysis in the present study showed a certain risk for postoperative retear in anteroposterior cuff tears, no significant factors were noted in the multivariate analysis. Studies on these points are now underway at our institution.

Although most tears occurred in the supraspinatus tendon, tearing in this tendon did not influence retear after surgery in group PS and APE. Mochizuki et al. [27, 28] reported that the footprint of the supraspinatus tendon on the greater tuberosity is much smaller than previously believed, and this area of the greater tuberosity is actually occupied by a substantial amount of the infraspinatus tendon. This may mean that during surgery, infraspinatus tendon repair rather than supraspinatus tendon repair may be closely associated not only with the footprint coverage at the greater tuberosity, but also with retear after surgery at the site.

The limitations of the present study were its retrospective cohort, short-term follow up, and small sample size, especially in group PS and APE in comparison with group AS. Further studies with longer follow-up and larger cohorts are needed to address these limitations. However, the strength of this study was that we clearly demonstrated that decreased active eternal range is a risk factor for large and massive tears, especially in PS and APE cuff tears.

Conclusions

Although multivariate analysis failed to detect significant risk factor for retear in patients with anterosuperior large/massive cuff tears who undergo ARCR, it demonstrated

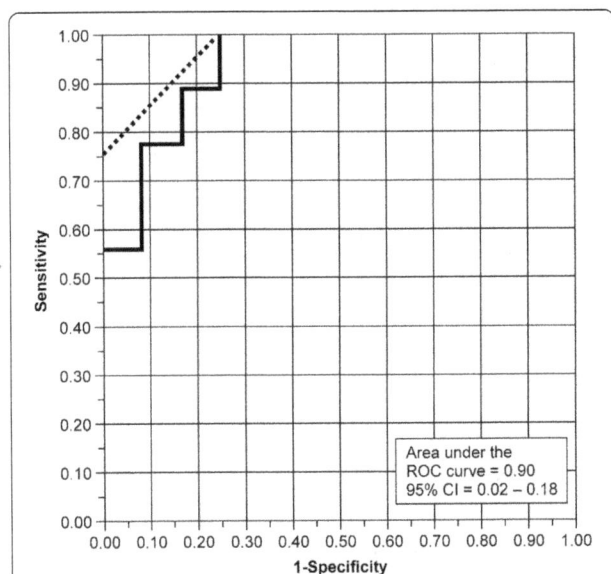

Fig. 1 Receiver operating characteristic (ROC) curve analysis to calculate the cutoff value for preoperative active external rotation range. AUC area under the curve, CI confidence interval

Area under the ROC curve = 0.90
95% CI = 0.02 – 0.18

Table 7 Correlation between active external rotation range (AERR) and its related variables

		Correlation coefficient (r)	P Value
Preoperative ER	Preoperative ER MS	0.3	0.06
Preoperative ER	ISP FD	−0.36	0.04
Preoperative ER	Goutallier ISP	−0.154	0.37
ISP FD	Preoperative ER MS	−0.0154	0.93
ISP FD	Goutallier ISP	0.82	< 0.001
Goutallier ISP	Preoperative ER MS	0.05	0.77

ER external rotation, MS muscle strength, ISP infraspinatus

that active external rotation less than 25° before surgery is a significant risk factor in those with posterosuperior large/massive tears. This study may help surgeons understand the results of arthroscopic surgery in patients with large/massive tears.

Abbreviations
AERR: Active external rotation range; ARCR: Arthroscopic rotator cuff repair; AUC: Area under the curve; ERS: External rotation strength; FD: fatty degeneration; GFDI: The Global Fatty Degeneration Index; JOA: Japanese Orthopedic Association; MA: Muscle atrophy; MRI: Magnetic resonance imaging; RCTs: Rotator cuff tears; ROC: Receiver-operating characteristic; ROM: Range of motion; UCLA: The University of California, Los Angeles

Acknowledgements
We thank Tatsuyuki Kakuma PhD from the Department of Bio-Statistical Center, Kurume University for his help with the statistical analysis.

Funding
We have no funding.

Authors' contributions
HS planned the study's design, data acquisition, analysis, and interpretation of data, and wrote the manuscript. MG supervised the study design, data analysis, and manuscript writing. YM, TO, and NS supervised the study design and data analysis. HH and HN carried out data acquisition and analysis. TK carried out the statistical data analysis. All authors read and approved the final manuscript.

Competing interests
The authors declare that they have no competing interests.

Author details
[1]Department of Orthopaedic Surgery, Kurume University School of Medicine, 67 Asahi-machi, kurume, Fukuoka 830-0011, Japan. [2]Department of Statistics, Kurume University School of Medicine, 67 Asahi-machi, kurume, Fukuoka 830-0011, Japan. [3]Department of Orthopaedic Surgery, Kurume University Medical Center, 155-1 Kokubu-machi Kurume, Fukuoka 839-0863, Japan.

References
1. Berth A, Neumann W, Awiszus F, Pap G. Massive rotator cuff tears: functional outcome after debridement or arthroscopic partial repair. J Orthop Traumatol. 2010;11:13–20.
2. Burkhart SS, Barth JR, Richards DP, Zlatkin MB, Larsen M. Arthroscopic repair of massive rotator cuff tears with stage 3 and 4 fatty degeneration. Arthroscopy. 2007;23:347–54.
3. Burkhart SS, Danaceau SM, Pearce CE Jr. Arthroscopic rotator cuff repair: Analysis of results by tear size and by repair technique-margin convergence versus direct tendon-to-bone repair. Arthroscopy. 2001;17:905–12.
4. Galatz LM, Ball CM, Teefey SA, Middleton WD, Yamaguchi K. The outcome and repair integrity of completely arthroscopically repaired large and massive rotator cuff tears. J Bone Joint Surg Am. 2004;86-A:219–24.
5. Lo IK, Burkhart SS. Arthroscopic revision of failed rotator cuff repairs: technique and results. Arthroscopy. 2004;20:250–67.
6. Yoo JC, Ahn JH, Koh KH, Lim KS. Rotator cuff integrity after arthroscopic repair for large tears with less-than-optimal footprint coverage. Arthroscopy. 2009;25:1093–100.
7. Saccomanno MF, Sircana G, Cazzato G, Donati F, Randelli P, Milano G. Prognostic factors influencing the outcome of rotator cuff repair: a systematic review. Knee Surg Sports Traumatol Arthrosc. 2015; https://doi.org/10.1007/s00167-015-3700-y.
8. Oh JH, Kim SH, Ji HM, Jo KH, Bin SW, Gong HS. Prognostic factors affecting anatomic outcome of rotator cuff repair and correlation with functional outcome. Arthroscopy. 2009;25:30–9.
9. Kim JR, Cho YS, Ryu KJ, Kim JH. Clinical and radiographic outcomes after arthroscopic repair of massive rotator cuff tears using a suture bridge technique: assessment of repair integrity on magnetic resonance imaging. Am J Sports Med. 2012;40:786–93.
10. Ueda Y, Sugaya H, Takahashi N, Matsuki K, Kawai N, Tokai M, et al. Rotator cuff lesions in patients with stiff shoulders: a prospective analysis of 379 shoulders. J Bone Joint Surg Am. 2015;97:1233–7.
11. Warner JJ, Higgins L, Parsons IM, Dowdy P. Diagnosis and treatment of anterosuperior rotator cuff tears. J Shoulder Elbow Surg. 2001;10:37–46.
12. DeOrio JK, Cofield RH. Results of a second attempt at surgical repair of a failed initial rotator-cuff repair. J Bone Joint Surg Am. 1984;66:563–7.
13. Miyoshi N, Suenaga N, Katayama K, Oizumi N, Yamaguchi H, Matsuno T. Radiological classification of glenoid deformity in rheumatoid arthritis. Int J Rheumatol. 2011;2011:239894.
14. Davidson JF, Burkhart SS, Richards DP, Campbell SE. Use of preoperative magnetic resonance imaging to predict rotator cuff tear pattern and method of repair. Arthroscopy. 2005;21:1428.
15. Mellado JM, Calmet J, Olona M, Esteve C, Camins A, Perez Del Palomar L, et al. Surgically repaired massive rotator cuff tears: MRI of tendon integrity, muscle fatty degeneration, and muscle atrophy correlated with intraoperative and clinical findings. AJR Am J Roentgenol. 2005;184:1456–63.
16. Lapner PL, Jiang L, Zhang T, Athwal GS. Rotator cuff fatty infiltration and atrophy are associated with functional outcomes in anatomic shoulder arthroplasty. Clin Orthop Relat Res. 2015;473:674–82.
17. Lee E, Choi JA, Oh JH, Ahn S, Hong SH, Chai JW, et al. Fatty degeneration of the rotator cuff muscles on pre- and postoperative CT arthrography (CTA): is the Goutallier grading system reliable? Skelet Radiol. 2013;42:1259–67.
18. Nakamura H, Gotoh M, Mitsui Y, Honda H, Ohzono H, Shimokobe H, et al. Factors affecting clinical outcome in patients with structural failure after arthroscopic rotator cuff repair. Arthroscopy. 2016;32:732–9.
19. Sugaya H, Maeda K, Matsuki K, Moriishi J. Repair integrity and functional outcome after arthroscopic double-row rotator cuff repair. A prospective outcome study. J Bone Joint Surg Am. 2007;89:953–60.
20. Choi S, Kim MK, Kim GM, Roh YH, Hwang IK, Kang H. Factors associated with clinical and structural outcomes after arthroscopic rotator cuff repair with a suture bridge technique in medium, large, and massive tears. J Shoulder Elbow Surg. 2014;23:1675–81.
21. Chung SW, Kim JY, Kim MH, Kim SH, Oh JH. Arthroscopic repair of massive rotator cuff tears: outcome and analysis of factors associated with healing failure or poor postoperative function. Am J Sports Med. 2013;41:1674–83.
22. Goutallier D, Postel JM, Bernageau J, Lavau L, Voisin MC. Fatty muscle degeneration in cuff ruptures. Pre- and postoperative evaluation by CT scan. Clin Orthop Relat Res. 1994;304:78–83.
23. Collin P, Matsumura N, Ladermann A, Denard PJ, Walch G. Relationship between massive chronic rotator cuff tear pattern and loss of active shoulder range of motion. J Shoulder Elbow Surg. 2014;23:1195–202.
24. Schnaser E, Toussaint B, Gillespie R, Lefebvre Y, Gobezie R. Arthroscopic treatment of anterosuperior rotator cuff tears. Orthopedics. 2013;36:e1394–400.
25. Maqdes A, Abarca J, Moraiti C, Boughebri O, Dib C, Leclere FM, et al. Does preoperative subscapularis fatty muscle infiltration really matter in anterosuperior rotator cuff tears repair outcomes? A prospective multicentric study. Orthop Traumatol Surg Res. 2014;100:485–8.
26. Ide J, Tokiyoshi A, Hirose J, Mizuta H. Arthroscopic repair of traumatic combined rotator cuff tears involving the subscapularis tendon. J Bone Joint Surg Am. 2007;89:2378–88.
27. Mochizuki T, Sugaya H, Uomizu M, Maeda K, Matsuki K, Sekiya I, et al. Humeral insertion of the supraspinatus and infraspinatus. New anatomical findings regarding the footprint of the rotator cuff. J Bone Joint Surg Am. 2008;90:962–9.
28. Mochizuki T, Sugaya H, Uomizu M, Maeda K, Matsuki K, Sekiya I, et al. Humeral insertion of the supraspinatus and infraspinatus. New anatomical findings regarding the footprint of the rotator cuff. Surgical technique. J Bone Joint Surg Am. 2009;91(Suppl 2 Pt 1):1–7.

14

An updated meta-analysis of the asporin gene D-repeat in knee osteoarthritis: effects of gender and ethnicity

Ruoxi Liu[1†], Xueling Yuan[1†], Jing Yu[2], Qi Quan[1], Haoye Meng[1], Cheng Wang[1], Aiyuan Wang[1], Quanyi Guo[1], Jiang Peng[1*] and Shibi Lu[1*]

Abstract

Background: Knee osteoarthritis (KOA) is the most prevalent form of knee joint disease and characterized by the progressive degeneration of articular cartilage. Although pathology of KOA remains unknown, genetic factors are considered to be the major cause. Asporin is a group of biologically active components of extracellular matrix (ECM) in articular cartilage, and asporin gene (ASPN) D-repeat polymorphism was reported to be associated with KOA. Thus, our meta-analysis is aimed at investigation of the association between asporin D-repeat polymorphism and susceptibility of KOA.

Methods: We gathered data from MEDLINE, Embase, OVID, and ScienceDirect to search relevant published epidemiological studies through April 2017. Compared with previous studies, our meta-analysis is the first study to investigate the association of ASPN D15, D16, and D17 alleles and KOA susceptibility by ethnic- and sex-stratified subgroup analysis.

Results: We found no significant association between D15 allele and susceptibility to KOA (OR = 1.05, 95% CI 0.95–1.17) in overall population. The same results were observed in the analysis of D16 (OR = 1.01, 95% CI 0.80–1.28) and D17 alleles (OR = 1.28, 95% CI 0.91–1.80). The ethnic- and sex-subgroup analyses did not alter the ORs. However, significant association was detected in the sensitivity analysis of D17 in overall population (OR = 1.05, 95% CI 0.95–1.17) and Asian population (OR = 1.78, 95% CI 1.02–3.11, $P < 0.05$).

Conclusion: Our results indicated that D-repeat polymorphism of ASPN may not play a major role in susceptibility of KOA in ethnic- and sex-specific analysis. Because of the limitations of the present meta-analysis, firm conclusions could not be drawn based on the current evidence, and further studies are required to detect genuine role of ASPN.

Keywords: Aspartic acid, Osteoarthritis, Knee, Gender, Ethnicity, Meta-analysis, Polymorphism

Background

Osteoarthritis (OA), which is characterized by the progressive degeneration of articular cartilage in joints, is one of the most common joint diseases that mainly affects the knees [1, 2]. Joint stiffness and pain appear to be the first symptoms, and joint swelling followed as the result of effusion and synovitis [3]. The knee osteoarthritis (KOA) has been identified of all ages and considered as the most common cause of disability after middle age [4].

However, current therapeutic methods only slow progression of KOA rather than prevent it [5]. The underlying mechanisms of KOA still remain unknown. Epidemiological studies had proved several risk factors associated with KOA, such as age, sex, obesity, kneeling, meniscal injuries, and mechanical forces [4]. Moreover, some previous studies uncovered several genetic linkage and candidate genes correlated with susceptibility to KOA [6, 7]. Taken together, KOA is considered as a polygenic disease controlled by both genetic and environmental factors.

* Correspondence: pengjiang301@126.com; lushibi301@126.com
†Equal contributors
[1]Institute of Orthopedics, Beijing Key Laboratory of Regenerative Medicine in Orthopedics, Key Laboratory of Musculoskeletal Trauma & War Injuries PLA, Chinese PLA General Hospital, FuXing Road 28th, Beijing 100853, China
Full list of author information is available at the end of the article

One conventional viewpoint is that KOA is produced by an imbalance between synthesis and degradation of the extracellular matrix (ECM) controlled by chondrocytes [8]. Asporin, which consists of 380 amino acids, belongs to small leucin-rich proteoglycans (SLRPs), a group of biologically active components of ECM in many tissues [9]. Compared with normal cartilage, the expression of asporin is increased in KOA cartilage. It directly binds to transforming growth factor-β (TGF-β) and inhibits tumor necrosis factor (TNF)-β-mediated expression of cartilage genes [10]. The asporin gene (ASPN), which locates in human chromosome 9q22-9q21.3, contains a triplet repeat coding for a polymorphic stretch of aspartic acid residues (D-repeat) in the N-terminal region of the protein [11]. The number of D-repeats varies from 9 (D9) to 20 (D20), and different number of D-repeats may play a different role in KOA onset and development [9, 12]. A positive association between the D14 allele and KOA susceptibility was first reported by Kizawa et al. in a cohort and a case-control study in Japanese population; they also found that D14 allele was upregulated while D13 allele was downregulated in KOA patients [13]. However, relevant meta-analysis yielded inconsistent results. Nakamura et al. reported a positive relation between ASPN D14 allele and KOA susceptibility in Asian population, and results have ethnic differences [14]. But recently, two meta-analyses both demonstrated that ASPN D13 and D14 alleles were not associated with the occurrence of KOA in Asian and European population [15, 16].

There may be two reasons for the abovementioned different results. First, there was a gender difference in the occurrence and pathology of KOA. Women usually have a higher incidence of KOA, and postmenopausal women tend to suffer more severe KOA [17]. Anterior cruciate ligament (ACL) injuries are one of the major causes of KOA in athletes and are more likely to occur in female athletes than in men [18–20]. Besides, it has been reported that females have greater pain intensity, functional limitations, and inflammatory reaction [21, 22]. Second, the incidence and symptoms of KOA have racial differences. Compared with Europeans, the prevalence and severity of KOA are higher in African–Americans [23, 24]. Moreover, Chinese women were reported to suffer more severe radiographic KOA than Caucasian women [25]. In this context, it is reasonable to hypothesize that the association between ASPN and KOA have gender and ethnic differences.

Here, we performed a meta-analysis of recent studies to investigate the association between ASPN D15, D16, and D17 alleles and susceptibility to KOA.

Methods
Search strategy and select criteria
We gathered data from MEDLINE, Embase, OVID, and ScienceDirect to search published epidemiological studies through April 2017 that were designed to explore the association between ASPN D-repeat polymorphism and KOA susceptibility. Combinations of keywords used in the search were ("ASPN" or "asporin"), ("polymorphism" or "polymorphisms"), and ("osteoarthritis" or "OA"). No restrictions including languages were imposed on our search.

To be consistent with other previous meta-analysis protocols, we included observational studies that recruited both KOA patients and healthy controls. The diagnostic criteria of KOA should be based on clinical symptoms, radiographic evidence, or joint replacement. Eligible studies should assess the association between ASPN D-repeat polymorphism and KOA susceptibility and had enough genetic frequency to extract. Interim analyses, overlapping study populations, and comparisons of laboratory methods were excluded. Potential studies for the eligibility criteria were reviewed by two independent readers (Liu and Yuan), with a third reviewer (Peng) to settle any discrepancies.

Date extraction
For all eligible published studies, data were independently extracted from full text with the use of a standard data extraction form by two authors (Liu and Yuan). The standard data extraction form contained information of title, authors, year of publication, study design, sample size, gender, ethnicity, allele count, and allele frequency in KOA patients and healthy controls.

Statistical analysis
We used the software Review Manager 5.3 (The Nordic Cochrane Center, Copenhagen, Denmark) and STATA 14.0 (Statacorp, College Station, TX, USA) for all the calculations of statistical analysis. The D15, D16, and D17 alleles vs others alleles combined were evaluated respectively because of no specific genotype distribution reported in the included original articles. Thus, we performed meta-analyses of the ASPN D15, D16, and D17 alleles and KOA susceptibility to investigate their association respectively by calculating odds ratios (ORs) and 95% confidence intervals (CIs).

Q-statistic was used to assess between-study heterogeneity, and $P < 0.1$ was considered statistically significant. The recently developed measure I^2 was also applied to test heterogeneity; values of $I^2 = 25$, 50, and 75% were considered low, moderate, and high, respectively [26].

Data are shown as ORs with a 95% CI, and statistical significance was defined as $P < 0.05$ (two-tailed). When heterogeneity was low, the ORs were obtained by fixed effects models [27, 28]. Otherwise, random effects models were used to estimate the ORs [29]. The fixed effects model assumes that genetic factors have similar effects on KOA susceptibility across all included studies and that observed variations among studies result from chance alone [30]. The random effects model assumes that different studies exhibit substantial diversity and assesses both within-study sampling error and between-study variance [29]. A sensitivity analysis was carried out to determine the effect of sample size by omitting one or more studies and assessing the change in the results of the meta-analysis. To test for publication bias, we performed Egger's linear regression analysis and Begg's test using the software package STATA 14.0 (Statacorp, College Station, TX, USA) [31].

Results

Search results and demographic characteristics

The preliminarily literature search yielded 257 articles fulfilling the search criteria of which 51 described case–control studies. Then, we excluded 13 studies for not KOA articles, 23 studies for not ASPN articles, and 5 studies for unusable data. A total of 10 studies fulfilled all inclusion and none of the exclusion criteria (Fig. 1). Noticeably, one of the included articles contained a case–control analysis and a cohort analysis; thus, they were investigated respectively. A total of 11 separate comparisons, with a total of 2745 KOA patients and 3621 controls, which involved 5 Caucasian, 4 Asian, and 2 Latin American populations, were included in this review. Additionally, Of the 11 separate comparisons, 5 sex-stratified comparisons were composed of 1528 females and 1186 males. The recruit criterion of KOA patients was according to symptoms or radiographic evidence in 7 articles and joint replacement in the rest of articles. Characteristics of included articles in the meta-analysis are presented in Table 1.

Results of meta-analysis

Table 2 showed the summary of association between D-repeat polymorphism and susceptibility to KOA. The detailed result is that the pooled OR for the D15 allele vs other alleles combined and its 95% CI included 1 (OR = 1.05, 95% CI 0.95–1.17) (Fig. 2), demonstrating that D15 allele had no significant relationship with susceptibility to KOA in the overall populations included in this review. The results of the combined meta-analysis showed that the D16 allele is not associated with the risk of KOA (OR = 1.01, 95% CI 0.80–1.28) (Fig. 3). The same results were also observed in the analysis of D17 allele (OR = 1.28, 95% CI 0.91–1.80) (Fig. 4), and no significant association was detected between D17 allele and occurrence of KOA.

For ethnic-specific analysis, no association was observed between D15 polymorphism and susceptibility to KOA in the Asian (OR = 0.93, 95% CI 0.69–1.27), Caucasian (OR = 1.11, 95% CI 0.98–1.26), or Latin American (OR = 0.81, 95% CI 0.46–1.42) populations (Fig. 5).

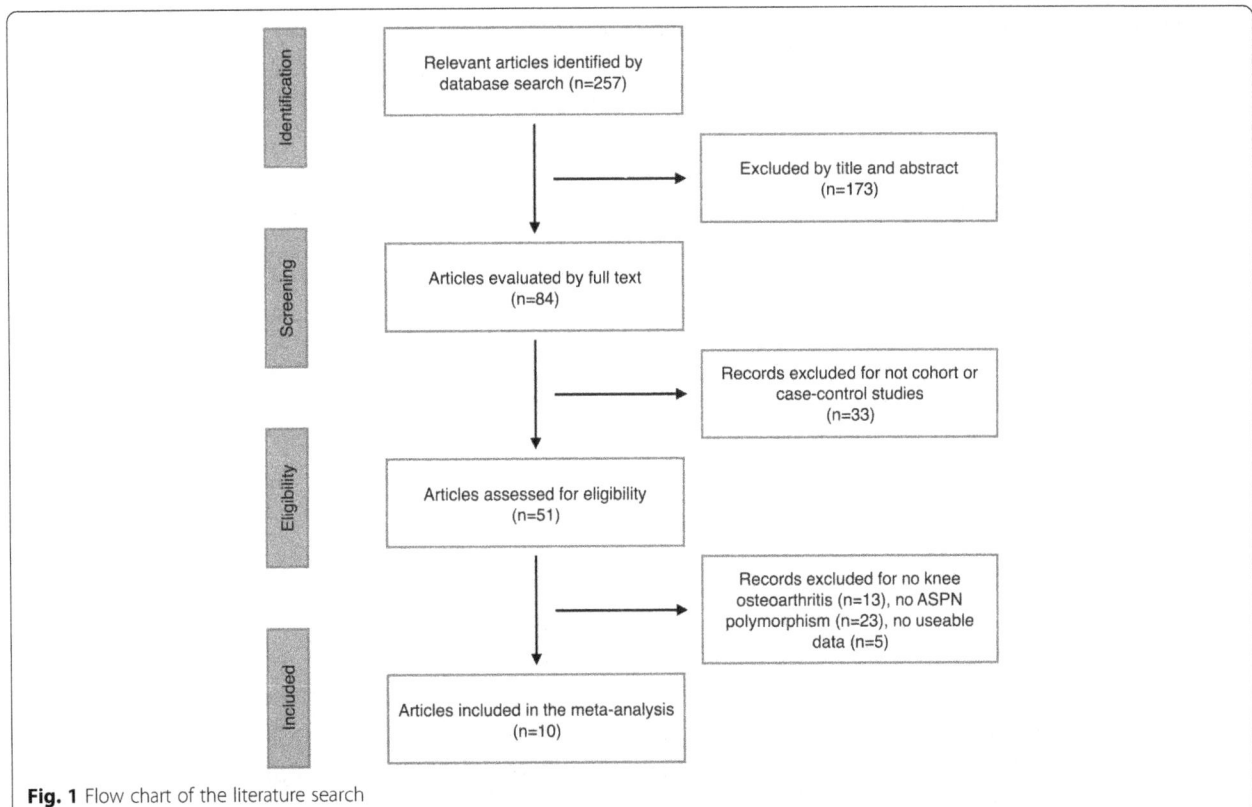

Fig. 1 Flow chart of the literature search

Table 1 Features of the included articles

Study	Ethnicity	Country	Study design	Gender (female/male)		Participants (number)	
				Case	Control	Case	Control
Jiang et al. [37]	Asian	China	Case control	NA	NA	218	454
Kizawa et al. [13]	Asian	Japan	Case control	NA	NA	393	374
Kizawa et al. [13]	Asian	Japan	Cohort	NA	NA	137	234
Song et al. [16]	Asian	Korea	Case control	152/38	154/222	190	376
Atif et al. [36]	Caucasian	USA	Case control	NA	NA	775	511
Jazayeri et al. [35]	Caucasian	Iran	Case control	72/28	72/28	100	100
Kaliakatsos et al. [34]	Caucasian	Greece	Case control	NA	NA	155	190
Mustafa et al. [32]	Caucasian	UK	Case control	158/120	392/356	278	748
Rodriguez-Lopez et al. [33]	Caucasian	Spain	Case control	153/35	115/179	188	294
Arellano et al. [21]	Latin American	Mexico	Case control	130/88	130/92	218	222
González-Huerta et al. [38]	Latin American	Mexico	Case control	NA	NA	93	118
Total				665/309	863/877	2745	3621

NA not available

The same results were also observed in the analysis of D16 and D17 alleles (Fig. 5). Similarly, none of the alleles showed significant sex-specific association with susceptibility to KOA (Fig. 5).

Sensitivity analysis and publication bias

Because of the high heterogeneity found in D16 and D17 allele analysis for overall and Asian population, we performed the sensitivity analysis to identify the results by removing the case–control study of Kizawa et al. [13] which induced heterogeneity. The results of sensitivity analysis showed the pooled OR of D17 allele vs other alleles combined exceeded 1 (OR = 1.43, 95% CI 1.09–1.89, $P < 0.05$) (Table 3), indicating a significant positive relationship between D17 allele and susceptibility to KOA after sensitivity analysis. The same results were also observed in D17 allele sensitivity analysis for Asian population (OR = 1.78, 95% CI 1.02–3.11, $P < 0.05$)

Table 2 Summary ORs, 95% CIs, and heterogeneity of the D-repeat polymorphism and the susceptibility to KOA

Polymorphism	Overall or subgroup (population or gender)	No. of studies	Test of association			Test of heterogeneity		
			OR	95% CI	P value	Model	P value	I^2 (%)
D15 versus Others	Overall	11	1.05	0.95–1.17	0.33	Fixed	0.37	8
	Asian	4	0.93	0.69–1.27	0.66	Fixed	0.93	0
	Caucasian	5	1.11	0.98–1.26	0.09	Fixed	0.35	10
	Latin American	2	0.81	0.46–1.42	0.46	Random	0.08	68
	Female	5	1.08	0.87–1.33	0.49	Fixed	0.18	36
	Male	5	0.94	0.71–1.24	0.66	Fixed	0.43	0
D16 versus Others	Overall	10	1.00	0.79–1.27	1.00	Random	0.03	51
	Asian	4	0.89	0.56–1.41	0.62	Random	0.03	66
	Caucasian	4	0.96	0.75–1.22	0.73	Fixed	0.24	29
	Latin American	2	1.23	0.55–2.73	0.85	Random	0.05	75
	Female	5	0.89	0.59–1.34	0.58	Random	0.10	48
	Male	5	0.82	0.56–1.21	0.32	Fixed	0.90	0
D17 versus Others	Overall	10	1.28	0.91–1.80	0.16	Random	0.07	44
	Asian	4	1.30	0.68–2.50	0.43	Random	0.08	56
	Caucasian	4	1.37	0.94–2.02	0.10	Fixed	0.25	26
	Latin American	2	1.32	0.38–4.57	0.66	Random	0.04	77
	Female	5	1.57	0.95–2.59	0.08	Fixed	0.65	0
	Male	5	1.77	0.87–3.60	0.11	Fixed	0.86	0

NA not available

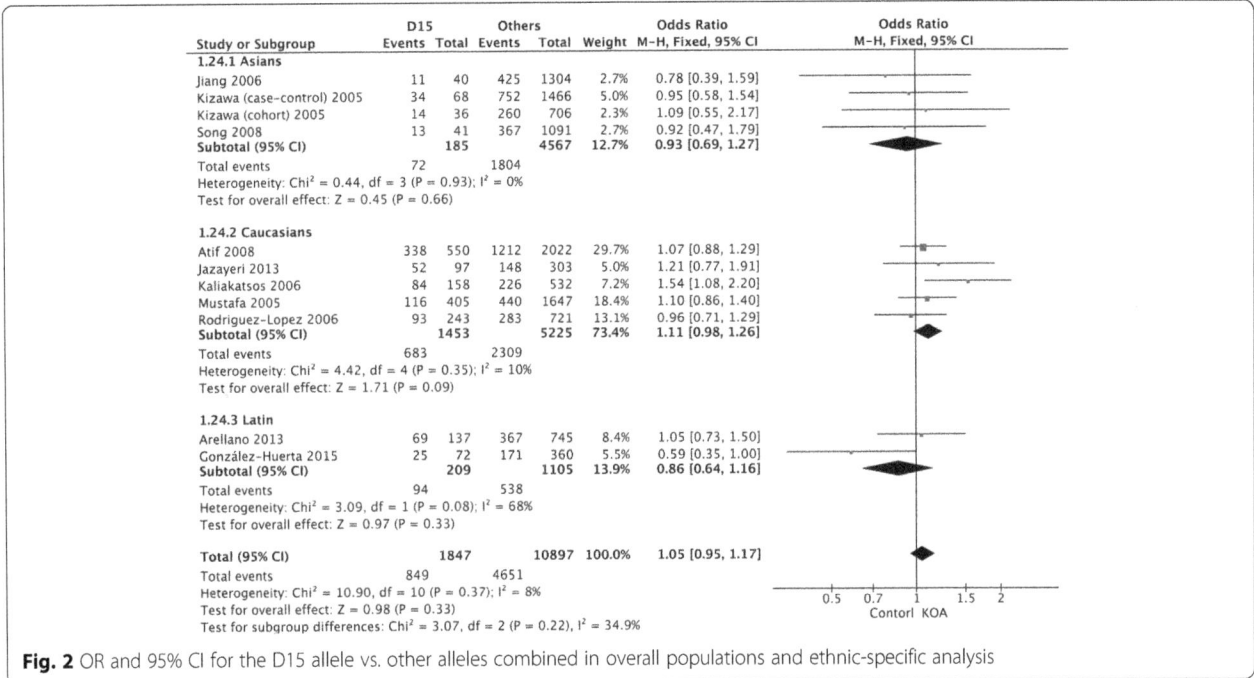

Fig. 2 OR and 95% CI for the D15 allele vs. other alleles combined in overall populations and ethnic-specific analysis

(Table 3). These results differed greatly from previous results without removing the article.

We estimated potential publication bias by Egger's regression test and Begg's test. The *P* value for Egger's and Begg's test of the asporin D15 allele analysis was 0.354 and 0.213, revealing no proof of publication bias. There was also no significant publication bias in analyses of D16 and D17 alleles (Egger's and Begg's test *P* > 0.1).

Discussion

In the current study, ten published articles (11 comparisons) were included with a total of 2745 KOA and 3621 controls from Caucasian, Asian, and Latin American populations to examine the relationship between ASPN D-repeat polymorphism and KOA susceptibility by ethnic- and sex-specific meta-analysis. We observed that D15, D16, and D17 alleles had no effect on KOA

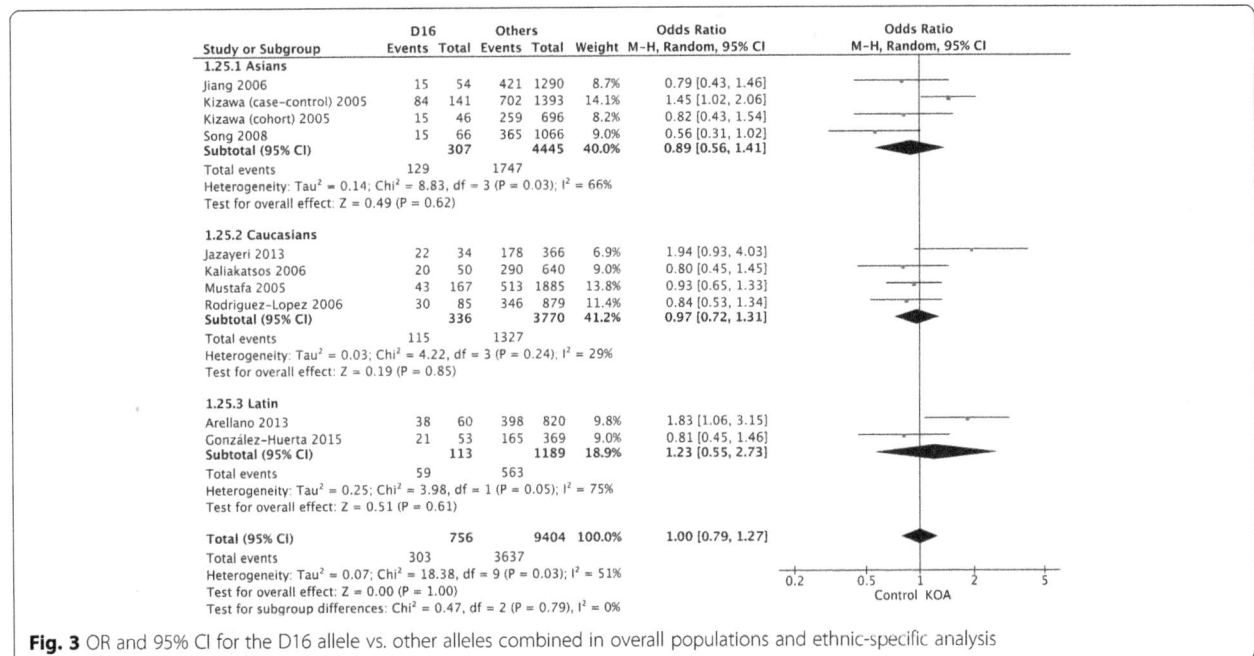

Fig. 3 OR and 95% CI for the D16 allele vs. other alleles combined in overall populations and ethnic-specific analysis

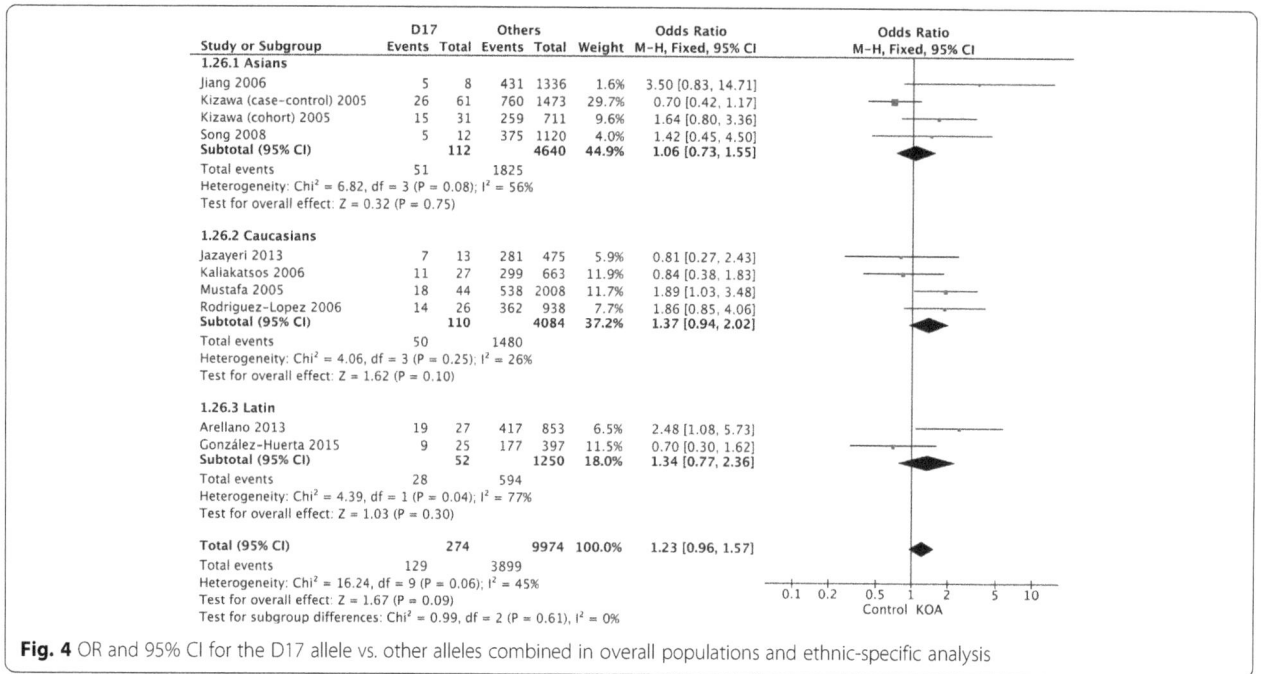

Fig. 4 OR and 95% CI for the D17 allele vs. other alleles combined in overall populations and ethnic-specific analysis

susceptibility with significant heterogeneity in overall population and subgroups mentioned above.

OA is the most common form of joint disorder, leading to physical disability in middle age around the world [4]. The pathogenesis of OA is complex and is still unclear at present, but the effects of genetic polymorphisms on OA susceptibility have attracted increasing attention [6, 7]. Some candidate genes coding for the proteins responsible for the maintenance of articular cartilage have already been reported. Among them, ASPN is an important biologically active component of ECM and a number of evidence demonstrates its role in OA pathogenesis [12]. Patients with OA have an increased expression of ASPN in contrast with healthy controls. One potential mechanism is that ASPN may suppress chondrogenesis by inhibiting TGF-β signaling pathway in the development of OA [10]. The number of D-repeats in N-terminal region of ASPN varies from 9 (D9) to 20(D20) [9]. However, the association between D-repeat polymorphism and KOA susceptibility remains controversial and needs to be further explored.

A positive association (OR = 2.49, 95% CI 1.4–4.4, $P < 0.01$) between the D14 allele and KOA susceptibility was first reported by Kizawa et al. in a cohort sample (394 cases and 374 controls) and a case–control study (137 cases and 234 controls) in Japanese population [13]. However, subsequent studies, which were carried out in different populations worldwide, showed inconsistent results. In UK cases and controls (278 cases and 748 controls), Mustafa et al. reported that ASPN D-repeat polymorphism had little effect on KOA susceptibility ($P > 0.1$) [32]. Another case–control study (188 cases

and 294 controls) in Spanish population yielded the same results ($P > 0.1$) [33]. Kaliakatsos et al. indicated that the D15 allele, but not the D14 allele, was found to be associated with increased risk of KOA (OR = 1.54, 95% CI 1.07–2.2, $P < 0.03$) in a Greek case–control study (155 cases and 190 controls) [34]. Similarly, Jazayeri et al. found that D15 allele could be considered as a risk allele only for women in the Iranian population (OR = 1.73, 95% CI 1.01–2.94, $P < 0.05$) [35]. Moreover, in Mexican Mestizo population, D16 allele was observed as a risk factor of KOA in females (OR = 2.226, 95% CI 1.064–3.151, $P < 0.03$), whereas male carriers of D17 allele were more susceptible to KOA (OR = 3.803, 95% CI 1.010–14.317, $P < 0.05$) [21]. There were a number of reasons for these confusing results. Differences in inclusion criteria might be one of them. Some studies recruited KOA patients according to symptoms or radiographic evidence [13, 21, 35–38], whereas the others according to joint replacement [32–34, 39]. Additionally, ethnic and gender differences might be another important reason as well.

Compared with the previous meta-analysis, there are three differences in the present study. First, it is the first study to investigate the association of ASPN D15, D16, and D17 alleles and KOA susceptibility. Second, our report enrolled five sex-stratified studies [32, 33, 35, 37, 39], and it is the first meta-analysis aimed at investigating the association between asporin D-repeat polymorphism and occurrence of KOA in gender-specific approach. Moreover, it included two new references, a new Iranian study [35]and a study in Mexican Mestizo population [38].

Study or Subgroup	D15 Events	Total	Other Events	Total	Weight	Odds Ratio M-H, Fixed, 95% CI
1.11.1 Female						
Jazayeri 2013	41	68	103	220	11.6%	1.72 [0.99, 3.00]
Jiang 2006	4	20	298	860	6.5%	0.47 [0.16, 1.42]
Mustafa 2005	72	235	244	865	43.6%	1.12 [0.82, 1.54]
Rodriguez-Lopez 2006	79	139	227	397	30.6%	0.99 [0.67, 1.46]
Song 2008	9	22	295	590	7.6%	0.69 [0.29, 1.64]
Subtotal (95% CI)		484		2932	100.0%	1.08 [0.87, 1.33]
Total events	205		1167			

Heterogeneity: Chi² = 6.20, df = 4 (P = 0.18); I² = 36%
Test for overall effect: Z = 0.69 (P = 0.49)

1.11.2 Male						
Jazayeri 2013	11	29	45	83	14.3%	0.52 [0.22, 1.23]
Jiang 2006	7	20	127	444	7.0%	1.34 [0.52, 3.45]
Mustafa 2005	44	170	196	782	51.2%	1.04 [0.71, 1.53]
Rodriguez-Lopez 2006	14	104	56	324	23.2%	0.74 [0.40, 1.40]
Song 2008	4	19	72	473	4.3%	1.49 [0.48, 4.60]
Subtotal (95% CI)		342		2106	100.0%	0.94 [0.71, 1.24]
Total events	80		496			

Heterogeneity: Chi² = 3.84, df = 4 (P = 0.43); I² = 0%
Test for overall effect: Z = 0.44 (P = 0.66)

Test for subgroup differences: Chi² = 0.58, df = 1 (P = 0.45), I² = 0%

Study or Subgroup	D16 Events	Total	Other Events	Total	Weight	Odds Ratio M-H, Fixed, 95% CI
1.23.1 Female						
Jazayeri 2013	16	24	128	264	6.9%	2.13 [0.88, 5.14]
Jiang 2006	11	39	291	853	17.7%	0.76 [0.37, 1.55]
Mustafa 2005	25	81	291	1019	28.7%	1.12 [0.68, 1.82]
Rodriguez-Lopez 2006	26	52	280	484	26.3%	0.73 [0.41, 1.29]
Song 2008	11	33	293	579	20.4%	0.49 [0.23, 1.02]
Subtotal (95% CI)		229		3199	100.0%	0.89 [0.67, 1.18]
Total events	89		1283			

Heterogeneity: Chi² = 7.74, df = 4 (P = 0.10); I² = 48%
Test for overall effect: Z = 0.79 (P = 0.43)

1.23.2 Male						
Jazayeri 2013	6	10	50	102	6.1%	1.56 [0.42, 5.86]
Jiang 2006	4	15	130	449	10.6%	0.89 [0.28, 2.85]
Mustafa 2005	18	86	222	866	54.3%	0.77 [0.45, 1.32]
Rodriguez-Lopez 2006	4	33	66	395	15.3%	0.69 [0.23, 2.02]
Song 2008	4	33	72	487	13.7%	0.80 [0.27, 2.33]
Subtotal (95% CI)		177		2299	100.0%	0.82 [0.56, 1.21]
Total events	36		540			

Heterogeneity: Chi² = 1.09, df = 4 (P = 0.90); I² = 0%
Test for overall effect: Z = 0.99 (P = 0.32)

Test for subgroup differences: Chi² = 0.12, df = 1 (P = 0.73), I² = 0%

Study or Subgroup	D17 Events	Total	Other Events	Total	Weight	Odds Ratio M-H, Fixed, 95% CI
1.27.1 Female						
Jazayeri 2013	5	11	139	277	23.7%	0.83 [0.25, 2.77]
Jiang 2006	3	4	299	876	2.8%	5.79 [0.60, 55.90]
Mustafa 2005	10	25	306	1075	34.2%	1.68 [0.74, 3.77]
Rodriguez-Lopez 2006	14	21	292	515	31.3%	1.53 [0.61, 3.85]
Song 2008	4	6	300	606	8.0%	2.04 [0.37, 11.22]
Subtotal (95% CI)		67		3349	100.0%	1.57 [0.95, 2.59]
Total events	36		1336			

Heterogeneity: Chi² = 2.47, df = 4 (P = 0.65); I² = 0%
Test for overall effect: Z = 1.77 (P = 0.08)

1.27.2 Male						
Jazayeri 2013	2	2	142	198	6.8%	1.98 [0.09, 41.94]
Jiang 2006	2	4	132	460	10.9%	2.48 [0.35, 17.82]
Mustafa 2005	8	19	232	933	51.3%	2.20 [0.87, 5.53]
Rodriguez-Lopez 2006	0	5	70	423	17.3%	0.46 [0.02, 8.34]
Song 2008	1	6	75	514	13.8%	1.17 [0.13, 10.16]
Subtotal (95% CI)		36		2528	100.0%	1.77 [0.87, 3.60]
Total events	13		651			

Heterogeneity: Chi² = 1.31, df = 4 (P = 0.86); I² = 0%
Test for overall effect: Z = 1.58 (P = 0.11)

Test for subgroup differences: Chi² = 0.07, df = 1 (P = 0.79), I² = 0%

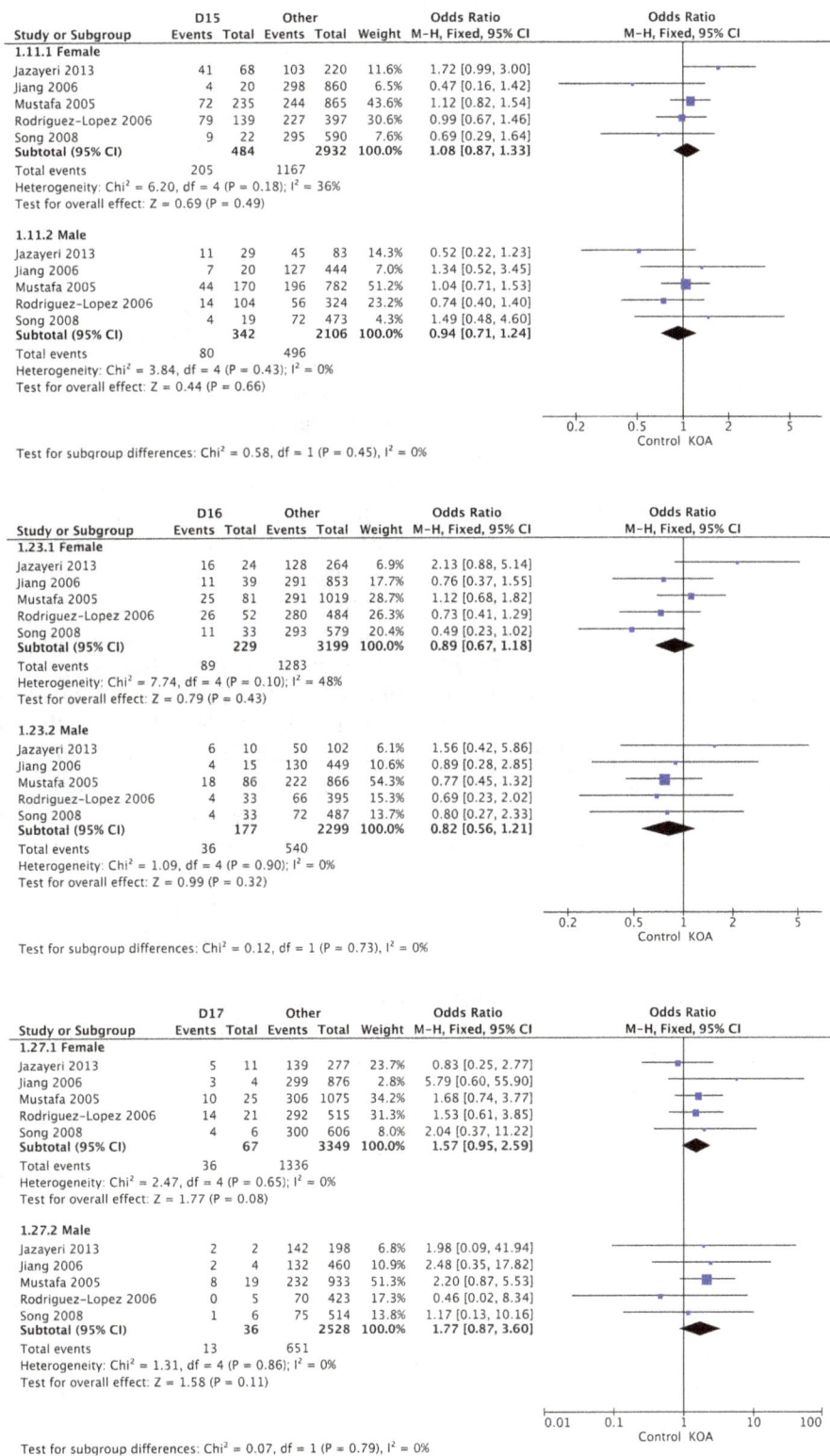

Fig. 5 OR and 95% CI for the D15, D16, and D17 alleles vs. other alleles combined in gender-specific analysis

Table 3 Sensitivity analysis of the association between D-repeat polymorphism and KOA susceptibility

Polymorphism	Population	Participants(number)		No. of studies	Test of association			Test of heterogeneity		
		Case	Control		OR	95% CI	P value	Model	P value	I^2 (%)
D17 versus others	Overall	3237	5398	9	1.43	1.09–1.89	0.01	Fixed	0.26	21
D17 versus others	Asian	1090	2128	3	1.78	1.02–3.11	0.04	Fixed	0.59	0
D16 versus others	Asian	1090	2128	3	0.70	0.50–1.00	0.05	Fixed	0.64	0

Excludes the case–control study of Kizawa et al. [13]

In the present meta-analysis, we summarized different studies mentioned above to assess heterogeneity and association between D-repeat polymorphism and KOA susceptibility. The pooling results failed to prove significant associations between the D15, D16, and D17 alleles and KOA occurrence in Caucasians, Asians, and Latin Americans, and the same results were also observed in sex-specific subgroups.

The heterogeneity between separate studies might be caused by lots of complex factors, including age, gender, quality of included studies, diagnostic criteria, inclusion criteria, racial differences, and environmental factors. In our present study, ethnic- and sex-specific subgroup analyses were performed to reduce heterogeneity. In addition, a sensitivity analysis was performed to evaluate the stability of the association between the D16 and D17 alleles and KOA susceptibility in overall and subgroups. After omitting the case–control study of Kizawa et al. [13], a positive association was observed between the D17 allele frequency and increased susceptibility to KOA with low heterogeneity. And similar result was observed in the ethnic-stratified subgroup that D17 allele was a risk factor of KOA in Asians. These opposite results indicated that the pooling results may include a type II error, or false negative, and were lacking enough stability to come to the firm conclusion on association between the D17 allele and KOA susceptibility in overall and Asians group. However, due to the small sample size of D17 allele, this result should be considered with caution.

Several previous studies had demonstrated the gender differences for patients in allele frequencies [34–36, 39]. Although more sex-stratified studies were required because original data of each research cannot be acquired, our study was the first meta-analysis stratified by both gender and ethnicity. The present meta-analysis of the asporin gene D-repeat may not describe a significant difference in sex-specific subgroups, but they reduced the heterogeneity to a certain extent. Nevertheless, the heterogeneity of our study could not be appropriately solved, and some underlying reasons might account for the current predicament.

For instance, different inclusion criteria could be an essential factor for heterogeneity. The included studies were four studies recruiting patients undergone total knee arthroplasty (TKA) [32–34, 39], and six studies enrolled participants by assessing clinical and radiologic evaluation [13, 21, 35–38]. Consequently, the current meta-analysis may include patients with various pathological and radiographic grades. Moreover, the existence of heterogeneity might also be explained by genotype–environment interaction that reflecting different genes respond to environmental variations in different ways.

The limitations of the present meta-analysis were briefly discussed in the following section. First, despite the subgroup analyses performed by ethnicity and gender, the existence of heterogeneity could not be totally resolved. We were failed to apply more types of subgroup analysis stratified by personal conditions or clinical variables because lack of enough original data from included studies. Therefore, the result of our meta-analysis should be interpreted with caution. Second, the environmental and genetic factors remained unclear in the present study. Both of them were responsible for the heterogeneity as well. Third, insufficient including studies with enough raw data, particularly in ethnic- and gender-stratified analyses, influenced the statistical efficacy and caused the high heterogeneity. It is also the reason why meta-regression analysis cannot be performed and was failed to detect the cause of heterogeneity. To settle the problems mentioned above, further studies with more different ethnic populations, unified inclusion criteria, functional research of ASPN D-repeat, sufficient raw data, and environmental and genetic interaction are clearly needed.

Conclusion

In conclusion, we carried out a meta-analysis of the association between D-repeat polymorphism of ASPN and susceptibility to KOA in Asian, Caucasian, and Latin American populations. Overall, we found no significant relationship between KOA susceptibility and the D15, D16, or D17 alleles. However, results with significant heterogeneity lacked sufficient stability to provide an accurate conclusion on this study. Further studies are required to investigate the role of ASPN; these findings may help to elucidate the pathogenesis of OA and may inform the development of novel therapeutic strategies for OA.

Abbreviations

ACL: Anterior cruciate ligament; ASPN: Asporin gene; CI: Confidence interval; ECM: Extracellular matrix; KOA: Knee osteoarthritis; OA: Osteoarthritis; OR: Odds ratio; SLRPs: Small leucin-rich proteoglycans; TGF: Transforming growth factor; TKA: Total knee arthroplasty

Acknowledgements

Not applicable.

Funding

This study was supported by the National Natural Science Foundation of China (8157090664, 21134004), National Basic Research Program of China (973 Program, 2014CB542201, 2012CB518106), National High Technology Research and Development Program of China (863 Program, 2015AA020303), and National Science and Technology Major Project of China (2016YFC1102104).

Authors' contributions

RL and XY carried out the molecular genetic studies, participated in the sequence alignment, and drafted the manuscript. JY revised the manuscript. QQ, HM, and CW carried out the immunoassays. AW and QG participated in the sequence alignment. JP participated in the design of the study and performed the statistical analysis. SL conceived of the study, participated in its design and coordination, and helped to draft the manuscript. All authors read and approved the final manuscript.

Competing interests

The authors declare that they have no competing interests.

Author details

[1]Institute of Orthopedics, Beijing Key Laboratory of Regenerative Medicine in Orthopedics, Key Laboratory of Musculoskeletal Trauma & War Injuries PLA, Chinese PLA General Hospital, FuXing Road 28th, Beijing 100853, China. [2]Department of Kampo Medicine, Yokohama University of Pharmacy, 601 Matano-cho, Totsuka-ku, Yokohama-shi, Kanagawa-ken 245-0066, Japan.

References

1. Haq SA, Davatchi F. Osteoarthritis of the knees in the COPCORD world. Int J Rheum Dis. 2011;14(2):122–9.
2. Woolf AD, Pfleger B. Burden of major musculoskeletal conditions. Bull World Health Organ. 2003;81(9):646–56.
3. Glyn-Jones S, Palmer AJ, Agricola R, Price AJ, Vincent TL, Weinans H, et al. Osteoarthritis Lancet. 2015;386(9991):376–87.
4. Felson DT, Anderson JJ, Naimark A, Kannel W, Meenan RF. The prevalence of chondrocalcinosis in the elderly and its association with knee osteoarthritis: the Framingham study. J Rheumatol. 1989;16(9):1241–5.
5. Jevsevar DS. Treatment of osteoarthritis of the knee: evidence-based guideline, 2nd edition. J Am Acad Orthop Surg. 2013;21(9):571–6.
6. Loughlin J. Genetic contribution to osteoarthritis development: current state of evidence. Curr Opin Rheumatol. 2015;27(3):284–8.
7. Reynard LN, Loughlin J. Insights from human genetic studies into the pathways involved in osteoarthritis. Nat Rev Rheumatol. 2013;9(10):573–83.
8. Goldring MB, Goldring SR. Articular cartilage and subchondral bone in the pathogenesis of osteoarthritis. Ann N Y Acad Sci. 2010;1192:230–7.
9. Lorenzo P, Aspberg A, Onnerfjord P, Bayliss MT, Neame PJ, Heinegard D. Identification and characterization of asporin. a novel member of the leucine-rich repeat protein family closely related to decorin and biglycan. J Biol Chem. 2001;276(15):12201–11.
10. Nakajima M, Kizawa H, Saitoh M, Kou I, Miyazono K, Ikegawa S. Mechanisms for asporin function and regulation in articular cartilage. J Biol Chem. 2007; 282(44):32185–92.
11. Henry SP, Takanosu M, Boyd TC, Mayne PM, Eberspaecher H, Zhou W, et al. Expression pattern and gene characterization of asporin. a newly discovered member of the leucine-rich repeat protein family. J Biol Chem. 2001;276(15): 12212–21.
12. Ikegawa S. Expression, regulation and function of asporin, a susceptibility gene in common bone and joint diseases. Curr Med Chem. 2008;15(7): 724–8.
13. Kizawa H, Kou I, Iida A, Sudo A, Miyamoto Y, Fukuda A, et al. An aspartic acid repeat polymorphism in asporin inhibits chondrogenesis and increases susceptibility to osteoarthritis. Nat Genet. 2005;37(2):138–44.
14. Nakamura T, Shi D, Tzetis M, Rodriguez-Lopez J, Miyamoto Y, Tsezou A, et al. Meta-analysis of association between the ASPN D-repeat and osteoarthritis. Hum Mol Genet. 2007;16(14):1676–81.
15. Xing D, Ma XL, Ma JX, Xu WG, Wang J, Yang Y, et al. Association between aspartic acid repeat polymorphism of the asporin gene and susceptibility to knee osteoarthritis: a genetic meta-analysis. Osteoarthr Cartil. 2013;21(11): 1700–6.
16. Song GG, Kim JH, Lee YH. A meta-analysis of the relationship between aspartic acid (D)-repeat polymorphisms in asporin and osteoarthritis susceptibility. Rheumatol Int. 2014;34(6):785–92.
17. Srikanth VK, Fryer JL, Zhai G, Winzenberg TM, Hosmer D, Jones G. A meta-analysis of sex differences prevalence, incidence and severity of osteoarthritis. Osteoarthr Cartil. 2005;13(9):769–81.
18. Agel J, Arendt EA, Bershadsky B. Anterior cruciate ligament injury in national collegiate athletic association basketball and soccer: a 13-year review. Am J Sports Med. 2005;33(4):524–30.
19. Bien DP. Rationale and implementation of anterior cruciate ligament injury prevention warm-up programs in female athletes. J Strength Cond Res. 2011;25(1):271–85.
20. Hibberd EE, Kerr ZY, Roos KG, Djoko A, Dompier TP. Epidemiology of acromioclavicular joint sprains in 25 National Collegiate Athletic Association Sports: 2009-2010 to 2014-2015 academic years. Am J Sports Med. 2016; 44(10):2667–74.
21. Arellano RD, Hernandez F, Garcia-Sepulveda CA, Velasco VM, Loera CR, Arguello JR. The D-repeat polymorphism in the ASPN gene and primary knee osteoarthritis in a Mexican mestizo population: a case-control study. J Orthop Sci. 2013;18(5):826–31.
22. Zhang W, Nuki G, Moskowitz RW, Abramson S, Altman RD, Arden NK, et al. OARSI recommendations for the management of hip and knee osteoarthritis: part III: changes in evidence following systematic cumulative update of research published through January 2009. Osteoarthr Cartil. 2010; 18(4):476–99.
23. Jordan JM, Helmick CG, Renner JB, Luta G, Dragomir AD, Woodard J, et al. Prevalence of knee symptoms and radiographic and symptomatic knee osteoarthritis in African Americans and Caucasians: the Johnston County Osteoarthritis Project. J Rheumatol. 2007;34(1):172–80.
24. Dillon CF, Rasch EK, Gu Q, Hirsch R. Prevalence of knee osteoarthritis in the United States: arthritis data from the Third National Health and Nutrition Examination Survey 1991-94. J Rheumatol. 2006;33(11):2271–9.
25. Zhang Y, McAlindon TE, Hannan MT, Chaisson CE, Klein R, Wilson PW, et al. Estrogen replacement therapy and worsening of radiographic knee osteoarthritis: the Framingham study. Arthritis Rheum. 1998;41(10):1867–73.
26. Higgins JP, Thompson SG. Quantifying heterogeneity in a meta-analysis. Stat Med. 2002;21(11):1539–58.
27. Laird NM, Mosteller F. Some statistical methods for combining experimental results. Int J Technol Assess Health Care. 1990;6(1):5–30.
28. Mantel N, Haenszel W. Statistical aspects of the analysis of data from retrospective studies of disease. J Natl Cancer Inst. 1959;22(4):719–48.
29. DerSimonian R, Laird N. Meta-analysis in clinical trials. Control Clin Trials. 1986;7(3):177–88.
30. Egger M, Smith GD, Phillips AN. Meta-analysis: principles and procedures. BMJ. 1997;315(7121):1533–7.
31. Egger M, Davey Smith G, Schneider M, Minder C. Bias in meta-analysis detected by a simple, graphical test. BMJ. 1997;315(7109):629–34.
32. Mustafa Z, Dowling B, Chapman K, Sinsheimer JS, Carr A, Loughlin J. Investigating the aspartic acid (D) repeat of asporin as a risk factor for osteoarthritis in a UK Caucasian population. Arthritis Rheum. 2005;52(11): 3502–6.
33. Rodriguez-Lopez J, Pombo-Suarez M, Liz M, Gomez-Reino JJ, Gonzalez A. Lack of association of a variable number of aspartic acid residues in the asporin gene with osteoarthritis susceptibility: case-control studies in Spanish Caucasians. Arthritis Res Ther. 2006;8(3):R55.
34. Kaliakatsos M, Tzetis M, Kanavakis E, Fytili P, Chouliaras G, Karachalios T, et al. Asporin and knee osteoarthritis in patients of Greek origin. Osteoarthr Cartil. 2006;14(6):609–11.

35. Jazayeri R, Qoreishi M, Hoseinzadeh HR, Babanejad M, Bakhshi E, Najmabadi H, et al. Investigation of the asporin gene polymorphism as a risk factor for knee osteoarthritis in Iran. Am J Orthop (Belle Mead NJ). 2013;42(7):313–6.

36. Atif U, Philip A, Aponte J, Woldu EM, Brady S, Kraus VB, et al. Absence of association of asporin polymorphisms and osteoarthritis susceptibility in US Caucasians. Osteoarthr Cartil. 2008;16(10):1174–7.

37. Jiang Q, Shi D, Yi L, Ikegawa S, Wang Y, Nakamura T, et al. Replication of the association of the aspartic acid repeat polymorphism in the asporin gene with knee-osteoarthritis susceptibility in Han Chinese. J Hum Genet. 2006; 51(12):1068–72.

38. Gonzalez-Huerta NC, Borgonio-Cuadra VM, Zenteno JC, Cortes-Gonzalez S, Duarte-Salazar C, Miranda-Duarte A. D14 repeat polymorphism of the asporin gene is associated with primary osteoarthritis of the knee in a Mexican Mestizo population. Int J Rheum Dis. 2015;

39. Song JH, Lee HS, Kim CJ, Cho YG, Park YG, Nam SW, et al. Aspartic acid repeat polymorphism of the asporin gene with susceptibility to osteoarthritis of the knee in a Korean population. Knee. 2008;15(3):191–5.

15

A posterior versus anterior debridement in combination with bone graft and internal fixation for lumbar and thoracic tuberculosis

Yu Huang[1†], Jin Lin[2†], Xuanwei Chen[1*], Jianhua Lin[1], Yulan Lin[3] and Hongjie Zhang[1]

Abstract

Background: Surgery treatment is usually required for spinal tuberculosis. The aim of this study was to compare the clinical efficacy and outcomes of anterior and posterior surgical approach in combination with debridement, bone grafting, and internal fixation.

Methods: All patients with thoracic and lumbar tuberculosis who underwent either the anterior or posterior surgery in combination with debridement, bone grafting, and internal fixation from August 2009 to August 2016 were reviewed retrospectively.

Results: A total of 186 patients were recruited in the analyses, 37 of whom received the anterior approach and 149 treated with the posterior approach. In the entire study population, there was no statistically significant difference between the groups in terms of kyphosis Cobb's angle, VAS pain score, neurological status, operation duration, perioperative blood loss, and hospitalization days ($p > 0.05$). Good clinical outcomes were achieved in both treatment groups. In lumbar vertebra-affected patients, the average preoperative kyphosis Cobb's angle was 8. 7 ± 16.6° and − 5.6 ± 16.0° for the anterior and posterior groups, respectively, which were corrected to − 3.3 ± 13. 2° and − 10.1 ± 13.8° after surgery. For thoracic vertebra-affected patients, the corrected kyphosis Cobb's angle was 8.1 ± 9.7° and 10.3 ± 6.5°, respectively. After surgery, 32.4% of patients in the anterior group and 48.3% of patients in the posterior group claimed no pain ($p = 0.24$), while 83.8 and 85.9% recovered to Frankel grade E, respectively ($p = 0.85$).

Conclusions: The posterior debridement joint bone graft and internal fixation is an alternative procedure to treat lumbar and thoracic tuberculosis compared to the traditional anterior approach with similar clinical efficacy in terms of pain control, Cobb's angle, and neurological function. The posterior approach is sufficient for lesion debridement.

Keywords: Spinal tuberculosis, Anterior, Posterior, Debridement, Surgery

Background

According to the World Health Organization's Global tuberculosis report 2015, tuberculosis now ranks alongside HIV as a leading cause of death worldwide with 1.4 million deaths in 2014 [1]. Spinal tuberculosis is the most common encountered extrapulmonary form of the disease and accounts for around 50% of musculoskeletal tuberculosis cases [2]. Thoracic spine is the most commonly affected, and involvement of lumbar and lumbosacral region is less common [3, 4]. Spinal tuberculosis can cause severe neurological deficits, kyphotic deformities, and paraplegia. The effective antitubercular therapy has allowed disease cure in majority of patients with conservative management alone [5]. However, surgery is indicated in patients having disabling back pain or progressive neurological deficit despite conservative management [5].The aims of such treatment are to eradicate

---

* Correspondence: amy801231@163.com

†Equal contributors

¹Department of Spinal Surgery, The First Affiliated Hospital of Fujian Medical University, Fuzhou, Fujian 350005, China

Full list of author information is available at the end of the article

the tuberculosis lesion, relieve spinal nerve compression, reconstruct spinal stability, and correct spinal deformity. Surgical treatment options are available including anterior spinal fusion, anterior-posterior spinal fusion, posterior spinal fusion alone, and posterior fusion followed by anterior spinal fusion [6–8]. Anterior debridement joint interbody fusion and internal fixation is being widely used in the clinical setting for the treatment of spinal tuberculosis, particularly for spinal destruction in the anterior and middle columns [5]. However, this method is time-consuming, causes high volume of blood loss, and results in the spread of infection and other postoperative complications [9–11]. On the other hand, posterior approach has recently been suggested as an alternative to the anterior approach because it is less invasive, allows circumferential cord decompression, can be extended proximally and distally from the involved segment, and provides a stronger three column fixation through uninvolved posterior elements via pedicle screws [12–14].

There are however only few studies available comparing the clinical efficacy and outcome between the anterior and posterior approaches, and the results are still controversial [15, 16]. In the prospective study, the posterior approach performed better than the anterior approach in terms of incision length, operative time, blood loss, and correction of kyphosis Cobb's angle [16]. Whereas, in the respective study, no statistically significant differences were found on the clinical efficacies between the different approaches [15]. Hence, we carried out this paper to investigate and compare the clinical efficacy and feasibility of surgical methods such as posterior debridement joint bone fixation therapy and anterior debridement joint bone fixation therapy for the treatment of spinal tuberculosis with compression fracture in order to provide new evidence for clinical treatment using these therapies.

Methods
Study patients
All patients of spinal tuberculosis with lumbar or thoracic compression fracture were respectively selected from The First Affiliated Hospital of Fujian Medical University between August 2009 and August 2016. We recruited those patients who received debridement, bone graft, and internal fixation via anterior or posterior approach. The diagnosis of thoracic and lumbar tuberculosis was based on clinical symptom including fatigue, night sweats, low-grade fever, weight loss, dorsal spine pain, paraparesis, and gibbus, in combination with imaging result of MRC and CT. All patients received standard laboratory tests, Mantoux tuberculin skin test, and MRC and CT in order to exclude those with active tuberculosis. Patients were treated with chemotherapy regimen 4–6 weeks prior to surgery, which consisted of

isoniazid (300 mg/day), rifampicin (450 mg/day), ethambutol (750 mg/day), and pyrazinamide (750 mg/day). The surgery indications included the presence of neurological deficits, spinal deformities, epidural abscesses compressing the dural sac, large paravertebral abscesses, radicular or dural compression caused by granulation tissue and abscesses, sequestrum or disc fragments resulting in neurological deficits or severe pain, and nondiagnostic biopsy specimen. All patients were as much as possible managed to have hemoglobin ≥ 100 g/l, erythrocyte sedimentation rate (ESR) < 40 mm/l before entering the surgery. No patient consent was obtained as this is a retrospective study based on clinical records.

Operative procedures
For the posterior approach, patients were positioned in the prone position after general anesthesia. A vertical incision was made over the spinous process and the bilateral facet joints; outer parts of the lamina were exposed. Afterward, the tissues were peeled off layer by layer to expose the vertebral till vision included a vertebra and the upper and lower vertebrae. A unilateral facetectomy and pediculectomy or bilateral facetectomy and pediculectomy were performed with debridement of the affected vertebral body, infected tissue, pus, granulation tissue, sequestrum, and disc necrotic tissue using curettes. We performed debridement of the vertebral body and disc space through one or both pedicles according to the range of lesion. The affected spinal segments were stabilized using a transpedicular screw and rod system. When the screws could not be placed into the affected vertebra bilaterally, or when thoracolumbar junction involvement was present, two vertebrae above and one vertebra below the involved vertebra were incorporated into the instrumentation system to correct the kyphosis. Finally, an intervertebral bone autograft or a titanium cage with a cancellous bone from the iliac crest was used. Streptomycin (2–3 g) was sprayed onto the operation site, and a local drainage tube was inserted before the incision was closed.

The anterior approach combined with debridement, bone autografting, and instrumentation was performed in patients, as described by Hodgson et al. [17]. After anesthesia, left or right lateral position was chosen according to the position of the vertebral body. An incision was made in the thoracoabdominal region along the lower edge of the 12th rib. Then, the tissues were peeled off layer by layer to expose the vertebra till vision included a vertebra and the upper and lower vertebrae. Then, the intervertebral nutrient vessels were amputated to expose vertebral lesions. Curette was used to debride the lesion and liposuction, abscess drainage, and scrap of sclerotic bone lesions around Banda healthy bone which were all performed until there was no infectious debris or pus. With C-arm X-ray, the lesion adjacent of the normal vertebrae was inserted with pedicle screws. Then, a temporary fixation rod was placed on the lighter side of the lesion to evade spinal cord injury during decompression, and the kyphosis was slowly corrected. After this, according to the intervertebral height and angle, suitable titanium mesh filled with autologous bone was selected and inserted into the bone to stabilize the vertebral height and lock nail plate (rod) system. Streptomycin 1.0 g and isoniazid 0.2 g were administered locally, and a drainage tube was placed before incisions were sutured.

Postoperative care

After close postoperative observation of changes in patients, anti-inflammatory and antitubercular drugs (for 12 to 18 months) were provided to maintain airway patency. Blood pressure, respiration, pulse, drainage volume of incision, sense, and motor response of the lower extremities were monitored after surgery. All patients received antituberculosis chemotherapy for at least 12 months. The drainage tube was removed when the drainage volume < 50 ml/day. The patients were encouraged to stand up with a bracing apparatus 2 weeks after surgery until 3 months.

Clinical measurements

The sagittal profile was measured by Cobb's method as the angle between the upper end plate and the lower end plate of the infected level (Fig. 1). The neurological function was evaluated according to the Frankel grading system: grades A–E [18]. Ten-point visual analog scale (VAS) was used to evaluate back pain. Surgery time (minutes), blood loss during surgery (ml), in-patient hospitalization days, and number of fused segment were also recorded. After surgery, patients were followed up for up to 1 year to retrieve their updates in VAS score, Frankel scale, and vital status.

Statistical analysis

T test was used to compare the kyphosis Cobb's angle, VAS score, surgery time, blood loss during surgery, and in-patient hospitalization days. Fisher's test and χ^2 test were used to compare the Frankel grades and comorbidity. Analysis of clinical outcome comparisons was also stratified based on tuberculosis duration (< 6 months or ≥ 6 months) and affected vertebral (lumbar or thoracic). Two-sided $p < 0.05$ was regarded as having statistical significance. The SAS Statistical Package (version 9.3, SAS Institute, Gary, NC) was used for all analyses.

Results

Baseline

There were 37 patients treated with the anterior approach and 149 patients with the posterior approach

(Table 1). The sex distribution was similar between the two approaches ($t = 0.61$, $p = 0.44$) with 20 males (54.1%) and 17 females (45.9%) in the anterior approach and 91 (61.1%) males and 58 females (38.9%) in the posterior approach. The overall average tuberculosis duration was 12.0 ± 18.4 months, with mean age of 50.0 ± 17.9 years in the entire study population. Patients in the two groups had similar age, duration of disease, and drug treatment duration after surgery ($p < 0.05$). The affected vertebrae were both nearly half lumbar (Fig. 2) and half thoracic (Fig. 3) in the two treatment groups. Patients in the anterior group (19.4 ± 7.7 days) received more days of postoperative chemotherapy than the posterior group (15.8 ± 6.7 days), with statistical significance ($t = 2.69$, $p = 0.01$). No statistically significant differences were observed for preoperative chemotherapy treatment ($t = -1.33$, $p = 0.19$).

Clinical efficacy comparison

Before surgery, the kyphosis Cobb's angle was found to be different between the anterior (12.2 ± 16.2°) and posterior (4.6 ± 17.6°) debridement groups ($t = 2.52$, p = 0.01) (Table 2). After surgery, Cobb's angle was corrected to 2.3 ± 12.9° in the anterior group and 0.2 ± 14.8° in the posterior group, respectively. No statistically significant differences were however found ($t = 0.83$, $p = 0.41$). Patients in the anterior group had higher VAS pain score (4.5 ± 1.3) before surgery than those in the posterior group (3.7 ± 1.2) ($t = 3.97$, $p = 0.0001$). After surgery, patients had the similar pain scores ($p = 0.42$). During the follow-up period, majority of patients had no pain. Most of the patients were graded with Frankel grade E (64.9 and 51.7% in the anterior and posterior groups, respectively) before surgery, which was improved to 83.8 and 85.9% after surgery. During follow-up, more than 90% of patients reported their neurological function in Frankel grade E. The average surgery times were similar in the posterior group (224.0 ± 84.0 min) than in the anterior group (212.8 ± 72.2 min) ($p = 0.42$). And the blood loss during surgery was also similar in the posterior group (748.7 ± 727.5 ml) and the anterior group (723.2 ± 544.8) ($p = 0.84$). The average number of fused segment was 2.22 ± 0.48 in the anterior group and 2.24 ± 0.66 in the posterior group ($p = 0.84$). However, no statistically significant differences were found for these clinical outcome measurements ($p > 0.05$). When analysis was stratified based on tuberculosis duration (< 6 months, ≥ 6 months), no differences of Cobb's angle were found ($p > 0.05$) (Table 3). No statistically significant differences were found for postoperative VAS pain score, Frankel grading, surgery time, blood loss volume during surgery, and comorbidity between different surgery approaches ($p > 0.05$).

Among patients with the lumbar vertebra affected, those who received anterior surgery had different Cobb's

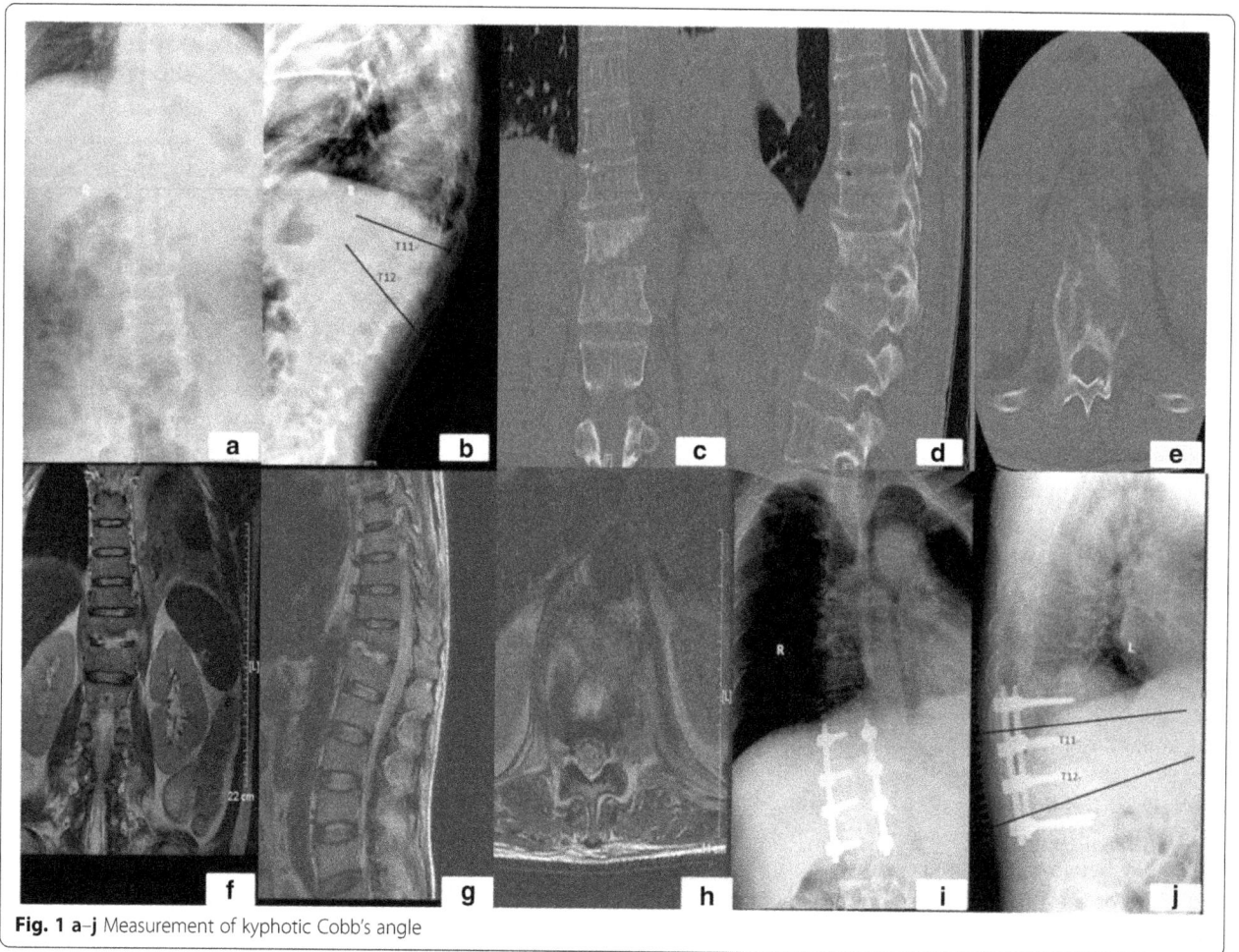

Fig. 1 a–j Measurement of kyphotic Cobb's angle

angle both before and after surgery, in comparison with those who received posterior surgery ($p < 0.05$) (Table 4). Anterior surgery has corrected Cobb's angle from an average $8.7 \pm 16.6°$ to $-3.3 \pm 13.2°$ (difference $-11.9 \pm 17.0°$, data not shown), in contrast to a corrected angle from $-5.6 \pm 16.0°$ to $-10.1 \pm 13.8°$ (difference $-4.5 \pm 16.3°$, data not shown) by posterior treatment. The corrected angles were not significant between the two surgeries ($p = 0.07$, data not shown). Patients under anterior surgery had more serious pain, no matter with the lumbar or thoracic vertebra affected before surgery treatment ($p < 0.05$). After surgery treatment, no pain differences were observed. In groups of the lumbar vertebra affected, patients receiving anterior surgery had better preoperative neurological function compared to those who received posterior surgery ($p = 0.01$). Among lumber vertebra-affected patients who received anterior surgery, 3 (15.8%) had Frankel grade D and 16 (84.2%) had grade E. In comparison, among those lumber vertebra-affected patients receiving posterior surgery, 1 was graded as C (1.4%), 36 were D (49.3%), and 36 were E (49.3%). However, no significant differences were observed for postoperative neurological

function ($p = 0.58$). In the lumber vertebra-affected group, the blood loss volume was higher in the posterior group (732.3 ± 846.7 ml) compared to the anterior group (671.6 ± 458.9 ml). Meanwhile, in the thoracic vertebra-affected group, longer surgery time was taken for the posterior approach (236.0 ± 90.0 min) compared to the anterior approach (200.1 ± 73.4 min). However, none of these differences were statistically significant ($p > 0.05$). The prevalence of comorbidity was 31.6% for lumbar vertebra-affected patients receiving anterior surgery, while only 19.2% in the posterior group suffered from comorbidity after surgery ($p = 0.35$).

Discussion

Our study indicates that both anterior or posterior debridement joint bone graft and internal fixation could achieve similar favorable clinical efficacy regarding pain, Cobb's angle, and neurological function. No statistically significant differences were found for surgery duration, perioperative blood loss, comorbidity, and hospitalization days.

The diagnosis of spinal tuberculosis is difficult and it commonly presents at an advanced stage, which lead to

Table 1 Baseline characteristics of the 186 spinal tuberculosis patients receiving anterior or posterior debridement joint bone graft and internal fixation

	Total	Anterior	Posterior	p value[a]
No. of individuals	186	37	149	
Sex				
Male	111 (59.7%)	20 (54.1%)	91 (61.1%)	0.44
Female	75 (40.3%)	17 (45.9%)	58 (38.9%)	
Age (years)	50.0 ± 17.9	46.6 ± 17.3	50.9 ± 18.0	0.19
Duration of disease (months)	12.0 ± 18.4	13.2 ± 21.6	11.7 ± 17.6	0.70
Vertebra affected				0.80
Lumbar	92 (49.5%)	19 (51.4%)	73 (49%)	
Thoracic	94 (50.5%)	18 (48.6%)	76 (51%)	
Chemotherapy duration (days)				
Preoperative	14.0 ± 10.9	11.9 ± 7.7	14.5 ± 11.5	0.19
Postoperative	16.5 ± 7.5	19.4 ± 9.7	15.8 ± 6.7	0.01
Vital status				
Dead	2 (1.1%)	1 (2.7%)	1 (0.7%)	0.47
Alive	117 (62.9%)	22 (59.5%)	95 (63.8%)	
Unknown	67 (36.0%)	14 (37.8%)	53 (35.5%)	

[a]*T* test used to compare continuous variables; chi-square and Fisher's tests used to compare the categorical variables

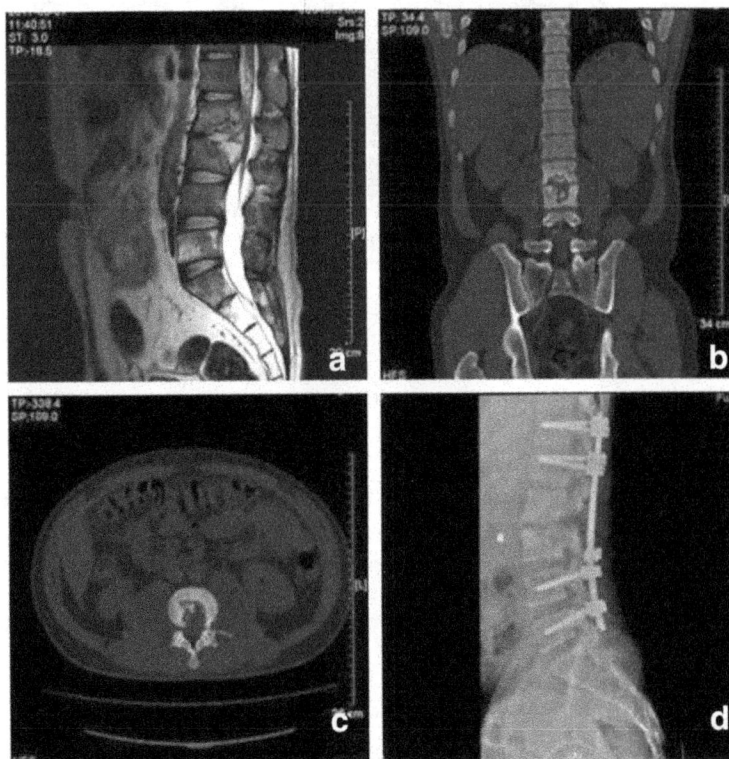

Fig. 2 A 30-year-old male patient presented with lumbar kyphosis due to destructive tubercular spondylodiscitis at L2–3 with a paravertebral abscess (**a–c**). After posterior debridement, this defect after the sagittal profile reconstruction and posterior instrumentation was bridged using an autologous iliac bone grafting (**d**)

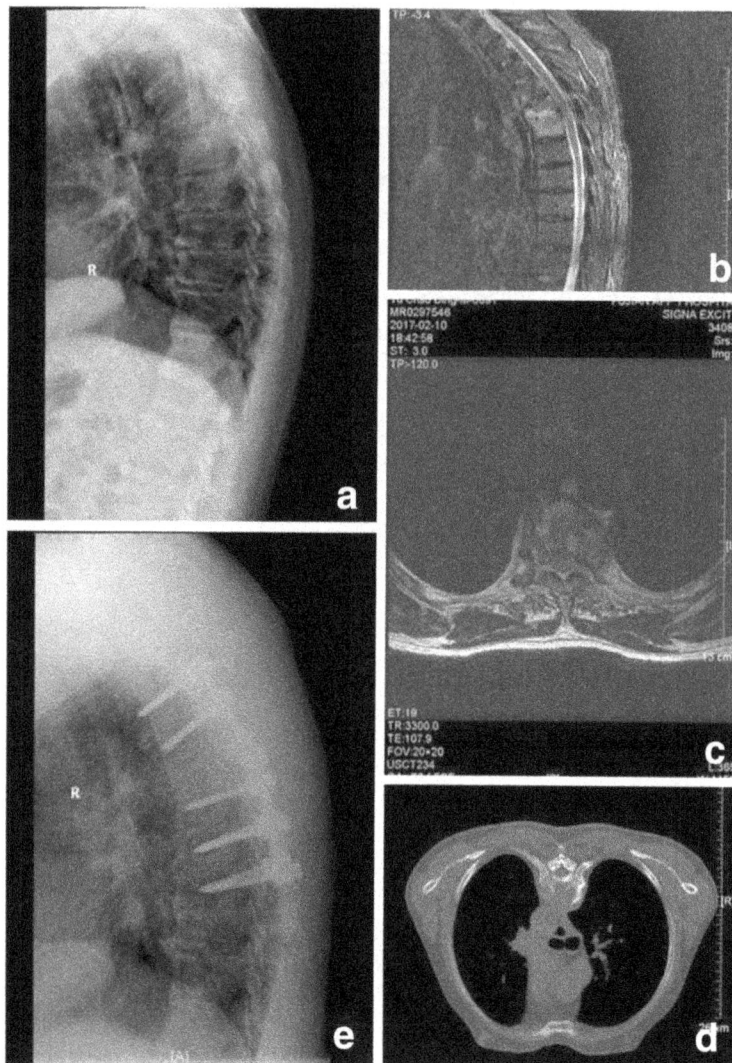

Fig. 3 A 69-year-old male patient presented with thoracic kyphosis due to destructive tubercular spondylodiscitis at T5–6 with a paravertebral abscess (**a**–**d**). After posterior debridement, this defect after the sagittal profile reconstruction and posterior instrumentation was bridged using an autologous iliac bone grafting (**e**)

higher rates of complications such as spinal cord compression and spinal deformity.

Since the 1960s, when Stock and Hodgson suggested spinal tuberculosis patients be treated with removal of lesion and an anterior interbody fusion surgical treatment, the anterior approach has been widely regarded as the gold standard [17]. An anterior approach allows for direct access to the lesion, adequate visualization of the lesion, and complete decompression of the spinal cord [19]. Since the introduction of the anterior approach, majority of surgeons favor it due to the concern over the safety of the posterior approach [20, 21]. However, this method is time-consuming, needs constant changing of surgery position, causes trauma to tissues such as the pleura and peritoneum, and results in the spread of infection and other postoperative complications [9].

Infection usually occurs more frequently in the anterior surgery compared to the posterior approach, mainly due to the deeper surgical approach, and is more likely to damage the blood vessels. In fact, in the current study, infection rates were 16.2% (6 out of 37 patients) for anterior surgery and 17.5% (26 out of 149 patients) for posterior surgery, respectively (data not shown). Furthermore, anterior decompression might be too drastic for elderly patients and children [16]. In recent years, one-stage posterior debridement combined with bone graft and internal fixation is more frequently applied in the clinic due to its advantages, such as lesser trauma, single incision, excision of lesions successfully completed in a period, bone implant and reconstruction of spinal stability, no need of changing the patient's position, easy examination of spinal fractures with fewer complications

Table 2 Clinical outcome of spinal tuberculosis patients using anterior or posterior debridement joint bone graft and internal fixation

	Total	Anterior	Posterior	p value[a]
Cobb's angle				
Preoperative	6.1 ± 17.5	12.2 ± 16.2	4.6 ± 17.6	0.01
Postoperative	0.6 ± 14.5	2.3 ± 12.9	0.2 ± 14.8	0.41
VAS score				
Preoperative				0.0003
0	1 (0.5%)	0	1 (0.7%)	
2	9 (4.8%)	0	9 (6.0%)	
3	93 (50.0%)	12 (3.4%)	81 (54.4%)	
4	16 (8.6%)	2 (5.4%)	14 (9.4%)	
5	53 (28.5%)	17 (46.0%)	36 (24.2%)	
6	8 (4.3%)	3 (8.1%)	5 (3.4%)	
7	6 (3.2%)	3 (8.1%)	3 (2.0%)	
Mean	3.8 ± 1.2	4.5 ± 1.3	3.7 ± 1.2	0.0001
Postoperative				0.24
0	84 (45.2%)	12 (32.4%)	72 (48.3%)	
1	76 (40.9%)	21 (56.8%)	55 (36.9%)	
2	25 (13.4%)	4 (10.8%)	21 (14.1%)	
3	0	0	0	
4	0	0	0	
5	1 (0.5%)	0	1 (0.7%)	
Mean	0.7 ± 0.8	0.8 ± 0.6	0.7 ± 0.8	0.42
Frankel score				
Preoperative				0.75
A	3 (1.6%)	0	3 (2.0%)	
B	7 (3.8%)	1(2.7%)	6 (4.0%)	
C	9 (4.8%)	2 (5.4%)	7 (4.7%)	
D	65 (35.0%)	10 (27.0%)	55 (36.9%)	
E	101 (54.3%)	24 (64.9%)	77 (51.7%)	
Postoperative				0.85
A	0	0	0	
B	1 (0.5%)	0	1 (0.7%)	
C	4 (2.2%)	1 (2.7%)	3 (2.0%)	
D	22 (11.8%)	5 (13.5%)	17 (11.4%)	
E	159 (85.5%)	31 (83.8%)	128 (85.9%)	
Surgery duration (minutes)	221.8 ± 81.8	212.8 ± 72.2	224.0 ± 84.0	0.42
Perioperative blood loss (ml)	743.7 ± 693.7	723.2 ± 544.8	748.7 ± 727.5	0.84
Comorbidity				
Yes	45 (24.2%)	11 (29.7%)	34 (22.8%)	0.38
No	141 (75.8%)	26 (70.3%)	115 (77.2%)	
Hospitalization (days)	20.5 ± 29.0	19.8 ± 8.2	20.7 ± 32.1	0.87
Fused segment	2.23 ± 0.62	2.22 ± 0.48	2.24 ± 0.66	0.84

[a]T test used to compare continuous variables; chi-square and Fisher's tests used to compare the categorical variables

Table 3 Clinical outcome of spinal tuberculosis patients using anterior or posterior debridement joint bone graft and internal fixation by stratification of disease duration

| | Tuberculosis duration | | | | | |
| | < 6 months | | | | ≥ 6 months | |
	Anterior	Posterior	p value[a]	Anterior	Posterior	p value[a]
No. of individuals	20	11		17	78	
Cobb's angle						
Preoperative	10.1 ± 11.4	4.1 ± 16.2	0.07	14.7 ± 20.5	5.1 ± 18.8	0.09
Postoperative	− 0.9 ± 12.4	− 0.4 ± 15.1	0.90	6.0 ± 12.8	0.8 ± 14.6	0.20
VAS score						
Preoperative	4.4 ± 1.2	3.4 ± 1.0	0.002	4.8 ± 1.3	4.0 ± 1.2	0.04
Postoperative	0.7 ± 0.6	0.6 ± 0.8	0.40	0.9 ± 0.6	0.8 ± 0.8	0.61
Follow-up	0.4 ± 0.5	0.2 ± 0.4	0.43	NA	0.2 ± 0.4	0.20
Frankel score						
Preoperative			0.51			0.96
A	0	2 (2.8%)		0	1 (1.3%)	
B	1 (5.0%)	3 (4.2%)		0	1 (1.3%)	
C	2 (10.0%)	4 (5.6%)		0	3 (3.9%)	
D	4 (20.0%)	26 (36.6%)		6 (35.3%)	29 (37.2%)	
E	13 (65.0%)	36 (50.7%)		11 (64.7%)	41 (52.6%)	
Postoperative			0.66			0.78
A	0	0		0	0	
B	0	1 (1.4%)		0	0	
C	1 (5.0%)	1 (1.4%)		0	2 (2.6%)	
D	3 (15.0%)	10 (14.1%)		2 (11.8%)	7 (9.0%)	
E	16 (80.0%)	59 (83.1%)		15 (88.2%)	69 (88.5%)	
Surgery duration (minutes)	197.2 ± 62.1	213.8 ± 89.8	0.30	231.1 ± 80.5	233.4 ± 77.8	0.90
Perioperative blood loss (ml)	660.0 ± 446.5	659.3 ± 582.5	1.00	797.6 ± 648.2	830.1 ± 833.5	0.90
Comorbidity						
Yes	7 (35.0%)	17 (23.9%)	0.39	4 (23.5%)	17 (21.8%)	1.00
No	13 (65.0%)	54 (76.1%)		13 (76.5%)	61 (78.2%)	
Hospitalization (days)	23.2 ± 9.6	22.8 ± 44.0	0.97	15.8 ± 3.2	18.7 ± 14.7	0.42
Fused segment	2.09 ± 0.29	2.19 ± 0.62	0.30	2.40 ± 0.63	2.30 ± 0.71	0.60

[a]T test used to compare continuous variables; chi-square and Fisher's tests used to compare the categorical variables

during correction, short operation time, and shorter hospitalization period [22–24]. Therefore, the discussion of decision of an appropriate surgery approach has drawn wide attention in recent years, but only a few studies have compared the clinical efficacy and outcomes [15, 16]. A recent study prospectively compared 27 spinal tuberculosis patients with lumbar compression fracture who underwent a posterior debridement joint bone fixation therapy versus 22 patients who underwent an anterior approach [15]. Operation time and perioperative blood loss were significantly lower in the posterior group than in the anterior group ($p < 0.05$), and the former group had lower prevalence of postoperative complications (18.5 vs. 28.6%). However, in a respective

study, patients with thoracic and lumbar tuberculosis who underwent posterior debridement, interbody autografting, and instrumentation ($n = 25$) and anterior approach ($n = 22$) were compared [16]. No statistically significant differences were observed for operation time, perioperative blood loss, perioperative and postoperative complications, neurological status, and the kyphosis Cobb's angle, which was in line with our study [16].

Our study has some limitations that should be described. A major concern is Cobb's angle and VAS pain score differences before surgery between the anterior and posterior groups, which might have attenuated the true association. It shall be mentioned that during 2009–2012, the patients were mainly chosen for different

Table 4 Clinical outcome of spinal tuberculosis patients using anterior or posterior debridement joint bone graft and internal fixation by stratification of the vertebra

	Vertebra affected					
	Lumbar			Thoracic		
	Anterior	Posterior	p value [a]	Anterior	Posterior	p value [a]
No. of individuals	19	73		18	76	
Cobb's angle						
Preoperative	8.7 ± 16.6	− 5.6 ± 16.0	0.002	15.9 ± 15.3	14.4 ± 12.7	0.70
Postoperative	− 3.3 ± 13.2	− 10.1 ± 13.8	0.05	8.1 ± 9.7	10.3 ± 6.5	0.25
VAS score						
Preoperative	4.6 ± 1.3	3.8 ± 1.2	0.01	4.4 ± 1.3	3.6 ± 1.2	0.01
Postoperative	0.6 ± 0.5	0.7 ± 0.7	0.78	0.9 ± 0.7	0.7 ± 0.9	0.22
Follow-up	0.2 ± 0.4	0.3 ± 0.5	0.55	0.3 ± 0.5	0.2 ± 0.4	0.54
Frankel score						
Preoperative			0.01			0.81
A	0	0		0	3 (4.0%)	
B	0	0		1 (5.6%)	6 (7.9%)	
C	0	1 (1.4%)		2 (11.1%)	6 (7.9%)	
D	3 (15.8%)	36 (49.3%)		7 (38.9%)	19 (25.0%)	
E	16 (84.2%)	36 (49.3%)		8 (44.4%)	41 (54.0%)	
Postoperative			0.58			0.49
A	0	0		0	0	
B	0	0		0	1 (1.3%)	
C	0	0		1 (5.6%)	3 (4.0%)	
D	0	5 (6.9%)		5 (27.8%)	12 (15.8%)	
E	19 (100%)	68 (93.1%)		12 (66.7%)	60 (79.0%)	
Surgery duration (minutes)	224.8 ± 70.8	211.6 ± 75.9	0.48	200.1 ± 73.4	236.0 ± 90.0	0.08
Perioperative blood loss (ml)	671.6 ± 458.9	732.3 ± 846.7	0.76	777.8 ± 632.0	764.5 ± 596.3	0.94
Comorbidity						
Yes	6 (31.6%)	14 (19.2%)	0.35	5 (27.8%)	20 (26.3%)	1.00
No	13 (68.4%)	59 (80.8%)		13 (72.2%)	56 (73.7%)	
Hospitalization (days)	18.5 ± 7.5	17.4 ± 8.7	0.61	21.2 ± 8.8	23.8 ± 44.1	0.64
Fused segment	2.16 ± 0.37	2.11 ± 0.40	0.67	2.28 ± 0.57	2.36 ± 0.83	0.70

[a] T test used to compare continuous variables; chi-square and Fisher's tests used to compare the categorical variables

surgery approaches based on the location of their tuberculosis focus in the front or back of the body. Since year 2012, most patients were operated by the posterior approach regardless of location of tuberculosis focus. Another concern is the limited sample size in the anterior group, which might also have attenuated the outcome comparison.

Conclusions

In conclusion, good clinical outcomes were achieved in both groups, which indicate that the posterior approach could be used as an alternative procedure to treat thoracic and lumbar tuberculosis patients in terms of pain control, Cobb's angle, and neurological function. No statistically significant differences were found for surgery duration, perioperative blood loss, comorbidity, and hospitalization days among two alternative surgical approaches.

Acknowledgements
Not applicable.

Funding
This project was funded by the National Natural Science Foundation of Fujian Province (13151039); Medical Innovation Subject in Fujian Province (2014-CX-22); Key Clinical Specialty Discipline Construction Program of Fujian, People's Republic of China; and Young and Middle-aged Teachers Education Scientific Research Project in Fujian Province (JAT160796).

Authors' contributions
The authors' contributions to this study were as follows. YH, JL, YLL, and XYC contributed to the study design. YH and JL contributed to the data collection. YH, JL, and YLL contributed to the statistical analysis. All authors wrote the manuscript. All authors read and approved the final manuscript.

Competing interests
The authors declare that they have no competing interests.

Author details
[1]Department of Spinal Surgery, The First Affiliated Hospital of Fujian Medical University, Fuzhou, Fujian 350005, China. [2]Department of Basic Medical Science, Fujian Medical College, Fuzhou, Fujian, China. [3]Public Health School, Fujian Medical University, Fuzhou, Fujian, China.

References
1. Powles T, Staehler M, Ljungberg B, Bensalah K, Canfield SE, Dabestani S, Giles R, Hofmann F, Hora M, Kuczyk MA, et al. Updated EAU guidelines for clear cell renal cancer patients who fail VEGF targeted therapy. Eur Urol. 2016;69(1):4–6.
2. Trecarichi EM, Di Meco E, Mazzotta V, Fantoni M. Tuberculous spondylodiscitis: epidemiology, clinical features, treatment, and outcome. Eur Rev Med Pharmacol Sci. 2012;16(Suppl 2):58–72.
3. Turgut M. Spinal tuberculosis (Pott's disease): its clinical presentation, surgical management, and outcome. A survey study on 694 patients. Neurosurg Rev. 2001;24(1):8–13.
4. Nussbaum ES, Rockswold GL, Bergman TA, Erickson DL, Seljeskog EL. Spinal tuberculosis: a diagnostic and management challenge. J Neurosurg. 1995;83(2):243–7.
5. Lee TC, Lu K, Yang LC, Huang HY, Liang CL. Transpedicular instrumentation as an adjunct in the treatment of thoracolumbar and lumbar spine tuberculosis with early stage bone destruction. J Neurosurg. 1999;91(2 Suppl):163–9.
6. Zhang HQ, Lin MZ, Li JS, Tang MX, Guo CF, Wu JH, Liu JY. One-stage posterior debridement, transforaminal lumbar interbody fusion and instrumentation in treatment of lumbar spinal tuberculosis: a retrospective case series. Arch Orthop Trauma Surg. 2013;133(3):333–41.
7. Machino M, Yukawa Y, Ito K, Nakashima H, Kato F. A new thoracic reconstruction technique "transforaminal thoracic interbody fusion": a preliminary report of clinical outcomes. Spine. 2010;35(19):E1000–5.
8. Zaveri GR, Mehta SS. Surgical treatment of lumbar tuberculous spondylodiscitis by transforaminal lumbar interbody fusion (TLIF) and posterior instrumentation. J Spinal Disord Tech. 2009;22(4):257–62.
9. Huang QS, Zheng C, Hu Y, Yin X, Xu H, Zhang G, Wang Q. One-stage surgical management for children with spinal tuberculosis by anterior decompression and posterior instrumentation. Int Orthop. 2009;33(5):1385–90.
10. Klockner C, Valencia R. Sagittal alignment after anterior debridement and fusion with or without additional posterior instrumentation in the treatment of pyogenic and tuberculous spondylodiscitis. Spine. 2003;28(10):1036–42.
11. Yau AC, Hsu LC, O'Brien JP, Hodgson AR. Tuberculous kyphosis: correction with spinal osteotomy, halo-pelvic distraction, and anterior and posterior fusion. J Bone Joint Surg Am. 1974;56(7):1419–34.
12. Moon MS, Woo YK, Lee KS, Ha KY, Kim SS, Sun DH. Posterior instrumentation and anterior interbody fusion for tuberculous kyphosis of dorsal and lumbar spines. Spine. 1995;20(17):1910–6.
13. Sundararaj GD, Behera S, Ravi V, Venkatesh K, Cherian VM, Lee V. Role of posterior stabilisation in the management of tuberculosis of the dorsal and lumbar spine. J Bone Joint Surg Br. 2003;85(1):100–6.
14. Chen X, Lin J, Chen L, Chen F, Xu W, Wei C. One-stage posterior debridement, bone graft, and internal fixation for thoracic tuberculosis. Zhongguo Xiu Fu Chong Jian Wai Ke Za Zhi. 2011;25(10):1172–5.
15. Yu WY, Lou C, Liu FJ, He DW. Clinical efficacy of one stage posterior debridement joint graft fixation for lumbar vertebral fractures in spinal tuberculosis patients with compression. Eur Rev Med Pharmacol Sci. 2016;20(15):3161–7.
16. Pu X, Zhou Q, He Q, Dai F, Xu J, Zhang Z, Branko K. A posterior versus anterior surgical approach in combination with debridement, interbody autografting and instrumentation for thoracic and lumbar tuberculosis. Int Orthop. 2012;36(2):307–13.
17. Hodgson AR, Stock FE, Fang HS, Ong GB. Anterior spinal fusion. The operative approach and pathological findings in 412 patients with Pott's disease of the spine. Br J Surg. 1960;48:172–8.
18. Frankel HL, Hancock DO, Hyslop G, Melzak J, Michaelis LS, Ungar GH, Vernon JD, Walsh JJ. The value of postural reduction in the initial management of closed injuries of the spine with paraplegia and tetraplegia. I. Paraplegia. 1969;7(3):179–92.
19. Guven O. Posterior instrumentation and anterior interbody fusion for tuberculous kyphosis of dorsal and lumbar spines. Spine. 1996;21(15):1840–1.
20. Tuli SM. Tuberculosis of the spine: a historical review. Clin Orthop Relat Res. 2007;460:29–38.
21. Jain AK. Tuberculosis of the spine: a fresh look at an old disease. J Bone Joint Surg Br. 2010;92(7):905–13.
22. Talu U, Gogus A, Ozturk C, Hamzaoglu A, Domanic U. The role of posterior instrumentation and fusion after anterior radical debridement and fusion in the surgical treatment of spinal tuberculosis: experience of 127 cases. J Spinal Disord Tech. 2006;19(8):554–9.
23. Guzey FK, Emel E, Bas NS, Hacisalihoglu S, Seyithanoglu MH, Karacor SE, Ozkan N, Alatas I, Sel B. Thoracic and lumbar tuberculous spondylitis treated by posterior debridement, graft placement, and instrumentation: a retrospective analysis in 19 cases. J Neurosurg Spine. 2005;3(6):450–8.
24. Lee JS, Moon KP, Kim SJ, Suh KT. Posterior lumbar interbody fusion and posterior instrumentation in the surgical management of lumbar tuberculous spondylitis. J Bone Joint Surg Br. 2007;89(2):210–4.

16

Open versus minimally invasive fixation of a simulated syndesmotic injury in a cadaver model

Adam C. Shaner[1], Norachart Sirisreetreerux[1,2], Babar Shafiq[1], Lynne C. Jones[1] and Erik A. Hasenboehler[1,3*]

Abstract

Background: Malreduction of unstable syndesmotic ankle fractures is common. This study compared the reduction quality of an anterolateral open technique (OT) versus a conventional minimally invasive technique (MIT).

Methods: Fourteen fresh-frozen lower torso specimens with 28 matched lower extremities underwent computed tomography (CT) to measure syndesmosis position before dissection. Reduction was performed using direct visualization and fluoroscopy for the OT group (right-sided specimens) and fluoroscopy only for the MIT group (left-sided specimens). Fixation was achieved with 2 cortical screws. Measurements were repeated with postfixation CT scans. Statistical analysis used a two-tailed t test ($a = 0.05$).

Results: Mean posterior fibula-tibia distance decreased after OT by 0.3 ± 0.5 mm and increased after MIT by 0.7 ± 0.6 mm ($P = 0.025$ for difference between techniques). Mean anterior fibula-tibia distance decreased after OT by 0.4 ± 0.2 mm ($P = 0.007$) and did not change significantly after MIT (− 0.01 ± 0.4 mm ($P = 0.686$). Mean anterior translation after OT was 0.04 ± 0.4 mm ($P = 0.856$), and mean posterior translation after MIT was 0.3 ± 0.7 mm ($P = 0.434$). Mean medialization after OT was 0.3 ± 0.4 mm ($P = 0.132$), and mean lateralization after MIT was 0.2 ± 0.6 mm ($P = 0.446$).

Conclusions: Both techniques produced near-anatomic reduction of the fibula, with MIT producing significantly more internal rotation malreduction than OT. OT appears to restore near-anatomic fibula position, although this did not differ significantly from the results of MIT. We conditionally recommend OT when closed reduction of the syndesmosis cannot be obtained.

Keywords: Ankle, Fibula, Minimally invasive technique, Open technique, Syndesmotic injury

Background

Unstable rotational ankle fractures with associated syndesmotic disruption are common, with approximately 20% of operatively treated fractures requiring syndesmosis fixation [1]. Achieving anatomic syndesmosis reduction intraoperatively is important but challenging. The optimal method for treating these injuries is debated in the literature, in regard to proper implant selection (screws versus suture), positioning of the ankle during repair, and initiation of postoperative weightbearing. Further, the number of fixation cortices (3 versus 4) is also debated because instrumentation loosening or failure can occur, respectively. Hence, a "gold standard" of treatment for these injuries has yet to be described [2, 3]. Despite advanced imaging modalities and fixation techniques [4, 5], malreduction risks remain high, with a reported rate of > 50% [6–8]. Suboptimal clamp position during open or closed reduction can lead to malreduction and may not be apparent with standard intraoperative imaging [9–13].

Intraoperative 3D fluoroscopy can be used to assist with assessment of ankle reduction [4]. Franke et al. [14] assessed syndesmosis reduction quality intraoperatively, comparing 3D fluoroscopy with standard fluoroscopy in 2286 ankle fractures. This comparison resulted in a revision of the reduction in 33% of cases, improving it in 31% of cases [14]. However, advanced intraoperative

* Correspondence: editorialservices@jhmi.edu
[1]Department of Orthopaedic Surgery, The Johns Hopkins University, 600 N Caroline Street, Baltimore, MD 21287, USA
[3]Department of Orthopaedic Surgery, The Johns Hopkins University/Johns Hopkins Bayview Medical Center, 4940 Eastern Ave., #A667, Baltimore, MD 21224-2780, USA
Full list of author information is available at the end of the article

imaging is expensive, not always available, and associated with a higher radiation dose compared with standard fluoroscopy. Furthermore, Davidovitch et al. [15] showed that intraoperative 3D fluoroscopy did not decrease the rate of syndesmosis malreduction in 36 patients.

Anatomic variation presents another challenge to reduction. Studies by Nault et al. [16] and Shah et al. [17] have shown significant anatomic variation of the distal tibiofibular joint, which has been described for both standard fluoroscopic measurements, as well as axial computed tomography (CT) imaging [18]. Mukhopadhyay et al. [19] showed that when comparing the injured ankle with the contralateral (uninjured) ankle fluoroscopically, syndesmosis diastasis can be improved significantly by using fluoroscopy, as opposed to standard reduction methods alone. These studies emphasize the importance of evaluating the anatomic position of the uninjured ankle and using an individualized approach to intraoperative reduction assessment.

Recent studies evaluating open reduction of the syndesmosis have shown improved reduction quality [20, 21], potentially reducing the need for advanced intraoperative imaging. The purpose of this study was to compare the reduction quality of two reduction techniques, an anterolateral open technique (OT) versus a conventional minimally invasive technique (MIT) for a syndesmotic injury. Using a simulated syndesmotic cadaveric model, we measured the width and reduction of the syndesmotic joint with preinjury and postreduction CT scans. We hypothesized that an anterolateral open approach with direct visualization of the syndesmosis would result in a lower rate of malreduction compared with a standard closed reduction and clamping technique using 2D fluoroscopy.

Methods

Fourteen fresh-frozen lower torso specimens (3 females) with 28 matched lower extremities were obtained from the Maryland State Anatomy Board. Dual-energy X-ray absorptiometry scans were obtained for all specimens to ensure adequate bone quality. Specimens had a mean T score of -0.39 (range, -2.2 to 2.3) and a mean Z score of 0.71 (range, -0.9 to 3.5) [22]. The mean age at the time of death was 77 ± 13 years. None of the specimens had a history of surgery in either ankle. All specimens underwent bilateral lower extremity CT scans with 1.5 mm cuts to measure the anatomic syndesmosis position (Fig. 1). The picture archiving and communication system software used for all CT scans (Emageon, Inc., UltraVisual Medical Systems, Birmingham, AL) allowed us to obtain precise measurements up to the fifth decimal place.

Measurements of the distal tibiofibular joint were obtained from the axial view at 1 cm from the distal tibial articular surface and were performed according to the techniques described below (Fig. 2).

Method of Tang et al. [23]

The center of the distal tibial metaphysis was established, and the distance (in cm) from this point was measured to the anterior (A) and posterior (B) fibular cortices. The ratio of A:B reflects the relative rotation of the fibula with values of < 1.0 cm indicating relative internal rotation and values > 1.0 cm representing relative external rotation.

Method of Elgafy et al. [24]

The distance (in mm) was measured between the closest point on the anterior tubercle of the tibia and the point

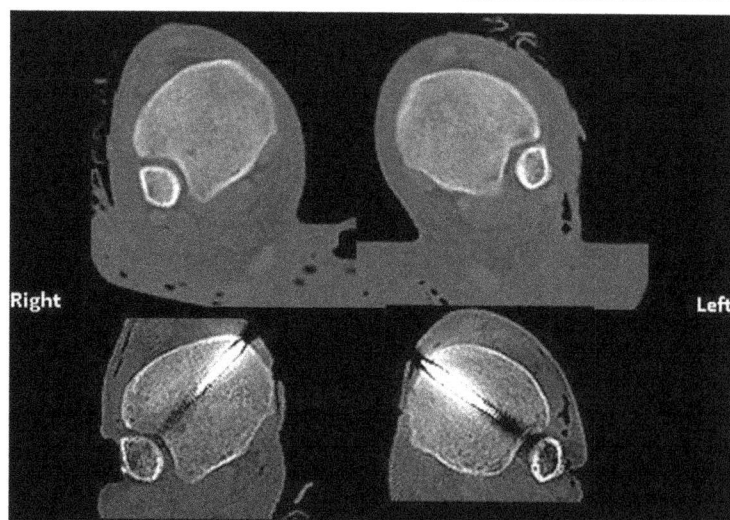

Fig. 1 Example of computed tomography scan axial images before and after reduction with open technique (right side) and minimally invasive technique (left side). Reduction appears to be almost identical to the predissection condition for both techniques

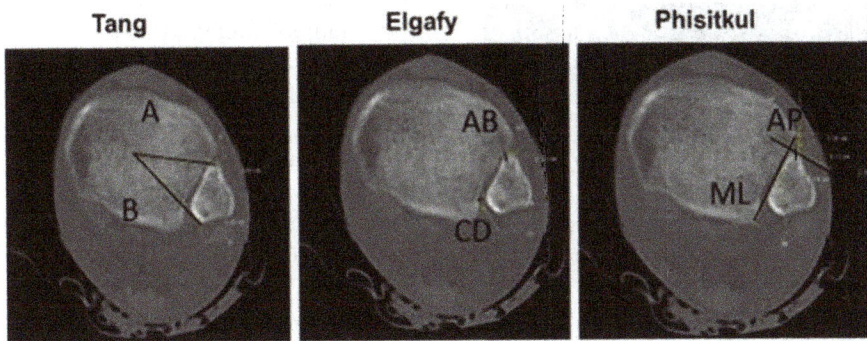

Fig. 2 UltraVisual imaging software (Emageon, Inc., UltraVisual Medical Systems, Birmingham, AL) was used to perform measurements on the axial computed tomography scan view at 1 cm above the distal tibia articular surface. Tang et al. [23], ratio of A:B distance reflects fibular rotation. Elgafy et al. [24] and Phisitkul et al. [25] methods, direct measurements of anterior (AB and AP) and posterior (CD and ML) tibial-fibular distance, represent fibular translation in the coronal and sagittal planes, respectively

on the fibula closest to that location (AB). A second measurement (in mm) was obtained between the point on the fibula that is midway between the medial-most and the posterior-most points, and the location on the tibia that is closest to that location (CD). Both the mean of the anterior and posterior measurements, as well as the difference between the anterior and posterior values (AB − CD) were calculated. A positive value indicates greater anterior distance (relative external rotation). A negative value indicates greater posterior distance (relative internal rotation).

Method of Phisitkul et al. [25]

The medial-lateral distance was measured (in mm) from the medial-most border of the fibula to a line connecting the anterior and posterior tubercles of the tibia. The anterior-posterior distance was measured between a line perpendicular to the tubercular line at the anterior tubercle and the anterior-most point of the fibula. Positive numbers denote posterior translation, and negative numbers denote anterior translation. For medial-lateral translation, positive numbers denote medial translation, and negative numbers denote lateral translation.

Injury simulation

Specimens underwent dissection and syndesmosis ligamentous division to simulate an unstable ankle injury using a previously described method [26]. All right-sided lower extremities underwent open dissection with an anterolateral approach to the anterior syndesmosis (Fig. 3a). The anterior inferior tibiofibular ligament (AITFL) was visualized directly and divided, along with the interosseous ligament and the distal 3 cm of the interosseous membrane. The fibula was then translated laterally using a lamina spreader, and the posterior inferior tibiofibular ligament (PITFL) was visualized and fully transected through the syndesmosis. The deep deltoid ligaments were then divided completely through a second longitudinal medial malleolus incision (Fig. 3b). Instability of the ankle with syndesmosis widening was confirmed using an external rotation stress test under direct and fluoroscopic visualization (Fig. 3c).

All left-sided lower extremities underwent ligamentous division using minimally invasive techniques with separate incisions anterior and posterior to the syndesmosis to divide the AITFL, PITFL, and interosseous membrane (Fig 4a). A medial malleolus incision was used to divide the deep deltoid ligaments (Fig. 3b, similarly as for OT).

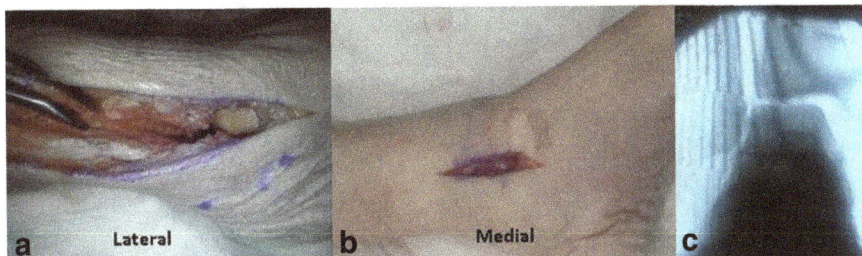

Fig. 3 a Anterolateral skin incision over the distal fibula and syndesmosis carried out more proximally to allow dissection of the interosseous membrane. The lamina spreader was used to visualize the PITFL and transect it. **b** Medial skin incision was made to transect the deltoid ligament. **c** External rotation stress view confirming instability

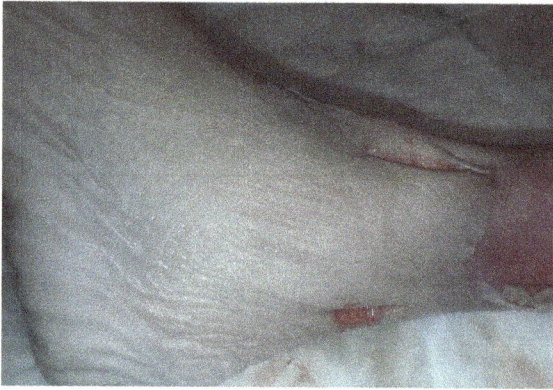

Fig. 4 For the minimally invasive technique, two incisions were made (anterior and posterior) over the AITFL and PITFL. Similar to Fig. 3, a medial skin incision was made over the medial malleolus to transect the deltoid ligament. A stress view was taken after preparation and under fluoroscopy, as shown in Fig. 3

An external rotation stress test using fluoroscopy was performed to verify instability (Fig. 3c). A large Weber clamp was used to obtain reduction in both techniques.

Syndesmosis reduction
Open approach
For the open approach, the syndesmosis was reduced under direct visualization, ensuring reduction of the fibular articulation with the tibia and position at the anterior incisura. Weber clamp tines were placed approximately 1 cm above the plafond, on the lateral malleolar ridge of the fibula and over the center of the anteroposterior width of the tibia medially. This allowed coaxial compression in the plane of the syndesmosis. Clamp position was verified and adjusted as needed using fluoroscopy (Figs. 1 and 5a, b). The clamp was adjusted to 4–5 clicks to standardize the amount of compression while holding the foot in neutral dorsiflexion. Subsequently, quadricortical trans-syndesmosis fixation was placed in classic fashion using 3.5-mm cortical screws (DePuy Synthes, Paoli, PA) from lateral to medial, after

predrilling with a 2.5-mm drill bit. Quadricortical fixation is the authors' preferred method because this technique can provide better syndesmotic stability versus tricortical fixation, which can lead to instrumentation loosening. Two parallel 3.5-mm cortical screws were placed approximately 0.5 and 1.5 cm above and parallel to the tibial plafond and approximately 30° from posterior to anterior in the horizontal plane. Proper position was verified using fluoroscopy (Fig. 5b).

Minimally invasive approach
For the minimally invasive approach, a 3-cm lateral incision was made over the distal fibula at the level of the tibiofibular joint. To obtain coaxial compression at the level of the syndesmosis, we placed Weber clamp tines similarly to the open approach (1 cm above the plafond on the lateral malleolar ridge of the fibula and over the center of the anteroposterior width of the tibia medially). Clamp position was verified and adjusted as needed using fluoroscopy, and reduction was judged using standard anteroposterior/mortise and perfect lateral fluoroscopic views. The clamp was adjusted to 4–5 clicks to standardize the amount of compression. Syndesmosis fixation was performed in a similar fashion to the OT, through a small lateral incision (Figs. 1 and 5a, b).

Postfixation CT scans were performed for all ankles, and measurements were obtained again using all three methods. Pre- and postdissection measurements were compared to evaluate reduction.

Statistical analysis
The data were collected and analyzed using an electronic spreadsheet (Excel 2007, Microsoft, Redmond, WA). Mean values and differences with 95% confidence intervals were calculated. To compare anatomic differences with regard to laterality on the same cadaver, we used an unpaired two-tailed t test for the predissection measurements of the left versus right side. The position of the fibula within the incisura before and after fixation was compared between the OT and MIT groups for all

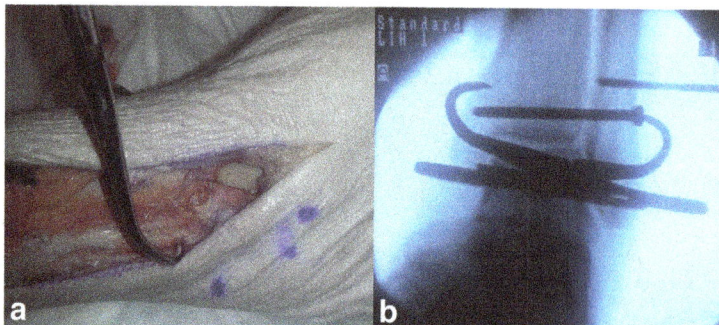

Fig. 5 a Clamp position with direct visualization of syndesmosis reduction anteriorly. **b** Fluoroscopic verification of clamp position, reduction of syndesmosis on mortise view, and placement of two 3.5-mm quadricortical screws

specimens using an unpaired two-tailed t test. A paired two-tailed t test was used to compare differences between pre- and postfixation measurements for the same specimen. P values less than 0.05 were considered statistically significant.

Results

No significant differences in preinjury fibular anatomic position were found between right and left lower extremities from the same cadaver (Table 1).

Using the measurement technique of Tang et al. [23], and comparing postdissection versus predissection values for the same limb, we found that MIT produced a mean decrease in the distance from the tibial center to the anterior fibular cortex of 0.2 ± 0.5 mm, and OT produced a mean decrease of 0.2 ± 0.7 mm. The posterior distance increased by a mean of 0.1 ± 0.9 mm using MIT compared with 0.4 ± 1.1 mm using OT. Neither difference was statistically significant when compared with preinjury anatomic position, nor was the difference between techniques significant. Both MIT and OT resulted in relative decreases in the ratio of anterior to posterior

distance of 0.01 ± 0.02 mm and 0.02 ± 0.03 mm, respectively. This indicates net internal rotation of the fibula with both methods (Table 1). The difference between methods was not statistically significant.

Using the method of Elgafy et al. [24], we observed a narrowing of the anterior syndesmosis of 0.4 ± 0.2 mm ($P = 0.007$) with OT. This was a significant difference compared with preinjury measurements but was not significantly different between techniques ($P = 0.071$). Conversely, MIT resulted in shortening of the anterior syndesmosis space by 0.01 ± 0.4 mm, but this was not statistically significant ($P = 0.686$). Measurement of the posterior syndesmosis distance showed a decrease of 0.3 ± 0.5 mm with OT, which was not a significant change ($P = 0.338$). MIT showed an increase in this distance of 0.7 ± 0.6 mm. This was significant not only compared with the prefixation anatomic fibular position ($P = 0.044$) but also compared with OT ($P = 0.025$). When analyzing the change in overall distance using the difference between the anterior and posterior measurements, neither OT (0.1 ± 0.6 mm, $P = 0.709$) nor MIT (0.6 ± 0.8 mm, $P = 0.133$)

Table 1 Computed tomography-based measurements of 14 matched-pair cadaveric ankles before dissection and after fixation of a simulated syndesmotic injury using OT versus MIT

Measure	Predissection measurements (mean ± SD), mm		P value	Postfixation difference (mean ± SD), mm				P value for OT versus MIT
	Right ankles	Left ankles		OT	P value	MIT	P value	
Tang et al. [23]								
A[a]	29 ± 1.1	28 ± 1.1	0.338					
B[b]	30 ± 1.4	30 ± 1.4	0.749					
A:B[c]	0.97 ± 0.03	0.95 ± 0.03	0.412					
Change in A				− 0.2 ± 0.7	0.54	− 0.2 ± 0.5	0.50	0.937
Change in B				0.4 ± 1.1	0.45	0.1 ± 0.9	0.81	0.644
Change in A:B				− 0.02 ± 0.03	0.17	− 0.01 ± 0.02	0.39	0.485
Elgafy et al. [24]								
AB[d]	1.7 ± 0.3	1.4 ± 0.3	0.266					
CD[e]	3.0 ± 0.5	2.9 ± 0.5	0.871					
AB − CD[f]	− 1.2 ± 0.6	− 1.4 ± 0.4	0.614					
Change in AB				− 0.4 ± 0.2	0.007	− 0.01 ± 0.4	0.686	0.071
Change in CD				− 0.3 ± 0.5	0.338	0.7 ± 0.6	0.044	0.025
Change in AB − CD				0.1 ± 0.6	0.709	0.6 ± 0.8	0.133	0.288
Phisitkul et al. [25]								
Anteroposterior[g]	2.0 ± 0.3	2.1 ± 0.4	0.634	− 0.04 ± 0.4	0.856	0.3 ± 0.7	0.434	0.434
Mediolateral[h]	2.2 ± 0.5	2.2 ± 0.4	0.966	− 0.3 ± 0.4	0.132	0.2 ± 0.6	0.446	0.151

MIT minimally invasive technique, *OT* open technique, *SD* standard deviation

[a]"A" represents distance from center of distal tibial metaphysis to anterior fibular cortices

[b]"B" represents distance from center of distal tibial metaphysis to posterior fibular cortices

[c]The ratio of A:B reflects the relative rotation of the fibula

[d]"AB" represents distance between closest point on anterior tubercle of tibia and point on fibula closest to that location

[e]"CD" represents distance between point on fibula midway between medial-most and posterior-most points, and location on tibia closest to that location

[f]"AB − CD" represents difference between mean anterior and posterior values

[g]Medial-lateral distance from medial-most border of fibula to a line connecting anterior and posterior tubercles of the tibia

[h]Anterior-posterior distance between a line perpendicular to the tubercular line at the anterior tubercle and the anterior-most point of the fibula

significantly changed the overall position of the fibula, with a comparative P value of 0.288 (Table 1).

Lastly, using the measurement method of Phisitkul et al. [25], we found that OT produced 0.04 ± 0.4 mm of anterior translation compared with preinjury position ($P = 0.856$), whereas MIT produced posterior translation of 0.3 ± 0.7 mm ($P = 0.434$), with no difference between groups ($P = 0.434$). Measurement of medial-lateral translation resulted in a net 0.3 ± 0.4 mm ($P = 0.132$) of medialization using OT and a relative lateralization of 0.2 ± 0.6 mm ($P = 0.446$) with MIT. Again, there was no significant difference between groups ($P = 0.151$).

Discussion

Syndesmotic ankle injuries are challenging to treat, with patients having pain and radiographic widening at 5-year follow-up in as many as 60% of cases [27]. Malreduction of the syndesmosis has been consistently shown to result in poor long-term outcomes, with ankle stiffness and poor functional outcome scores [1, 7].

With both techniques, we were able to restore the syndesmosis to near-anatomic (predissection) position. The quality of reduction was acceptable in the MIT and OT groups, with no malreductions > 0.2 mm using any of the measurement techniques. However, even with direct visualization of the AITFL and anterior incisura and proper clamp positioning using appropriate visualization and fluoroscopy, there was a propensity for a decrease in the anterior fibula-incisura distance of up to 0.4 mm. This was the only significant difference we found with OT, and it did not occur with increased anterior-posterior translation or posterior fibular rotation. This suggests that there was a net compression effect or medial translation, rather than rotational malreduction. This finding is consistent with studies by Haynes et al. [28] and Cherney et al. [29] that showed overcompression was likely during reduction clamping of the syndesmosis, with a mean of 1 mm of overcompression and 5° of external rotation. Similar results were found in a cadaveric study by Phisitkul et al. [25], which showed a mean syndesmosis displacement of 0.1 ± 0.77 mm in all degrees of instability and overcompression of 0.93 ± 0.70 mm during clamping, with the clamp in the neutral anatomical axis.

Use of intraoperative imaging to assess reduction quality is challenging. A cadaver study by Marmor et al. [10] showed that as much as 30° of external rotation may be undetectable using intraoperative fluoroscopy. Franke et al. [14] used intraoperative 3D fluoroscopy scanning to assess reduction performed under fluoroscopy and found malreduction in 33% (82 of 251) of cases. Even with the use of intraoperative 3D scanning, Davidovitch et al. [15] showed a 31% (5 of 16) malreduction rate, compared with a 25% (5 of 20) malreduction rate with standard fluoroscopic imaging [30].

Alternative fixation methods such as a suture endobutton have been described. Although this technique may improve reduction by allowing physiologic motion at the syndesmosis, this method has not been shown to prevent syndesmosis malreduction completely [30]. Further, other than avoiding removal of instrumentation after 1 year or secondary to instrumentation failure or loosening as seen with screw fixation, clinical and radiographic outcomes at 1 year have not shown statistically significant differences between endobutton and screw fixation [31, 32].

Recently, open reduction and debridement of the syndesmosis has been shown to result in improved reduction rates. However, a greater amount soft tissue dissection is necessary for this approach [7, 21].

Miller et al. [20] reported a decreased rate of malreduction using direct visualization of the PITFL and posterior malleolus. A 16% malreduction rate (24 of 149 ankles) was found in ankles in which the posterior syndesmosis and posterior malleolus were fixed with direct visualization, compared with a 52% (13 of 24) malreduction rate in ankles fixed with indirect and fluoroscopic reduction only. In our cadaver model, the PITFL was divided completely but not repaired because no posterior malleolus fragment was present. This may have contributed to the similar results for the OT and MIT groups in our study.

Open reduction of the anterior syndesmosis was superior to the MIT in preventing overall internal rotation malreduction of the fibula based on the increase in posterior fibula-incisura distance. The MIT produced an increase in this distance of 0.7 ± 0.6 mm, which was significant not only compared with the anatomic (prefixation) fibular position ($P = 0.044$) but also compared with OT ($P = 0.025$). With no associated net change in the anterior fibula-incisura distance, this represents a purely internal rotation malreduction of the fibula, similar to that found by Davidovitch et al. [15].

This type of malreduction likely results from improper clamp positioning during reduction [11, 25, 33]. Clamp overcompression could also be a reason for malreduction, and using a calibrated clamping device during reduction, with or without the aid of advanced intraoperative imaging, might be necessary. We attempted to standardize this by limiting compression to 4–5 clicks with the clamp. However, the clinical relevance of this possible overtensioning has yet to be determined.

Our study has several strengths. We were able to reliably simulate a syndesmotic injury with a reproducible amount of instability using a cadaver model. Furthermore, pre- and postdissection CT scans allowed for accurate assessment of patient anatomy for determining quality of reduction after fixation. The precision of the measurements obtained through the software we used (Emageon UltraVisual) might not be clinically relevant; however, we believe that such precision increases the reliability of our reduction methods. We controlled for anatomic variability by using matched-pair cadaver ankles.

This study also has several limitations. Dissection and fixation were performed in cadaveric ankles, in which bone density and the quality of skin, tendon, and articular tissues differ from the in vivo state. This may influence measurements and affect the validity of our model; however, bone density was verified and controlled for with pre-evaluation dual-energy X-ray absorptiometry scanning. The type of reduction clamp (e.g., large Weber, peri-articular, or collinear) is a surgeon-specific choice. We used a larger, pointed Weber clamp because of the thin habitus of our specimens. Another weakness of our study is that our model reflected a purely ligamentous injury of the ankle without associated high fibular fracture as typically seen in the clinical setting. Syndesmotic injuries with associated fibular fractures can be difficult to reduce because any malreduction of the fibula increases the likelihood of syndesmosis malreduction. That said, anatomic fibula reduction is usually achieved for distal fibula shaft fractures, whereas more proximal fractures are left unreduced because displacement is minimal and considered to be clinically unimportant. On the basis of this consideration, we chose a purely ligamentous injury model, as used in previous ankle studies. This model was easily reproducible, thereby eliminating the variability of fracture size, location, and fixation options. The absence of a repaired PITFL in our model may also have affected overall reduction because anatomic reduction of the posterior malleolus or direct reduction of PITFL injuries has been shown to restore rotational fibular stability similar to syndesmosis fixation [21, 34].

Conclusion

Our study indicates that the quality of syndesmosis reduction achieved using MIT (with conventional 2D fluoroscopy) is comparable to that achieved using OT (with direct visualization). MIT produced more internal rotation malreduction of the fibula compared with OT. However, there was no significant difference in fibula reduction between the two techniques. Therefore, we can only conditionally recommend OT for the reduction of the syndesmosis. This technique might be useful when reduction of the syndesmosis cannot be obtained using MIT (e.g., in cases of interposition of soft tissue). Randomized clinical trials are needed to validate these findings and to provide further insight into optimal treatment of these challenging injuries.

Abbreviations

AITFL: Anterior inferior tibiofibular ligament; CT: Computed tomography; MIT: Minimally invasive technique; OT: Open technique; PITFL: Posterior inferior tibiofibular ligament

Acknowledgements
The authors thank Stephen Belkoff, PhD, and Demetries Boston at Johns Hopkins Bayview Medical Center for their assistance with study organization and cadaver resources.

Funding
Study was supported by a DePuy Synthes research grant for the hardware and specimens only.

Authors' contributions
ACS and NS prepared the specimens and performed the fixations and CT scans. ACS wrote the manuscript and performed the data analysis. LCJ assisted with the data analysis and interpretation and reviewed the manuscript. NS and BS reviewed the manuscript and contributed to manuscript drafting and correction. EAH supervised the entire project, reviewed the data, and corrected the manuscript. All authors read and approved the final manuscript.

Competing interests
EAH provides consultancy for the DePuy Synthes and received grants for research and research fellow. The other authors declare that they have no competing interests.

Author details
[1]Department of Orthopaedic Surgery, The Johns Hopkins University, 600 N Caroline Street, Baltimore, MD 21287, USA. [2]Department of Orthopaedics, Faculty of Medicine, Ramathibodi Hospital, Mahidol University, 270 Rama VI Rd, Ratchathewi, Bangkok 10400, Thailand. [3]Department of Orthopaedic Surgery, The Johns Hopkins University/Johns Hopkins Bayview Medical Center, 4940 Eastern Ave., #A667, Baltimore, MD 21224-2780, USA.

References
1. Egol KA, Pahk B, Walsh M, Tejwani NC, Davidovitch RI, Koval KJ. Outcome after unstable ankle fracture: effect of syndesmotic stabilization. J Orthop Trauma. 2010;24:7–11.
2. Zalavras C, Thordarson D. Ankle syndesmotic injury. J Am Acad Orthop Surg. 2007;15:330–9.
3. Heim D, Heim U, Regazzoni P. Malleolar fractures with ankle joint instability—experience with the positioning screw. Unfallchirurgie. 1993;19: 307–12.
4. Ebinger T, Goetz J, Dolan L, Phisitkul P. 3D model analysis of existing CT syndesmosis measurements. Lowa Orthop Jl. 2013;33:40–6.
5. Knops SP, Kohn MA, Hansen EN, Matityahu A, Marmor M. Rotational malreduction of the syndesmosis: reliability and accuracy of computed tomography measurement methods. Foot Ankle Int. 2013;34:1403–10.
6. Gardner MJ, Demetrakopoulos D, Briggs SM, Helfet DL, Lorich DG. Malreduction of the tibiofibular syndesmosis in ankle fractures. Foot Ankle Int. 2006;27:788–92.
7. Sagi HC, Shah AR, Sanders RW. The functional consequence of syndesmotic joint malreduction at a minimum 2-year follow-up. J Orthop Trauma. 2012;26:439–43.
8. Pelton K, Thordarson DB, Barnwell J. Open versus closed treatment of the fibula in Maissoneuve injuries. Foot Ankle Int. 2010;31:604–8.
9. Koenig SJ, Tornetta P III, Merlin G, Bogdan Y, Egol KA, Ostrum RF, Wolinsky PR. Can we tell if the syndesmosis is reduced using fluoroscopy? J Orthop Trauma. 2015;29:e326–30.
10. Marmor M, Hansen E, Han HK, Buckley J, Matityahu A. Limitations of standard fluoroscopy in detecting rotational malreduction of the syndesmosis in an ankle fracture model. Foot Ankle Int. 2011;32:616–22.
11. Miller AN, Barei DP, Iaquinto JM, Ledoux WR, Beingessner DM. Iatrogenic syndesmosis malreduction via clamp and screw placement. J Orthop Trauma. 2013;27:100–6.
12. Rasi AM, Kazemian G, Omidian MM, Nemati A. Syndesmotic malreduction after ankle ORIF: is radiography sufficient? Arch Bone Joint Surg. 2013;1:98–102.
13. Warner SJ, Fabricant PD, Garner MR, Schottel PC, Helfet DL, Lorich DG. The measurement and clinical importance of syndesmotic reduction after

operative fixation of rotational ankle fractures. J Bone Joint Surg Am Vol. 2015;97:1935–44.

14. Franke J, von Recum J, Suda AJ, Grutzner PA, Wendl K. Intraoperative three-dimensional imaging in the treatment of acute unstable syndesmotic injuries. J Bone Joint Surg Am Vol. 2012;94:1386–90.

15. Davidovitch RI, Weil Y, Karia R, Forman J, Looze C, Liebergall M, Egol K. Intraoperative syndesmotic reduction: three-dimensional versus standard fluoroscopic imaging. J Bone Joint Surg Am Vol. 2013;95:1838–43.

16. Nault ML, Hebert-Davies J, Laflamme GY, Leduc S. CT scan assessment of the syndesmosis: a new reproducible method. J Orthop Trauma. 2013;27:638–41.

17. Shah AS, Kadakia AR, Tan GJ, Karadsheh MS, Wolter TD, Sabb B. Radiographic evaluation of the normal distal tibiofibular syndesmosis. Foot Ankle Int. 2012;33:870–6.

18. Dikos GD, Heisler J, Choplin RH, Weber TG. Normal tibiofibular relationships at the syndesmosis on axial CT imaging. J Orthop Trauma. 2012;26:433–8.

19. Mukhopadhyay S, Metcalfe A, Guha AR, Mohanty K, Hemmadi S, Lyons K, O'Doherty D. Malreduction of syndesmosis—are we considering the anatomical variation? Injury. 2011;42:1073–6.

20. Miller AN, Carroll EA, Parker RJ, Boraiah S, Helfet DL, Lorich DG. Direct visualization for syndesmotic stabilization of ankle fractures. Foot Ankle Int. 2009;30:419–26.

21. Schottel PC, Baxter J, Gilbert S, Garner MR, Lorich DG. Anatomic ligament repair restores ankle and syndesmotic rotational stability as much as syndesmotic screw fixation. J Orthop Trauma. 2016;30:e36–40.

22. Nordin BE. The definition and diagnosis of osteoporosis. Calcif Tissue Int. 1987;40:57–8.

23. Tang CW, Roidis N, Vaishnav S, Patel A, Thordarson DB. Position of the distal fibular fragment in pronation and supination ankle fractures: a CT evaluation. Foot Ankle Int. 2003;24:561–6.

24. Elgafy H, Semaan HB, Blessinger B, Wassef A, Ebraheim NA. Computed tomography of normal distal tibiofibular syndesmosis. Skelet Radiol. 2010;39:559–64.

25. Phisitkul P, Ebinger T, Goetz J, Vaseenon T, Marsh JL. Forceps reduction of the syndesmosis in rotational ankle fractures: a cadaveric study. J Bone Joint Surg Am Vol. 2012;94:2256–61.

26. Ebramzadeh E, Knutsen AR, Sangiorgio SN, Brambila M, Harris TG. Biomechanical comparison of syndesmotic injury fixation methods using a cadaveric model. Foot Ankle Int. 2013;34:1710–7.

27. van Vlijmen N, Denk K, van Kampen A, Jaarsma RL. Long-term results after ankle syndesmosis injuries. Orthopedics. 2015;38:e1001–6.

28. Haynes J, Cherney S, Spraggs-Hughes A, McAndrew CM, Ricci WM, Gardner MJ. Increased reduction clamp force associated with syndesmotic overcompression. Foot Ankle Int. 2016;37:722–9.

29. Cherney SM, Haynes JA, Spraggs-Hughes AG, McAndrew CM, Ricci WM, Gardner MJ. In vivo syndesmotic overcompression after fixation of ankle fractures with a syndesmotic injury. J Orthop Trauma. 2015;29:414–9.

30. Summers HD, Sinclair MK, Stover MD. A reliable method for intraoperative evaluation of syndesmotic reduction. J Orthop Trauma. 2013;27:196–200.

31. Laflamme M, Belzile EL, Bedard L, van den Bekerom MP, Glazebrook M, Pelet S. A prospective randomized multicenter trial comparing clinical outcomes of patients treated surgically with a static or dynamic implant for acute ankle syndesmosis rupture. J Orthop Trauma. 2015;29:216–23.

32. Westermann RW, Rungprai C, Goetz JE, Femino J, Amendola A, Phisitkul P. The effect of suture-button fixation on simulated syndesmotic malreduction: a cadaveric study. J Bone Joint Surg Am Vol. 2014;96:1732–8.

33. Kennedy MT, Carmody O, Leong S, Kennedy C, Dolan M. A computed tomography evaluation of two hundred normal ankles, to ascertain what anatomical landmarks to use when compressing or placing an ankle syndesmosis screw. Foot (Edinburgh, Scotland). 2014;24:157–60.

34. Miller AN, Carroll EA, Parker RJ, Helfet DL, Lorich DG. Posterior malleolar stabilization of syndesmotic injuries is equivalent to screw fixation. Clin Orthop. 2010;468:1129–35.

17

A comparison of clinical efficacy between different surgical approaches for popliteal cyst

Bo Yang[*†] , Fengchun Wang[†], Yanhua Lou[†], Juan Li, Lei Sun, Lei Gao and Feng Liu

Abstract

Background: A popliteal cyst is a benign swelling with synovial fluid located behind the knee joint. Popliteal cysts are often asymptomatic; however, symptomatic cysts may cause pain and may need surgery interventions. Here, we performed a perspective study to compare the clinical efficacy of different surgical approaches, including traditional open excision and advanced arthroscopic treatment.

Methods: A total of 76 patients with popliteal cysts were assigned into three groups by a randomized complete block design. Group A included 32 patients (15 males and 17 females, age 55.3 ± 9.8 years) who received arthroscopic internal drainage of the cysts. Group B included 19 patients (9 males and 10 females, age 55.4 ± 7.6 years) who received open excision after arthroscopic treatment. Group C included 25 patients (11 males and 14 females, age 54.2 ± 8.5 years) who received open excision. All patients were followed up for an average of 13.7 ± 2.4 months. The following parameters were compared: the time of surgery, during surgery, the length of incision, the incision healing rate, the visual analog scale (VAS) for pain, the hospitalization time, the rate of recovery to level 0–1 cysts, the recurrence rate, and the Lysholm score.

Results: Group A exhibited significant better outcomes compared to groups B and C in the length of incision (1.6 ± 0.1 cm), the incision healing rate (100%), the postoperative VAS score (2.7 ± 1.2), the hospitalization time (7.8 ± 2.8 days), and the Lysholm score at the last follow-up (85.8 ± 5.2). The recurrence rate is significantly lower in groups A (3.1%) and B (5.2%) than group C (40%) ($P < 0.001$).

Conclusions: Arthroscopic treatment for popliteal cysts exhibited better clinical outcomes with minimal invasion and can be recommended for future clinical interventions.

Keywords: Arthroscopy, Popliteal cyst, Internal drainage, Open excision

Background

Popliteal cyst is a common knee joint disease and often seen in elderly patients with knee osteoarthritis or meniscus tear [1, 2]. Traditionally, treatment usually involves open excision from the posterior side of the knee. However, it requires a large incision and is associated with high recurrence rates [3, 4]. It is becoming a commonplace that understanding pathological progression underlying popliteal cysts is beneficial for the current treatment [5]. In recent years, minimally invasive arthroscopy has provided surgeons an alternative approach with prominent advantages [6, 7]. However, arthroscopic treatment alone may not be enough to address both the underlying pathology in the knee joint and the cyst [8]. On the other hand, the combination of arthroscopic treatment and open excision was rarely reported. It is difficult to suggest the best treatment for popliteal cysts because the direct comparison between different surgical approaches with long-term follow-ups are lacking. Here, we sought to compare three different surgical treatments of popliteal cyst: arthroscopic internal drainage, open excision after arthroscopic treatment, and open excision.

* Correspondence: yb_lxp@sina.com
†Equal contributors
Department of Orthopaedics, Tai'an Central Hospital, Tai'an, Shandong 271000, China

Methods

Ethics, consent, and permissions

This study was approved by the Ethics Committee of Tai'an Central Hospital. Written information consent to participate was obtained from all patients.

Patients

A total of 76 patients (35 males and 41 females, age 55.0 ± 8.8 years) with popliteal cysts were enrolled at Tai'an Central Hospital between April 2013 and February 2017. Preoperative magnetic resonance imaging (MRI) and X-ray radiography were conducted to confirm the diagnosis and classify the patients. All patients were scored according to Rauschning and Lindgren classification (RLC) and Kellgren-Lawrence system (K-L) [9]. Patients with K-L grade greater than III, patients with ligament injuries, and patients with recurrent popliteal cysts were excluded in the study. The patients were randomly assigned into three surgical groups using complete block design. Randomly generated numbers were assigned to each patient and divided by 3: remainder 1 was defined as group A, remainder 2 was defined as group B, and remainder 0 was defined as group C. Group A included 32 patients who received arthroscopic internal drainage of the cysts (15 males and 17 females, age 55.3 ± 9.8 years; RLC 20 grade II and 12 grade III; K-L 7 grade 0, 13 grade I, and 12 grade II; 2 patients had cyst only, 13 combined with meniscus injuries, 7 combined with cartilage injuries, 5 had both meniscus and cartilage injuries, 5 combined with synovitis). Group B included 19 patients who received open excision after arthroscopic treatment (9 males and 10 females, age 55.4 ± 7.6 years; RLC 1 grade I, 11 grade II, and 7 grade III; K-L 3 grade 0, 8 grade I, and 8 grade II; 7 patients combined with meniscus injuries, 5 combined with cartilage injuries, 6 had both meniscus and cartilage injuries, 1 combined with synovitis). Group C included 25 patients who received open excision of the cysts (11 males and 14 females, age 54.2 ± 8.5 years; RLC 1 grade I, 13 grade II, and 11 grade III; K-L 4 grade 0, 10 grade I, and 11 grade II; 1 patient had cyst only, 10 patients combined with meniscus injuries, 7 combined with cartilage injuries, 5 had both meniscus and cartilage injuries, 2 combined with synovitis). All procedures were performed by the same surgeon.

Surgical methods

Arthroscopic internal drainage (group A)

Patients were placed in supine position with routine anesthesia or epidural anesthesia. Tourniquet was applied to prevent bleeding during the procedure. However, in order to avoid deep vein thrombosis, tourniquet had to be removed after 1 h and re-applied 10 min later. The procedure was paused during the 10 min. If bleeding occurred, plasma knife was used to stop bleeding. After disinfection, 1–2 ml methylene blue was injected into the cyst to identify the valvular opening. An arthroscope was used to detect any meniscus or cartilage injuries and synovial hyperplasia. Next, an arthroscope was inserted through the anterolateral portal into the posteromedial compartment, via the space between the posterior cruciate ligament and the medial femoral condyle (Fig. 1a, b). Posteromedial compartments were visualized to confirm the position of medial gastrocnemius tendon and the transverse posteromedial synovial folds and the opening of the cyst (Fig. 1c, d). The posteromedial portal was then established under the light, and a shaver was inserted and placed next to the medial head of the gastrocnemius muscle to clean the joint space and the opening of the cyst (Fig. 1e). At this time, outflow of cyst fluid was visualized by methylene blue, and the opening was incised to at least 5×5 mm (Fig. 1f). If there existed meniscus or cartilage injuries, appropriate repair surgeries were performed immediately. A total of 18 patients received meniscus repairs and 12 received cartilage repairs. Finally, the joint capsule was thoroughly cleaned and flushed after hemostasis. Limb restraint was not necessary after the procedure. Quadriceps exercises started as early as 6 h postoperative time. Elastic bandages and ice cubes were applied at the surgical site and were removed after 2–3 days. Patients could start to walk after 3 days and were discharged after 5 to 7 days.

Open excision after arthroscopic treatment (group B)

Patients were placed in supine position with routine anesthesia or epidural anesthesia. An arthroscope was utilized to clean the joint space and check for any meniscus or cartilage injuries and synovial hyperplasia. A total of 13 patients received meniscus repairs, and 11 received cartilage repairs. Next, patients were switched to the prone position for open excision. An S-shaped incision (8 to 12 cm) was made in the medial popliteal area. The deep fascia was incised longitudinally to expose the cyst. Blunt dissection was used around the cyst close to the semimembranosus muscle, the medial gastrocnemius muscle, and the bursa. The cyst was kept intact to avoid vessel and nerve damage. The cyst was lifted and cut off at the root. If the cyst was connected to the joint space, suturing was performed. Thoroughly flushing and suturing were the final steps. Bandage with moderate pressure and a drainage tube were placed after the procedure. The knee was restrained in the extension position. Quadriceps exercises started the next day. Patients were able to walk with cane after 7 days when post-surgical pain was largely relieved and subject to knee exercises strengthening gradually. Sutures were removed after 12–14 days.

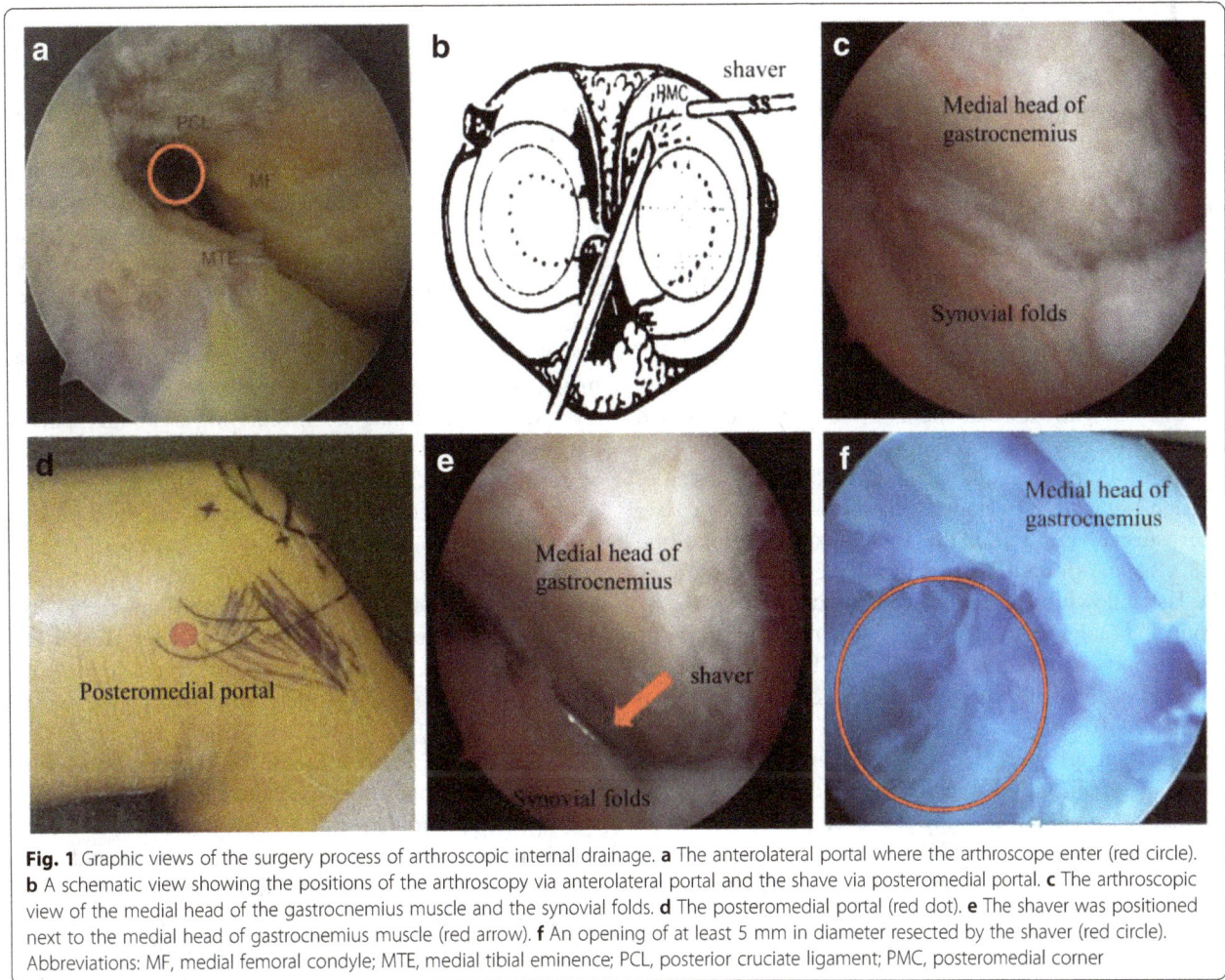

Fig. 1 Graphic views of the surgery process of arthroscopic internal drainage. **a** The anterolateral portal where the arthroscope enter (red circle). **b** A schematic view showing the positions of the arthroscopy via anterolateral portal and the shave via posteromedial portal. **c** The arthroscopic view of the medial head of the gastrocnemius muscle and the synovial folds. **d** The posteromedial portal (red dot). **e** The shaver was positioned next to the medial head of gastrocnemius muscle (red arrow). **f** An opening of at least 5 mm in diameter resected by the shaver (red circle). Abbreviations: MF, medial femoral condyle; MTE, medial tibial eminence; PCL, posterior cruciate ligament; PMC, posteromedial corner

Open excisions (group C)

Open excisions were performed in the same way as described in group B.

Follow-up visits

All functional evaluations during follow-up visits were performed by independent clinicians who were blinded to the treatment. Incision healing was assessed repeatedly on days 1, 2, 3, 5, 7, and 12 post surgery. The incision healing was evaluated as follows: grade 1, good healing with no adverse events; grade 2, redness, induration, and hematoma or fluid build-up around the incision; grade 3, suppuration around the incision that requires surgical drainage. The postoperative pain visual analog scale (VAS) score was assessed on the third day after surgeries. At the last follow-up visits, all patients underwent MRI scanning. The popliteal cysts were evaluated according to RLC, and knee functions were evaluated by Lysholm scores.

Statistics

Statistical analysis was performed using SPSS 18.0. The data were presented as mean ± standard deviation. Comparisons were done by one-way ANOVA with least significant difference post hoc test or chi-square test with chi-square partitioning. An α of 0.05 is considered as the cutoff for statistical significance.

Results

There was no significant difference in preoperative measurements among the three groups of patients, including age, gender, healing rate, preoperative Lysholm, and pain VAS scores (Table 1). The three groups were also no comparable in perioperative complications such as popliteal hematoma, neural or vascular injury, and symptomatic deep vein thrombosis (DVT) or pulmonary embolism (PE), as well as follow-up time. During arthroscopic treatment, those patients with co-existing injuries received repairing surgeries for management perspective. In total, 18 patients had meniscal surgery and 12 had chondral surgery in group A,

Table 1 Patient information

		Group A	Group B	Group C	F/x^2	P value
Age		55.3 ± 9.8	55.4 ± 7.6	54.2 ± 8.5	0.151	0.860
Gender	Male	15	9	11	0.064	0.968
	Female	17	10	14		
Preoperative Lysholm score		47.3 ± 5.7	47.3 ± 5.4	47.4 ± 4.7	0.001	0.999
Preoperative VAS score		6.5 ± 0.8	6.6 ± 0.9	6.2 ± 0.7	1.769	0.178
Perioperative complications		0	0	0		
Symptomatic DVT/PE	Yes	4	3	4	0.174	0.917
	No	28	16	21		
Follow-up time (months)		13.8 ± 2.7	13.7 ± 2.2	13.7 ± 2.3	0.006	0.994

whereas 13 patients had meniscal surgery and 11 had chondral surgery in group B.

Patients in group A did significantly better in terms of incision healing (100% grade 1), the pain VAS score 3 days after surgery (2.7 ± 1.2), the total hospitalization time (7.8 ± 2.8 days), and the Lysholm knee scaling score at the last follow-up (85.8 ± 5.2) compared to group B and group C (Table 2; $P < 0.05$). There was no significant difference between group B and group C (Table 3). Group A also had significantly shorter incision (1.6 ± 0.1 cm) than group C (10.6 ± 1.8), whereas group C was significantly shorter than group B (13.7 ± 2.7). As expected, group B required significantly longer operative duration (109.2 ± 25.4 min) compared to both group A (63.7 ± 12.7 min) and group C (62.5 ± 9.6 min).

In group A, we observed that the cysts started to shrink 2 months post surgery in 13 patients (Fig. 2). In 8 patients, the cysts completely disappeared by 8 months under MRI. At the last follow-up visits, which were on average 13.7 months after the surgery, an independent clinician who was blinded to the treatment scored all patients according to the Rauschning and Lindgren classification. The patients in grade II and above were defined as recurrent patients. The recurrence rates were significantly lower in group A (3.1%) and group B (5.2%) than those in group C (40%).

Table 2 Surgery and post-surgery data

		Group A	Group B	Group C
Surgical time (min)		63.7 ± 12.7	109.2 ± 25.4	62.5 ± 9.6
Length of incision (cm)		1.6 ± 0.1	13.7 ± 2.7	10.6 ± 1.8
Incision healing	Grade 1	32	14	18
	Grade 2	0	5	7
Postoperative VAS score		2.7 ± 1.2	4.1 ± 0.7	3.8 ± 0.8
Hospitalization time (days)		7.8 ± 2.8	15.9 ± 3.4	15.9 ± 5.5
Recovery to grade 0 or I cysts		96.9%	94.8%	60%
Recurrence rate		3.1%	5.2%	40%
Lysholm score at last follow-up		85.8 ± 5.2	80.3 ± 3.9	78.9 ± 5.0

Discussion

Popliteal cysts, also called Baker's cysts, are often seen at the gastrocnemius-semimembranosus bursa behind the knee joint [10]. Although the exact mechanisms for popliteal cysts are not clear, it is widely accepted that they result from a one-directional flow of knee effusion into the bursa through a valvular opening [11, 12]. Most popliteal cysts are connected to the knee joint space and often associated with intra-articular pathology [11–13]. Traditional treatment for popliteal cysts is using open excision from a posterior incision. However, this surgery usually involves extensive exposures and risk of neural or vascular injuries. Patients are prone to scar formation after surgery, resulting in unsatisfying cosmetic appearance [14]. More importantly, open excision does not address the associated intra-articular pathology and has a high recurrence rate [4, 15]. Based on the one-way valve mechanism, we believe that the key to successful treatment of popliteal cysts is dealing with the associated intra-articular lesions and re-establishing the bi-directional communication between the bursa and the joint space [16]. Arthroscopic internal drainage for popliteal cysts has become widely accepted in the recent years [6, 7].

In this study, we compared three different surgical approaches for popliteal cysts: arthroscopic internal drainage, open excision after arthroscopic treatment, and open excision alone. Arthroscopic internal drainage and open excision required less surgical time. In four patients of group A, arthroscopic internal drainage can be achieved within 45 min. On the other hand, the combination treatment needed much longer time, among which two surgeries lasted more than 2.5 h. Arthroscopic internal drainage was significantly better than the other approaches in the following parameters: the incision length, the incision healing rate, VAS pain score after surgery, and the Lysholm score at the last follow-up. Importantly, more than 1 year after the surgeries, we only observed one case of recurring cysts in patients receiving arthroscopic or combination treatment respectively. The recurrence rate was 3.1% for arthroscopic internal drainage and 5.2% for combination treatment, compared to 40% for open excision. It was consistent with previous publications that open excision procedure without other interventions leads to a higher recurrence rate [4, 9].

Arthroscopic treatment requires the smallest incision and is more effective to improve knee functions. It is capable of cleaning lesions inside the knee joint while simultaneously re-establishing the bi-directional communication between the cyst and the joint capsule [10]. Additionally, arthroscopic treatment is more cost-efficient by significantly shortening the hospitalization time.

Arthroscopic approach requires sufficient sterile saline, which can flush out free radicals and inflammatory

Table 3 Surgery and post-surgery data (post hoc analysis)

	Group A vs B		Group A vs C		Group B vs C	
	t/x^2	P value	t/x^2	P value	t/x^2	P value
Surgical time (min)	− 45.523	< 0.001	1.208	0.779	46.731	< 0.001
Length of incision (cm)	− 12.109	< 0.001	− 9.012	< 0.001	3.097	< 0.001
Incision healing rate	9.336	0.002	10.214	0.001	0.015	0.901
Postoperative VAS score	− 1.449	< 0.001	− 1.104	< 0.001	0.345	0.228
Hospitalization time (days)	− 8.051	< 0.001	− 8.076	< 0.001	− 0.025	0.983
Recovery to grade 0 or I cysts	0.145	0.704	12.254	< 0.001	6.947	0.008
Recurrence rate	0.145	0.704	12.254	< 0.001	6.947	0.008
Lysholm score at last follow-up	5.581	< 0.001	6.964	< 0.001	1.383	0.349

cytokines, leading to reduced infection, inflammatory responses, and pain postoperatively. We did not encounter infection in the arthroscopic internal drainage group. In the combination group, patients needed to be turned over and disinfected again, resulting in much longer procedure time, with increased the risk of infection [17]. Therefore, although very good outcomes of the combination treatment were observed here and others [18], the shorter operation duration and low infection rates favored arthroscopic internal drainage. Additionally, because of less pain scores in arthroscopic internal drainage, patients were able to walk earlier, which effectively prevented vein thrombosis in lower limbs. This resulted in shorter hospitalization time, which was cost-efficient.

Conclusions

Our results suggest that it is critical to clear intra-articular pathology for the successful treatment of popliteal cyst, whereas the removal of the cyst is not the primary goal for surgical intervention. Arthroscopic internal drainage of the cyst not only treats the intra-

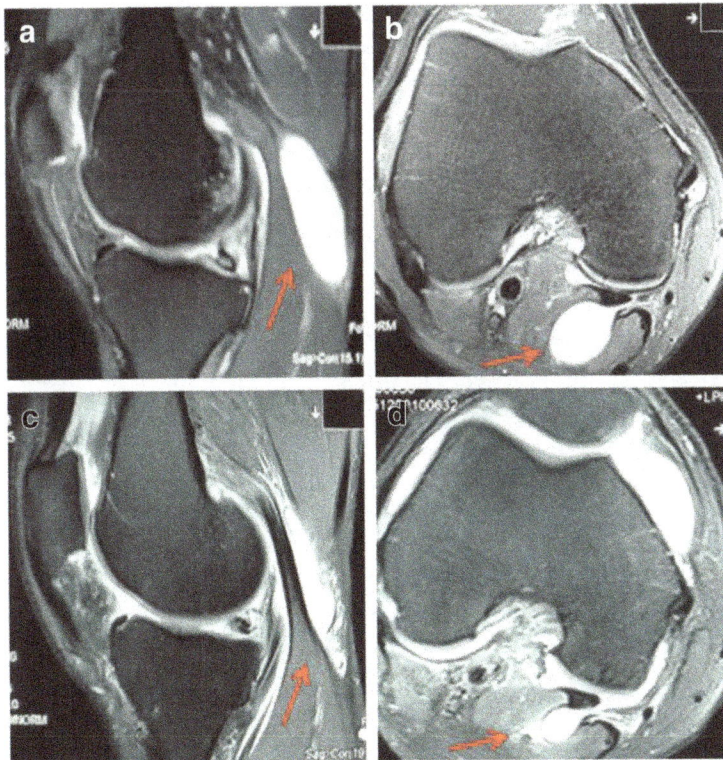

Fig. 2 Representative MRI images from group A patient, after receiving arthroscopic internal drainage. **a**, **b** Preoperative sagittal and axial views around the knee joint. **c**, **d** Postoperative sagittal and axial images at 2 months follow-up exhibited substantial shrinkage of the cyst. Red arrows indicate the popliteal cyst

articular lesions but also re-establishes the bi-directional communication between the bursa and the joint space. The minimally invasive procedure has small incision, quick recovery, good efficacy, and low recurrence rate. Although it may require a longer learning curve for the technique, we would recommend arthroscopic treatment for popliteal cysts in clinical practice.

Abbreviations
DVT: Deep vein thrombosis; PE: Pulmonary embolism; VAS: Visual analog score

Acknowledgements
We thank all the patients participating in this study. We thank SinoScript LLC for language proofreading.

Funding
Not applicable.

Authors' contributions
BY designed the study and randomly assigned the patient groups; BY, JL, LS, LG, and FL performed the procedures; FW and YL collected pre- and postoperative measurements and analyzed the data; BY, FW, and YL wrote the manuscript. All authors read and approved the final manuscript.

Competing interests
The authors declare that they have no competing interests.

References
1. Katz JN, Brownlee SA, Jones MH. The role of arthroscopy in the management of knee osteoarthritis. Best Pract Res Clin Rheumatol. 2014; 28(1):143–56.
2. Labropoulos N, Shifrin DA, Paxinos O. New insights into the development of popliteal cysts. Br J Surg. 2004;91(10):1313–8.
3. Takahashi M, Nagano A. Arthroscopic treatment of popliteal cyst and visualization of its cavity through the posterior portal of the knee. Arthroscopy. 2005;21(5):638.
4. Rupp S, Seil R, Jochum P. Long-term results after excision of a popliteal cyst. Unfallchirurg. 2001;104(9):847–51.
5. Malinowski K, Synder M, Sibinski M. Selected cases of arthroscopic treatment of popliteal cyst with associated intra-articular knee disorders primary report. Ortop Traumatol Rehabil. 2011;13(6):573–82.
6. Lie CW, Ng TP. Arthroscopic treatment of popliteal cyst. Hong Kong Med J. 2011;17(3):180–3.
7. Ohishi T, et al. Treatment of popliteal cysts via arthroscopic enlargement of unidirectional valvular slits. Mod Rheumatol. 2015;25(5):772–8.
8. Rupp S, et al. Popliteal cysts in adults. Prevalence, associated intraarticular lesions, and results after arthroscopic treatment. Am J Sports Med. 2002; 30(1):112–5.
9. Rauschning W, Lindgren PG. Popliteal cysts (Baker's cysts) in adults. I. Clinical and roentgenological results of operative excision. Acta Orthop Scand. 1979;50(5):583–91.
10. Kim KI, et al. Arthroscopic anatomic study of posteromedial joint capsule in knee joint associated with popliteal cyst. Arch Orthop Trauma Surg. 2014; 134(7):979–84.
11. Ko S, Ahn J. Popliteal cystoscopic excisional debridement and removal of capsular fold of valvular mechanism of large recurrent popliteal cyst. Arthroscopy. 2004;20(1):37–44.
12. Kim TW, Suh JT, Son SM, Moon TY, Lee IS, Choi KU, Kim JI. Baker's cyst with intramuscular extension into vastus medialis muscle. Knee Surg Relat Res. 2012;24(4):249–53.
13. Sansone V, et al. Popliteal cysts and associated disorders of the knee. Critical review with MR imaging. Int Orthop. 1995;19(5):275–9.
14. Bohensky MA, et al. Quantifying the excess cost and resource utilisation for patients with complications associated with elective knee arthroscopy: a retrospective cohort study. Knee. 2014;21(2):491–6.
15. Fritschy D, et al. The popliteal cyst. Knee Surg Sports Traumatol Arthrosc. 2006;14(7):623–8.
16. Sansone V, et al. An unusual cause of popliteal cyst. Arthroscopy. 2004;20(4): 432–4.
17. Pinkowsky GJ, Lynch S. Locked knee caused by lateral meniscal capsular disruption: verification by magnetic resonance imaging and arthroscopy. Am J Orthop (Belle Mead NJ). 2013;42(12):E116–7.
18. Saylik MGK. Treatment of baker cyst, by using open posterior cystectomy and supine arthroscopy on recalcitrant cases (103 knees). BMC Musculoskelet Disord. 2016;17:435.

18

Autologous platelet-rich plasma induces bone formation of tissue-engineered bone with bone marrow mesenchymal stem cells on beta-tricalcium phosphate ceramics

Tengbo Yu[1], Huazheng Pan[2], Yanling Hu[1*], Hao Tao[1], Kai Wang[1] and Chengdong Zhang[1]

Abstract

Background: The purpose of the study is to investigate whether autologous platelet-rich plasma (PRP) can serve as bone-inducing factors to provide osteoinduction and improve bone regeneration for tissue-engineered bones fabricated with bone marrow mesenchymal stem cells (MSCs) and beta-tricalcium phosphate (β-TCP) ceramics. The current study will give more insight into the contradictory osteogenic capacity of PRP.

Methods: The concentration of platelets, platelet-derived growth factor-AB (PDGF-AB), and transforming growth factor-β1 (TGF-β1) were measured in PRP and whole blood. Tissue-engineered bones using MSCs on β-TCP scaffolds in combination with autologous PRP were fabricated (PRP group). Controls were established without the use of autologous PRP (non-PRP group). In vitro, the proliferation and osteogenic differentiation of MSCs on fabricated constructs from six rabbits were evaluated with MTT assay, alkaline phosphatase (ALP) activity, and osteocalcin (OC) content measurement after 1, 7, and 14 days of culture. For in vivo study, the segmental defects of radial diaphyses of 12 rabbits from each group were repaired by fabricated constructs. Bone-forming capacity of the implanted constructs was determined by radiographic and histological analysis at 4 and 8 weeks postoperatively.

Results: PRP produced significantly higher concentration of platelets, PDGF-AB, and TGF-β1 than whole blood. In vitro study, MTT assay demonstrated that the MSCs in the presence of autologous PRP exhibited excellent proliferation at each time point. The results of osteogenic capacity detection showed significantly higher levels of synthesis of ALP and OC by the MSCs in combination with autologous PRP after 7 and 14 days of culture. In vivo study, radiographic observation showed that the PRP group produced significantly higher score than the non-PRP group at each time point. For histological evaluation, significantly higher volume of regenerated bone was found in the PRP group when compared with the non-PRP group at each time point.

Conclusions: Our study findings support the osteogenic capacity of autologous PRP. The results indicate that the use of autologous PRP is a simple and effective way to provide osteoinduction and improve bone regeneration for tissue-engineered bone reconstruction.

Keywords: Platelet-rich plasma, Tissue-engineered bone, Beta-tricalcium phosphate, Osteogenic, Scaffold, Autologous

* Correspondence: huyanlingqy@126.com
[1]Department of Orthopaedic Surgery, Affiliated Hospital of Qingdao University, Qingdao, Shandong 266000, People's Republic of China
Full list of author information is available at the end of the article

Background

Repair of bone defects remains a difficult challenge in orthopedic and maxillofacial surgery. A variety of strategies have been developed based on the dogma that the effectiveness of any successful bone graft material generally can be attributed to one or more of three properties: osteogenic cells, osteoconduction, and osteoinduction [1].

Nowadays, a tissue engineering strategy has appeared as one of the most promising approaches in regenerating damaged or diseased bones [2, 3]. The challenges of bone tissue engineering emphasize the need to provide osteoblast-like cells combined with growth factors in a biomechanically stable scaffold. Bone marrow mesenchymal stem cells (MSCs) have been demonstrated to be a very attractive cell source in tissue engineering due to their capacity to differentiate into lineages of the mesenchymal tissues, including the bone, the cartilage, and the muscle [4]. With regard to the scaffold used in bone tissue engineering, beta-tricalcium phosphate (β-TCP) ceramics have been extensively recognized as scaffolds because they possess satisfactory biocompatibility, osteoconductivity, and mechanical properties [5, 6]. However, they do not have osteoinductive capacity. This incapacity of inducing bone formation can be overcome by adding growth factors and cytokines onto ceramic scaffolds.

Platelet-rich plasma (PRP) is a concentration of platelets in a small volume of plasma. Because biological factors released by platelets have an effect on osteocompetent cells, scientists have proposed the delivery of a concentrate of platelets at the site of the injury as a successful strategy for fostering the regeneration pathway during bone wound healing [7, 8]. Autologous PRP has been used for the treatment of bone defects in maxillofacial surgery and orthopedics for accelerating bone formation [9, 10]. However, the effects of PRP on the enhancement of bone regeneration remain debated. Some studies have not observed any improvement in bone formation and maturation [11–14]. The contradictory PRP study outcomes remain to be elucidated. Furthermore, to the best of our knowledge, there are no studies that evaluated the performance of autologous PRP in combination with MSCs and β-TCP to repair segmental bone defects in vivo.

In the present study, a tissue-engineered bone using MSCs on a β-TCP scaffold in combination with autologous PRP was developed. The vitro proliferation, osteogenic differentiation of MSCs and in vivo bone-forming capacity in segmental bone defect models of the fabricated constructs were evaluated when in combination with autologous PRP or not.

The purpose of this study is to investigate whether autologous PRP can serve as bone-inducing factors to provide osteoinduction and improve bone regeneration for tissue-engineered bones fabricated with MSCs and β-

TCP ceramics. The current study will give more insight into the contradictory osteogenic capacity of PRP.

Methods

Animals and scaffold materials

Ten-month-old male New Zealand white rabbits weighing 2.0–2.5 kg were employed. The present research was approved by the Qingdao University Medical College Medical Ethics Committee. All experimental procedures were in compliance with the principles of International Laboratory Animal Care and with the European Communities Council Directive (86/809/EEC).

β-TCP scaffolds (Bio-lu Bio Materials Company Limited, China) were formed into cuboids (5 × 5 × 5 mm) for in vitro study and cylinders (diameter, 4 mm; length, 12 mm) for in vivo study. The scaffold had a high degree of porosity (75 ± 10%) and was completely interconnected. The average pore diameter was 530 ± 50 μm, and the interconnecting channels were 150 ± 50 μm in diameter. These parameters meet the criteria to act as scaffold material for bone regeneration [15, 16].

Isolation, expansion, and osteogenic differentiation of rabbit MSCs

Samples of MSCs were obtained from iliac bone marrow aspirates of New Zealand white rabbits. MSCs isolation and expansion were performed as reported by Liu H et al. [17]. Briefly, nucleated cells were isolated using the density gradient centrifugation method. Then, cells were cultured at 37 °C in a humidified atmosphere containing 5%CO_2, and medium was changed every 3 days. Upon reaching about 90% confluence, the cells were trypsinized and replated at 1×10^4 cells/cm^2 for further expansion. Cell passaging was performed and cells from the third passage were used in the following experiments. The MSCs from rabbits were cultured individually.

To induce osteogenic differentiation, the third passage cells were then cultured for up to 2 weeks in an osteogenic induction medium containing basic culture medium, with the addition of 100 nM dexamethasone, 50 μg/ml ascorbic acid-2-phosphate, and 10 mM β-glycerophosphate (all from Sigma). The culture medium was changed every 3 days. The osteogenic differentiation of MSCs was confirmed by positive results of alkaline phosphatase (ALP) and Alizarin red S staining.

Preparation of autologous PRP

Autologous PRP was prepared from the same rabbit as used for MSCs isolation as described by Ishida et al. [18]. Briefly, 10 ml of peripheral blood was drawn, via puncture of the central auricular artery, into a syringe containing 1 ml of acid citrate dextrose. The blood sample was initially centrifuged for 15 min at 800 rpm at 20 °C to separate the plasma containing the platelets from the red cells. The plasma was drawn off the top and centrifuged again for 15 min at 2000 rpm at 20 °C to separate the platelets. The platelet-poor plasma was then drawn off the top, leaving the PRP and buffy coat. Then, the buffy coat and PRP were re-suspended, and about 1 ml of PRP was produced.

In vitro study

Six New Zealand white rabbits were used for in vitro study. The undifferentiated MSCs and their autologous PRP were prepared from these rabbits.

Measurement of platelets and growth factors

The concentrations of platelets in PRP and whole blood were counted with an automated hematology analyzer (Nikon, Japan). To measure the concentrations of growth factors in PRP, thrombin (0.8IUactivity)-calcium chloride (1 M) solution (1:1) (Tissucol-Duo, Baxter, Germany) is used to activate the platelets. The fibrin gel was formed within 8 to 10 mins. The concentrations of platelet-derived growth factor-AB (PDGF-AB) and transforming growth factor-β1 (TGF-β1) secreted from activated PRP and whole blood were measured with commercial enzyme-linked immunosorbent assay (ELISA) kit (Cusabio Biotech Co. Ltd., China), according to the manufacturer's instructions.

Cell seeding and in vitro cultivation of constructs

The autologous PRP and cell suspension at a density of 1×10^7 cells/ml were mixed at a volume ratio of 4:1 to obtain cell-PRP mixture at a density of 2×10^6 cells/ml as reported by Tajima et al. [19]. One hundred microliters of cell-PRP mixture was evenly dripped onto each β-TCP scaffold (PRP group). Controls were established without the use of PRP. MSC suspensions at a density of 2×10^6 cells/ml were seeded into β-TCP scaffolds to fabricate constructs (non-PRP group). The constructs were incubated at 37 °C for 2 h to allow for cell diffusion and attachment. Then, 20 μl of thrombin (0.8IUactivity)-calcium chloride (1 M) solution (1:1) (Tissucol-Duo, Baxter, Germany) was added onto fabricated constructs. All constructs were cultured statically for up to 2 weeks in an osteogenic induction medium which contained basic culture medium, with the addition of 100 nM dexamethasone, 50 μg/ml ascorbic acid-2-phosphate, and 10 mM β-glycerophosphate (all from Sigma). The medium was changed every 3 days.

Cell proliferation assay

The proliferation of MSCs on fabricated constructs was measured by using the MTT (3-(4,5-dimethylthiazol-2yl)-2,5-diphenyl-2H-tetrazolium bromide) assay after 1, 7, and 14 days of culture as described by Wang H et al. [20]. The absorbance of the solution in each well was measured by a microplate reader (Bio-Tek, USA) at a wavelength of 570 nm.

Cell osteogenic differentiation assay

ALP and osteocalcin (OC) as the quantitative indices of osteogenic capability were measured after 1, 7, and 14 days of culture. To assess the ALP activity, cell lysates were prepared using the procedure described by Jiang et al. [21]. ALP activity assay is based on the conversion of p-nitrophenyl phosphate (P-NPP) into p-nitrophenol (P-NP) in the presence of ALP, where the rate of P-NP production is proportional to ALP activity. Protein concentrations of the cell lysates were determined by Bradford protein assay (Bio-Rad Laboratories, USA). The results of ALP activity were expressed as nmol/min/mg protein. OC content was measured by radioimmunoassay using an OC RIA Kit (Dongya, Beijing, China) in accordance with the manufacturer's instruction. OC content was normalized to protein concentration.

In vivo study

Twenty-four New Zealand white rabbits used for in vivo study were randomized into the PRP group and non-PRP group by coin flipping. Both groups were then randomly subdivided into two subgroups that were sacrificed after 4 and 8 weeks postoperatively. The osteogenically differentiated MSCs and their autologous PRP were obtained from these rabbits.

Preparation of implants

Following the above-mentioned cell seeding method, 200 μl of cell-PRP mixture or cell suspension was respectively dripped onto each cylindrical scaffold. Two hours later, 40 μl of thrombin (0.8IUactivity)-calcium chloride (1 M) solution (1:1) (Tissucol-Duo, Baxter, Germany) was added onto fabricated constructs.

Surgical procedures for implantation

The segmental bone defect model was prepared as described by Niemeyer P et al. [22]. Briefly, under sterile conditions, the left radial shaft was exposed through a 2-cm longitudinal incision over the radius. A 12-mm bone segment with periosteum was excised from the middle of the radial diaphysis. The ulna was left intact for mechanical stability. The fabricated constructs were implanted into bone defects according to the scheduled grouping. The middle point of the length for each implanted construct was labeled with a 3–0 suture for the accurate selection of histological sections of specimens. All rabbits were kept in separate cages, fed a standard diet, and allowed to move freely after surgery without plaster immobilization.

Radiographic evaluation

Six rabbits from each subgroup were subject to X-ray examination respectively at 4 and 8 weeks postoperatively. The exposure conditions were 45 kV, 125 mA, and 32 ms. The exposure distance was 100 cm. The films were analyzed and scored following Yang's method [23]. The scale was composed of four categories (Table 1). The proximal, central, and distal part of graft was scored individually, and a summarized score was calculated. Scoring was assessed under a double blinding protocol by two independent observers.

Histological evaluation

After the above-mentioned examination, the six rabbits from each subgroup were sacrificed. The implant site (12 mm) along with the host bone (5 mm from either side) of each animal was resected out from the whole bone. The specimens were fixed with 4% buffered paraformaldehyde, decalcified in 50 mM ethylenediaminetetraacetic acid, and embedded in paraffin. The sections (5 μm thick) at the interface region were longitudinally cut and stained with hematoxylin and eosin (HE) to evaluate bony union between host bone and implants. Furthermore, three levels of sections (5 μm thick) were transversely sliced at a quarter, half, and three-quarter of the length of each implanted construct and stained with HE to analyze new bone formation. Each section was

Table 1 Radiographic grading system [23]

Grading items	Score
Periosteal reaction[a]	
None	0
Minimal (localized to the gap)	1
Medium (extends over the gap; < 1/4)	2
Moderate (< 1/2 but > 3/4)	3
Full	4
Osteotomy site[a]	
Osteotomy line completely radiolucent	0
Osteotomy line partially radiolucent	2
Osteotomy line invisible	4
Remodeling[a]	
None apparent	0
Intramedullary space	1
Intracortical	2
Graft appearance[a]	
Unchanged/intact	0
Mild resorption	1
Moderate replacement	2
Mostly replaced	3
Fully reorganized	4

[a]Proximal, distal, and central part of graft scored individually

observed under light microscope by two independent observers, and 10 images were randomly obtained in one section. All images were transferred to a computer for image processing and analysis (Image-Pro Plus software, Media Cybernetics, USA). The tissue composition of the new bone, β-TCP, and connective tissue were presented as the percentage of bone area in relation to the view field area of each image. Based on the percentage of tissue composition of three representative sections from three levels, the average percentage per implanted construct was calculated.

Statistical analysis

Results are expressed as mean ± standard deviation. Statistical analysis to compare results between two groups was carried out by independent sample t test with SPSS for Windows 15.0 (SPSS, USA). Differences were considered to be significant if $p < 0.05$.

Results

Concentration of platelets and growth factors

The mean platelet count for PRP was $1056 ± 106 × 10^3$ platelets/μl, while that of whole blood was $201 ± 23 × 10^3$ platelets/μl (a 5.25-fold increase in platelets in PRP than in whole blood). Correspondingly, PRP produced 2.64-fold increase in PDGF-AB concentration and 3.54-fold increase in TGF-β1 concentration respectively. These values confirmed the presence of a sufficient concentration of platelets during the PRP preparation. The concentration of platelet, TGF-β1, and PDGF-AB were significantly higher in PRP than those in whole blood ($p < 0.05$, Table 2).

Cell proliferation in vitro

The absorbance values for two groups of MSCs increased with the length of the culture period. The PRP group demonstrated significantly higher absorbance values compared with the non-PRP group at all time points ($p < 0.05$), which indicates that autologous PRP has a stimulative effect on the MSCs proliferation (Fig. 1).

Cell osteogenic differentiation in vitro

The ALP activity of the two groups of MSCs increased with prolonged incubation period. At 1 day after seeding, there was no significant difference in ALP activity. However, significantly higher ALP activity was detected

Table 2 Concentration of platelets and growth factors in PRP and whole blood ($n = 6$, mean ± SD)

	Platelet(10^9/L)	PDGF-AB(ng/ml)	TGF-β1 (ng/ml)
Whole blood	201.57 ± 23.35	19.43 ± 0.92	36.32 ± 3.87
PRP	1056.28 ± 106.17*	51.25 ± 5.46*	128.62 ± 13.05*

*$p < 0.05$ compared with whole blood

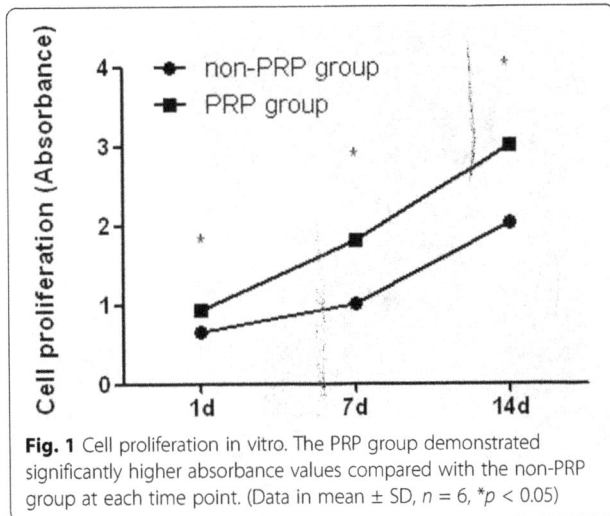

Fig. 1 Cell proliferation in vitro. The PRP group demonstrated significantly higher absorbance values compared with the non-PRP group at each time point. (Data in mean ± SD, n = 6, *p < 0.05)

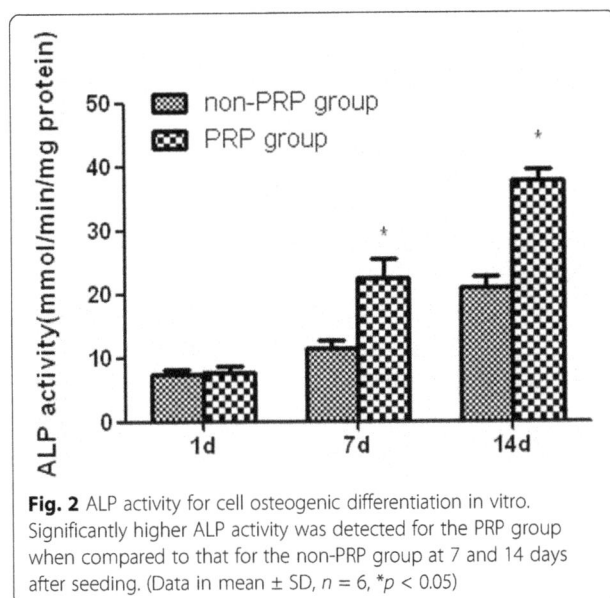

Fig. 3 OC content for cell osteogenic differentiation in vitro. The PRP group exhibited significantly higher OC content than the non-PRP group on days 7 and 14 after being cultured. (Data in mean ± SD, n = 6, *p < 0.05)

for the PRP group when compared to the non-PRP group at 7 and 14 days after seeding (p < 0.05, Fig. 2). As for OC content, no OC was detected for both groups at 1 day of cultivation. The PRP group exhibited significantly higher OC content than the non-PRP group on days 7 and 14 after being cultured (p < 0.05, Fig. 3). These results indicate that autologous PRP is effective for promoting osteogenic differentiation of MSCs.

Radiographic evaluation

At 4 weeks postoperatively, the high-density radioopaque areas of implants were clearly identified at bone defect sites in both groups and a distinct radiolucent zone at the interface between the implant and the host bone was visible. However, the boundary of implanted constructs in PRP group became more cloudy along with

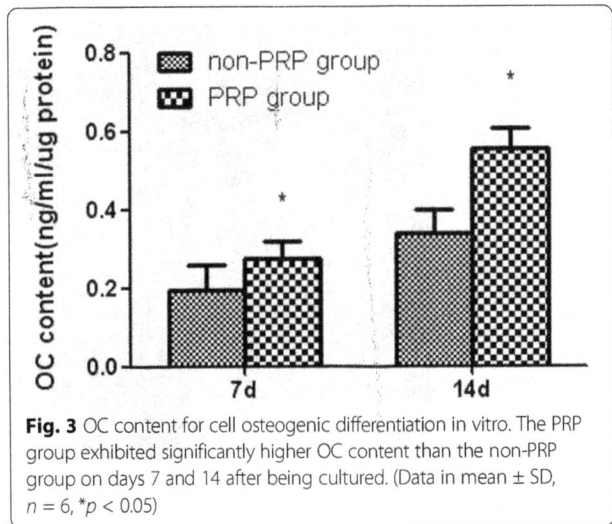

Fig. 2 ALP activity for cell osteogenic differentiation in vitro. Significantly higher ALP activity was detected for the PRP group when compared to that for the non-PRP group at 7 and 14 days after seeding. (Data in mean ± SD, n = 6, *p < 0.05)

degradation and more bone callus at the interfacial area was found. At 8 weeks postoperatively, the absence of this radiolucent zone was observed for both groups, which is considered as the union between the implant and host bone. PRP group achieved more osseous callus around the periphery of the implant (Fig. 4). The radiographic grading score at the proximal, central, and distal part of implants graft increased with implantation time in both groups. The PRP group showed significantly higher score than the non-PRP group at each time point (p < 0.05, Table 3). Correspondingly, summarized scores showed similar results, also reaching statistical significance (p < 0.05, Table 3).

Gross view and histological evaluation

All rabbits survived until the scheduled date of sacrifice without any evidence of inflammation or infection at the implantation site such as incision infection or skin necrosis. At 4 weeks after surgery, the entire implanted material could be identified for both groups, and the interface between the implant and the host bone was visible. At 8 weeks postoperatively, both groups achieved integration between implanted constructs and host bone on either side. The implanted material was still identifiable in the middle region of defect in Non-PRP group, while no apparent remnants of implanted material were found in PRP group.

Under a light microscope, the micro pores of the implanted constructs in both groups were filled with loose connective tissue at 4 weeks postoperatively. More newly formed bone tissues were deposited in PRP group. With the implantation prolonged, the new bone formation and the degradation of scaffolds were increasingly obvious. At 8 weeks postoperatively, the PRP group demonstrated more extensive bone formation with the degradation of most of the scaffolds compared with the

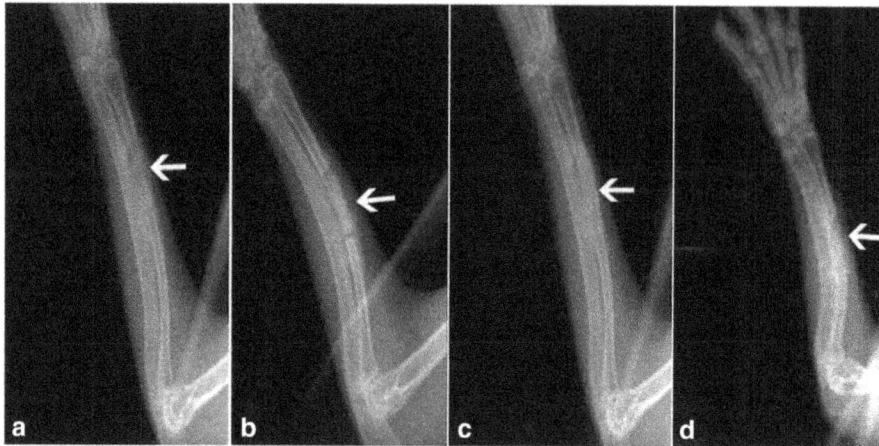

Fig. 4 Representative radiographs of critical-sized bone defects repair by PRP group constructs (**a**, **c**) and Non-PRP group constructs (**b**, **d**) at 4 weeks (**a**, **b**) and 8 weeks (**c**, **d**) postoperatively. At 4 weeks postoperatively, the radioopaque areas of implants and radiolucent zone at the interface between the implant and host bone was visible in both groups. However, the boundary of constructs in the PRP group became more cloudy. At 8 weeks postoperatively, a decrease in radiopacity related to the new bone formation and material degradation was more obvious in the PRP group. The radiolucent zone at the interfacial area almost disappeared in the PRP group. The arrow indicates the implanted construct

non-PRP group (Fig. 5). Furthermore, the amount of newly formed bone varied in the different locations of implants. New bone formation was more obvious in the peripheral regions of implants than that in the central regions at any time point. The percentage of new bone tissue in the defect region increased with time in both groups. The extent of new bone formation was significantly more obvious in the PRP group than that in the non-PRP group at each time point ($p < 0.05$, Table 4). For the amount of remaining β-TCP and connective tissue, inverse results were found, also reaching statistical significance ($p < 0.05$, Table 4). At the interfacial area between the implant and the host bone, newly formed bone grew and merged for both groups with prolonged implantation period. Although similar histological changes occurred, the amount and rate of new bone formation of the non-PRP group was less and slower than that of the PRP group (Fig. 6).

Discussion

The hypothesis for this study was that the introduction of autologous PRP may improve the osteogenic potential of tissue-engineered bones. In vitro study, MTT assay demonstrated that the MSCs in the presence of autologous PRP exhibited excellent proliferation at each time point. Osteogenic differentiation results showed significantly high levels of synthesis of ALP and OC by the MSCs in combination with autologous PRP after 7 and 14 days of culture. No OC was detected for both groups at 1 day of cultivation. This is probably because OC is a late marker of the maintenance of the osteoblastic phenotype. With regard to the bone-forming capacity in vivo, radiographic and histological observation showed that the PRP group constructs accelerated bone healing in rabbit segmental defects of radial diaphyses over the 8-week period, compared with the non-PRP group constructs. The radiographic observation showed that the PRP group produced significantly higher score than the Non-PRP group at each time point. For histological evaluation, significantly higher volume of regenerated bone was found in the PRP group when compared with the non-PRP group at each time point. Given these results, it is clear that the autologous PRP had a stimulative effect on in vitro proliferation and osteogenic differentiation, and in vivo bone formation of MSCs in our experimental setting.

PRP develops a fibrin gel network containing a myriad of growth factors after activation, such as platelet-

Table 3 X-ray scores at the proximal, central and distal location and summarized scores of implants ($n = 6$, mean ± SD)

Group	Time	Proximal	Central	Distal	summarized
Non-PRP group	4 weeks	2.667 ± 0.817	1.5 ± 1.049	3 ± 0.894	7.167 ± 1.835
PRP group	4 weeks	4.833 ± 1.472*	3 ± 0.894*	4.667 ± 1.211*	12.5 ± 2.811*
Non-PRP group	8 weeks	7.5 ± 1.049	3.667 ± 1.633	7 ± 1.549	18.167 ± 1.602
PRP group	8 weeks	10.5 ± 1.653*	6 ± 1.265*	11.833 ± 2.927*	28.333 ± 1.862*

*$p < 0.05$ compared with the non-PRP group

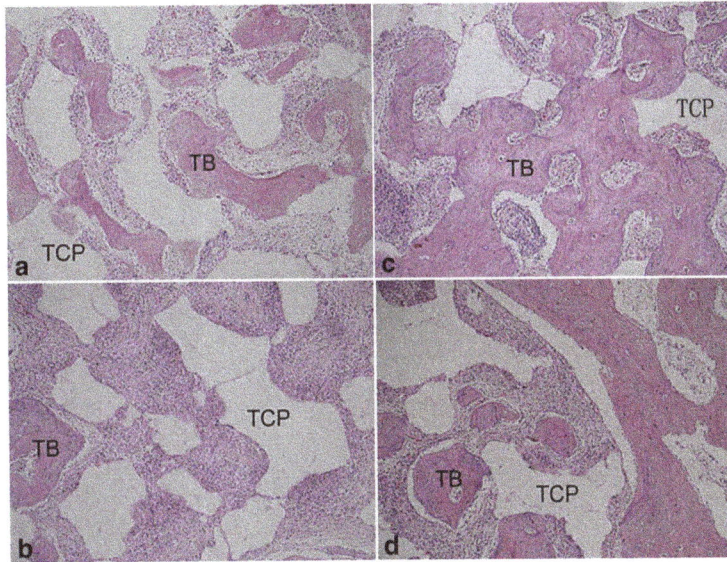

Fig. 5 Histological evaluation of regenerated bone of PRP group constructs (**a**, **c**) and non-PRP group constructs (**b**, **d**) at 4 weeks (**a**, **b**) and 8 weeks (**c**, **d**) postoperatively. The PRP group demonstrated more extensive bone formation with the degradation of implanted constructs than the non-PRP group at each time point. (HE staining × 100. TCP, tricalcium phosphate; TB, tissue-engineered bone)

derived growth factor (PDGF) and transforming growth factor (TGF). All these factors have a stimulating effect on bone defect healing via chemotactic and mitogenic effects on preosteoblastic and osteoblastic cells [7, 8, 24–26]. Thus, the possibility of delivering these matrix elements and growth factors within a bone defect is behind the theory of the use of PRP in bone reconstruction therapy. Since the local application of PRP was proposed by Marx et al. [27] to enhance and accelerate the maturity of corticocancellous grafts to repair continuity defects of the maxillofacial region in 1998, PRP has been widely used in preclinical and clinical applications for regeneration of the bone. However, its use has never produced consistent and reliable results in terms of bone regeneration. The inconsistency of results found in various studies may result from differences in platelet concentration, biology among species, bone defect models and bone grafting materials combined with PRP. It should be noticed that these studies should not be directly compared because the study designs were very different.

Platelet concentration of prepared PRP is one of the key factors that may help in understanding such controversial results about the effectiveness of PRP. Platelet count in PRP may vary according to the preparation technique, ranging from two to several folds above the physiological levels. It has been stated by Weibrich et al. [28] that advantageous biological effects seem to occur when PRP with a platelet concentration of approximately 1,000,000/µl is used. At lower concentrations, the effect is suboptimal, while higher concentrations might have a paradoxically inhibitory effect. It also has been suggested that PRP should achieve a two- to sixfold increase in platelet concentration over baseline [7, 8]. In the current study, PRP platelet count were $1056 \pm 106 \times 10^3$ platelets/µl, a measured increase of $525 \pm 36\%$ from whole blood. Correspondingly, PRP produced 2.64-fold increase in PDGF-AB concentration and 3.54-fold increase in TGF-β1. This may represent an explanation for the positive results of the present study.

With regard to grafting materials combined with PRP, several studies have evaluated the effect of PRP in combination with β-TCP materials. The study from Li H et al. [29] reported that the addition of PRP to β-TCP failed to improve bone healing in an anterior spinal

Table 4 Tissue composition by the new bone, β-TCP, and connective tissue of implants ($n = 6$, mean ± SD)

Group	Time	New bone (%)	β-TCP (%)	Connective tissue (%)
Non-PRP group	4 weeks	16.333 ± 2.16	41 ± 3.578	41.333 ± 3.011
PRP group	4 weeks	29.667 ± 1.366*	36 ± 3.847*	36 ± 4.243*
Non-PRP group	8 weeks	29.333 ± 1.75	36.5 ± 1.871	33.833 ± 2.858
PRP group	8 weeks	39.5 ± 1.871*	29.5 ± 1.049*	29.333 ± 2.582*

*$p < 0.05$ compared with the non-PRP group

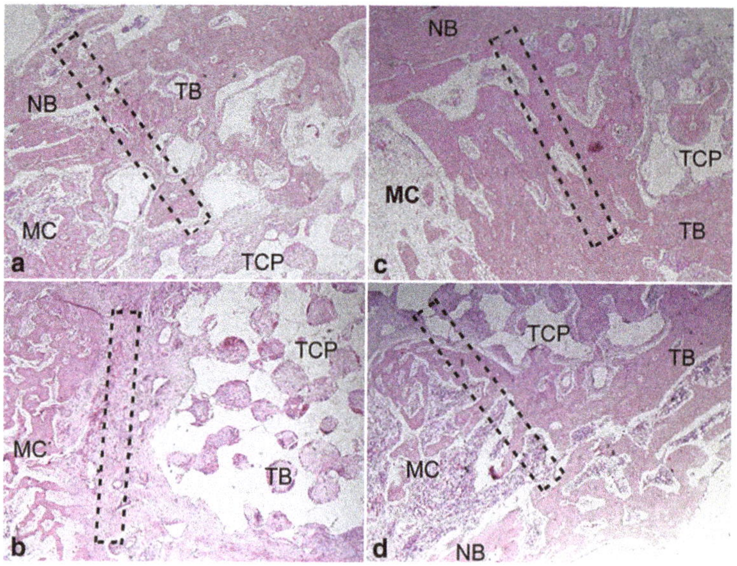

Fig. 6 Histological evaluation of interfacial area between the implant and the host bone of PRP group constructs (**a**, **c**) and non-PRP group constructs (**b**, **d**) at 4 weeks (**a**, **b**) and 8 weeks (**c**, **d**) postoperatively. The newly formed bone grew and merged at interfacial area for both groups with implantation period prolonging. However, the amount and rate of the new bone formation of the non-PRP group was less and slower than that of PRP group (HE staining; × 40. TCP, tricalcium phosphate; TB, tissue-engineered bone; NB, native bone; MC, medullary cavity. The dotted rectangles indicate the interfacial area)

fusion. The reason for the failure of PRP might be the absence of precursor cells. The study by Kasten P et al. [30] found that MSC/TCP failed to profit from the frozen PRP for ectopic bone formation. One possible explanation is that that frozen PRP has weaker osteogenic properties than fresh PRP. Nowadays, there is no data that proves that frozen PRP is equally effective as fresh PRP regarding osteogenesis. The beneficial effect of autologous PRP combined with β-TCP was reported by Long Bi et al. [31], who used a goat tibial cavity defect model.

In the present study, a segmental bone defect model in a rabbit radius was adapted for low regenerative potential and similarity to the clinical situation, which is of great interest for an orthopedic surgeon. Management of large segmental bone defects, particularly in diaphyseal bones, remains a considerable challenge for orthopedic surgeons. In recent years, tissue engineering has provided a promising method for repairing such bone defects [32]. However, the clinical application of these advances in the field of tissue engineering is still limited. Increasing research has found that the key factor contributing to poor repair with a tissue-engineered bone is poor vascularization [33, 34]. Several strategies for enhancing vascularization are currently under investigation. These include modification of the scaffold design, delivery of angiogenic factors, and prevascularization procedure [35]. Vascular endothelial growth factor (VEGF) as angiogenic factors can enhance regional vascularization by altering the responsiveness of local

endothelia cells to angiogenic stimuli [36, 37]. Furthermore, VEGF was demonstrated by Street et al. [38] to stimulate bone repair by promoting angiogenesis and bone turnover. When PRP is combined with TCP scaffolds, the platelet can release the VEGF. So the fabricated constructs possess angiogenic factors, which may improve the bone regeneration by increasing vascular growth. This may be one of the reasons for more effective repair of segmental bone defect models. The limitation of the current experimental design is that the blood vessel formation of tissue-engineered bone constructs was not investigated. This should be addressed in future studies.

At present, it is recognized that growth factors regulate fracture healing and physiological remodeling by inducing chemotaxis, differentiation, proliferation, and synthetic activity of bone cells. However, the combinations, concentrations, and application time points of various growth factors in reparative processes were poorly understood. Our findings support the use of autologous PRP as an easy and physiological way of application for growth factors in natural composition to improve bone regeneration. A combination of MSCs with PRP on biomechanically stable β-TCP scaffolds fulfills the requirements of ideal bone graft substitutes: progenitor cells for osteogenesis, scaffold material for osteoconduction, and growth factors for osteoinduction. All these may explain the success of fabricated tissue-engineered bone observed in our experimental setting. Furthermore, the advantages of autologous PRP also include its safety and its availability in an easy-to-develop manner.

Conclusions

Our study findings support the osteogenic capacity of autologous PRP. The results indicate that the use of autologous PRP is a simple and effective way to provide osteoinduction and improve bone regeneration for tissue-engineered bone reconstruction.

Abbreviations

ALP: Alkaline phosphatase; MSC: Marrow mesenchymal stem cell; OC: Osteocalcin; PDGF: Platelet-derived growth factor; PRP: Platelet-rich plasma; TGF: Transforming growth factor; β-TCP: Beta-tricalcium phosphate

Acknowledgements

The authors are grateful to Dr. Peng Zhao for the technical assistance with histology. We acknowledge all the staff in the animal experiment center of Qingdao University, who contributed great help on animal daily nursing care.

Funding

This study was supported by the High Education Development Foundation of Shandong Province, China (No. J11LF22).

Authors' contributions

TB Y, YL H, and HZ P made substantial contributions to the conception and design, acquisition of data, analysis and interpretation of data, and drafting of the manuscript; HT performed the statistical analysis. KW and CD Z participated in the design and coordination of the study, and assisted with drafting the manuscript. All authors carried out the analyses, read, and approved the final manuscript.

Competing interests

The authors declare that they have no competing interests.

Author details

[1]Department of Orthopaedic Surgery, Affiliated Hospital of Qingdao University, Qingdao, Shandong 266000, People's Republic of China.
[2]Department of Clinical Laboratory, Affiliated Hospital of Qingdao University, Qingdao, Shandong 266000, People's Republic of China.

References

1. Bauer TW, Muschler GF. Bone graft materials. An overview of the basic science. Clin Orthop Relat Res. 2000;371:10–27.
2. Schroeder JE, Mosheiff R. Tissue engineering approaches for bone repair: concepts and evidence. Injury. 2011;42(6):609–13.
3. Drosse I, Volkmer E, Capanna R, De Biase P, Mutschler W, Schieker M. Tissue engineering for bone defect healing: an update on a multi-component approach. Injury. 2008;39(Suppl 2):S9–20.
4. Pountos I, Giannoudis PV. Biology of mesenchymal stem cells. Injury. 2005; 36(Suppl 3):S8–12.
5. Fujibayashi S, Shikata J, Tanaka C, Matsushita M, Nakamura T. Lumbar posterolateral fusion with biphasic calcium phosphate ceramic. J Spinal Disord. 2001;14:214–21.
6. Kasten P, Beyen I, Niemeyer P, Luginbühl R, Bohner M, Richter W. Porosity and pore size of beta-tricalcium phosphate scaffold can influence protein production and osteogenic differentiation of human mesenchymal stem cells: an in vitro and in vivo study. Acta Biomater. 2008;4:1904–15.
7. Marx RE. Platelet-rich plasma: evidence to support its use. J Oral Maxillofac Surg. 2004;62(4):489–96.
8. Intini G. The use of platelet-rich plasma in bone reconstruction therapy. Biomaterials. 2009;30(28):4956–66.
9. Kitoh H, Kitakoji T, Tsuchiya H, Katoh M, Ishiguro N. Transplantation of culture expanded bone marrow cells and platelet rich plasma in distraction osteogenesis of the long bones. Bone. 2007;40(2):522–8.
10. Simon Z, Friedlich J. The use of autogenous bone grafting with platelet-rich plasma for alveolar ridge reconstruction: a clinical report. J Calif Dent Assoc. 2006;34(11):895–9.
11. Aghaloo TL, Moy PK, Freymiller EG. Investigation of platelet-rich plasma in rabbit cranial defects: a pilot study. J Oral Maxillofac Surg. 2002;60:1176–81.
12. Froum SJ, Wallace SS, Tarnow DP, Cho SC. Effect of platelet-rich plasma on bone growth and osseointegration in human maxillary sinus grafts: three bilateral case reports. Int J Periodontics Restorative Dent. 2002;22(1):45–53.
13. Choi BH, Im CJ, Huh JY, Suh JJ, Lee SH. Effect of platelet-rich plasma on bone regeneration in autogenous bone graft. Int J Oral Maxillofac Surg. 2004;33:56–9.
14. Gerard D, Carlson ER, Gotcher JE, Jacobs M. Effects of platelet-rich plasma on the healing of autologous bone grafted mandibular defects in dogs. J Oral Maxillofac Surg. 2006;64:443–51.
15. Karageorgiou V, Kaplan D. Porosity of 3D biomaterial scaffolds and osteogenesis. Biomaterials. 2005;26(27):5474–91.
16. Kamitakahara M, Ohtsuki C, Miyazaki T. Behavior of ceramic biomaterials derived from tricalcium phosphate in physiological condition. J Biomater Appl. 2008;23(3):197–212.
17. Liu H, Li H, Cheng W, Yang Y, Zhu M, Zhou C. Novel injectable calcium phosphate/chitosan composites for bone substitute materials. Acta Biomater. 2006;2:557–65.
18. Ishida K, Kuroda R, Miwa M, Tabata Y, Hokugo A, Kawamoto T, et al. The regenerative effects of platelet-rich plasma on meniscal cells in vitro and its in vivo application with biodegradable gelatin hydrogel. Tissue Eng. 2007;13(5):1103–12.
19. Tajima N, Sotome S, Marukawa E, Omura K, Shinomiya K. A three-dimensional cell-loading system using autologous plasma loaded into a porous β-tricalcium-phosphate block promotes bone formation at extraskeletal sites in rats. Mater Sci Eng C. 2007;27:625–32.
20. Wang H, Li Y, Zuo Y, Li J, Ma S, Cheng L. Biocompatibility and osteogenesis of biomimetic nano-hydroxyapatite/polyamide composite scaffolds for bone tissue engineering. Biomaterials. 2007;28(22):3338–48.
21. Jiang T, Abdel-Fattah WI, Laurencin CT. In vitro evaluation of chitosan/poly(lactic acid-glycolic acid) sintered microsphere scaffolds for bone tissue engineering. Biomaterials. 2006;27(28):4894–903.
22. Niemeyer P, Szalay K, Luginbühl R, Südkamp NP, Kasten P. Transplantation of human mesenchymal stem cells in a non-autogenous setting for bone regeneration in a rabbit critical-size defect model. Acta Biomater. 2010;6(3):900–8.
23. Yang CY, Simmons DJ, Lozano R. The healing of grafts combining freeze-dried and demineralized allogeneic bone in rabbits. Clin Orthop Relat Res. 1994;298:286–95.
24. Fiedler J, Roderer G, Gunther KP, Brenner RE. BMP-2, BMP-4, and PDGF-bb stimulate chemotactic migration of primary human mesenchymal progenitor cells. J Cell Biochem. 2002;87:305–12.
25. Baylink DJ, Finkelman RD, Mohan S. Growth factors to stimulate bone formation. J Bone Miner Res. 1993;8:565–72.
26. Bostrom MP, Saleh KJ, Einhorn TA. Osteoinductive growth factors in preclinical fracture and long bone defects models. Orthop Clin North Am. 1999;30:647–58.
27. Marx RE, Carlson ER, Eichstaedt RM, Schimmele SR, Strauss JE, Georgeff KR. Platelet-rich plasma: growth factor enhancement for bone grafts. Oral Surg Oral Med Oral Pathol Oral Radiol Endod. 1998;85(6):638–46.
28. Weibrich G, Hansen T, Kleis W, Buch R, Hitzler WE. Effect of platelet concentration in platelet-rich plasma on peri-implant bone regeneration. Bone. 2004;34:665–71.
29. Li H, Zou X, Xue Q, Egund N, Lind M, Bünger C. Anterior lumbar interbody fusion with carbon fiber cage loaded with bioceramics and platelet-rich plasma. An experimental study on pigs. Eur Spine J. 2004;13(4):354–8.
30. Kasten P, Vogel J, Luginbühl R, Niemeyer P, Weiss S, Schneider S, et al. Influence of platelet-rich plasma on osteogenic differentiation of mesenchymal stem cells and ectopic bone formation in calcium phosphate ceramics. Cells Tissues Organs. 2006;183(2):68–79.
31. Bi L, Cheng W, Fan H, Pei G. Reconstruction of goat tibial defects using an injectable tricalcium phosphate/chitosan in combination with autologous platelet-rich plasma. Biomaterials. 2010;31(12):3201–11.
32. Dumic-Cule I, Pecina M, Jelic M, Jankolija M, Popek I, Grgurevic L, et al. Biological aspects of segmental bone defects management. Int Orthop. 2015;39(5):1005–11.
33. Nakasa T, Ishida O, Sunagawa T, Nakamae A, Yasunaga Y, Agung M, et al. Prefabrication of vascularized bone graft using a combination of fibroblast growth factor-2 and vascular bundle implantation into a novel

interconnected porous calcium hydroxyapatite ceramic. J Biomed Mater Res A. 2005;75(2):350–5.

34. Kawamura K, Yajima H, Ohgushi H, Tomita Y, Kobata Y, Shigematsu K, et al. Experimental study of vascularized tissue-engineered bone grafts. Plast Reconstr Surg. 2006;117(5):1471–9.

35. Rouwkema J, Rivron NC, van Blitterswijk CA. Vascularization in tissue engineering. Trends Biotechnol. 2008;26(8):434–41.

36. Cao L, Arany PR, Wang YS, Mooney DJ. Promoting angiogenesis via manipulation of VEGF responsiveness with notch signaling. Biomaterials. 2009;30:4085–93.

37. Huang YC, Kaigler D, Rice KG, Krebsbach PH, Mooney DJ. Combined angiogenic and osteogenic factor delivery enhances bone marrow stromal cell-driven bone regeneration. J Bone Miner Res. 2005;20:848–57.

38. Street J, Bao M, de Guzman L, Bunting S, Peale FV Jr, Ferrara N, et al. Vascular endothelial growth factor stimulates bone repair by promoting angiogenesis and bone turnover. Proc Natl Acad Sci U S A. 2002;99(15):9656–61.

Repair of articular cartilage and subchondral defects in rabbit knee joints with a polyvinyl alcohol/nano-hydroxyapatite/polyamide 66 biological composite material

Tao Guo[1*], Xiaobin Tian[1], Bo Li[1], Tianfu Yang[2] and Yubao Li[3]

Abstract

Background: This study sought to prepare a new PVA/n-HA/PA66 composite to investigate the repair of articular cartilage and subchondral defects in rabbit knee joints.

Methods: A $5 \times 5 \times 5$ mm-sized defect was created in the patellofemoral joints of 72 healthy adult New Zealand rabbits. The rabbits were then randomly divided into three groups ($n = 24$): PVA/n-HA+PA66 group, polyvinyl alcohol (PVA) group, and control (untreated) group. Cylindrical PVA/n-HA+PA66, 5×5 mm, comprised an upper PVA layer and a lower n-HA+PA66 layer. Macroscopic and histological evaluations were performed at 4, 8, 12, and 24 weeks, postoperatively. Type II collagen was measured by immunohistochemical staining. The implant/cartilage and bone interfaces were observed by scanning electron microscopy.

Results: At 24 weeks postoperatively, the lower PVA/n-HA+PA66 layer became surrounded by cartilage, with no obvious degeneration. In the PVA group, an enlarged space was observed between the implant and the host tissue that had undergone degeneration. In the control group, the articular cartilage had become calcified. In the PVA/n-HA+PA66 group, positive type II collagen staining was observed between the composite and the surrounding cartilage and on the implant surface. In the PVA group, positive staining was slightly increased between the PVA and the surrounding cartilage, but reduced on the PVA surface. In the control group, reduced staining was observed throughout. Scanning electron microscopy showed increased bone tissue in the lower n-HA+PA66 layer that was in close approximation with the upper PVA layer of the composite. In the PVA group, the bone tissue around the material had receded, and in the control group, the defect was filled with bone tissue, while the superior aspect of the defect was filled with disordered, fibrous tissue.

Conclusion: The diphase biological composite material PVA/n-HA+PA66 exhibits good histocompatibility and offers a satisfactory substitute for articular cartilage and subchondral bone.

Keywords: Biological composite material, Articular cartilage, Subchondral bone, Repair

---

* Correspondence: drguotao04b@sina.com
[1]Department of Orthopedics, Guizhou Province People's Hospital, Guiyang, Guizhou province 550002, China
Full list of author information is available at the end of the article

Background

Articular cartilage is a type of hyaline cartilage characterized by low friction, good elasticity, and hypertonicity that has an important role in maintaining joint movement. Trauma and osteoarthritis are the two factors that can lead to articular surface defects, which eventually develop into joint dysfunction. Joint fusion or joint replacement is necessary to repair joint dysfunction, because articular cartilage itself lacks a regenerative capacity [1, 2]. Adult articular cartilage has a limited reparatory capability; that is, it can partially or totally repair itself when the defect diameter is less than 3 mm but not when the diameter exceeds 3 mm, in which case it will develop into arthritis [3]. Joint replacement is not ideal for young and middle-aged patients because the joint implant has a limited life expectancy. For this reason, an effective method for repairing articular cartilage defects is an emergent issue in the field of orthopedics.

Previous methods used to repair articular cartilage defects include enhancement of the articular cartilage healing capacity and biological repair by autologous or xenogenic tissue grafting. The latter method includes autologous periosteal, perichondrial, and osteochondral grafting as well as allogeneic osteochondral grafting. But the long-term therapeutic effects of these methods are not satisfactory [4]. With advances in tissue engineering technology, some progress has been made in the repair of articular cartilage defects. Nevertheless, repair of articular cartilage to a high standard, with satisfactory long-term therapeutic effects, has not been acquired in the clinic [5, 6]. At present, the artificial materials used in the treatment of advanced osteoarthrosis are made of metal, ceramics, and ultra-high molecular weight polyethylene, with increasing attention being paid to the postoperative complications caused by implant abrasion and loosening. Therefore, some researchers are investigating alternative artificial cartilage substitutes as a repair strategy [7].

Elastomeric materials with a similar biomechanical property to cartilage have been mostly selected as alternative materials for cartilage replacement therapies, such as silicon rubber, polyurethane, and polyvinyl alcohol (PVA) hydrogel. Silicon rubber is no longer a popular material choice, owing to its ease of abrasion and absorption of oil in the body [8]. Polyurethane, as a long-term implant material, requires an improvement in its degradation rate. Moreover, the hydrolysate of the curing agent diisocyanate is a potential carcinogenic substance [9]. Polyvinyl alcohol (PVA) hydrogel, on the other hand, is a porous material similar to natural cartilage and is considered by some to be an ideal alternative material to cartilage [10]. It is a water-soluble synthetic polymer hydrolyzed by polyvinyl acetate that has been widely used as artificial cartilage, drug delivery systems, artificial meniscus, heart valve, anti-thrombin materials, vascular grafts, and biomedical sponges in the field of biomedicine for its high elasticity, stable chemical property, ease of molding, absence of toxicity and adverse reactions, and good histocompatibility within the human body [11–16].

Despite its suitable properties, the use of the PVA hydrogel in an articular cartilage and subchondral bone defect remains a concern for orthopedists. Previously, the implanted PVA was fixed by sticking or sutures, which produced poor fixation and led to the formation of a gap between the PVA and the subchondral bone. Fabricating the PVA biomaterial into a cylinder, which can be inserted into the articular cartilage and subchondral bone, offers poor stability to the joint. Likewise, mechanical fixation and chemical fixation have also yielded unsatisfactory outcomes [17, 18]. Therefore, the application of PVA for the repair of articular cartilage defects is limited.

In this study, we prepared a novel artificial bone material comprising nano-hydroxyapatite (n-HA) and polyamide 66 (PA66) (n-HA+PA66) to form a base for insertion of the PVA hydrogel. This double-layered biomaterial PVA/n-HA+PA66 composite was prepared using the in situ synthesis and freeze-thaw cycle method. The upper layer of the biomaterial composite was made of PVA and used as a substitute for articular cartilage, while the lower layer was made of n-HA+PA66 and used to substitute for subchondral bone. The upper layer and lower layer were firmly connected prior to implantation in a rabbit patellofemoral defect model to assess its potential use as a therapeutic grafting substitute.

Methods

Materials

Biomaterial composites PVA/n-HA+PA66 and PVA were provided by the Nanometer Analytical and Testing Center, Sichuan University, China.

Animals

This study was performed at the Laboratory of Tissue Engineering, Department of Orthopedics, Huaxi Hospital, Sichuan University, China between July 2014 and July 2016. Seventy-two healthy adult New Zealand rabbits, aged 5–8 months, weighing 160–240 g, and with an equal number of males and females, were provided by the Laboratory Animal Center, Sichuan University, China.

Model preparation and group management

Seventy-two rabbits (36 male and 36 female) were randomly divided into three groups with 24 rabbits in each group: PVA/n-HA+PA66 implant (contains 11 male and 13 female), PVA implant (contains 14 male and 10 female), and control (contains 11 male and 13 female). Following anesthesia by an intraperitoneal injection of 30 g/L pentobarbital, an incision was made on the skin around the medial patella to expose the patellofemoral joint. The femoral bone joint was perforated (diameter 5 mm, depth 5 mm) to prepare models of articular cartilage and subchondral bone defects. The double-layer biomaterial composite PVA/n-HA+PA66 and simple PVA were implanted into the hole, respectively, and lightly pressed through the use of an inserter to stabilize the implant, the control group received no treatment. Each rabbit was intramuscularly injected with 40,000 units of penicillin per day for 3 days after surgery. After wound sutures, the operated limbs were not immobilized and allowed to move freely.

Gross observation
After surgery, the diet, activity level, wound healing, and range of motion were assessed for each rabbit. At a postoperative time period of 4, 8, 12, or 24 weeks, rabbits were sacrificed under anesthesia and the articular cavity was opened to examine the cartilage surrounding the implant, synovial membrane, and implant stability and compared with the contralateral joint surface.

Histomorphological observation
Eighteen rabbits were sacrificed at postoperative 4 weeks for histomorphological observation, 18 rabbits were sacrificed at postoperative 8 weeks, and 9 rabbits were sacrificed at 12 and 24 weeks postoperatively for histomorphological observation and immunohistochemical detection. Nine rabbits were sacrificed at 12 and 24 weeks postoperatively for scanning electron microscopy observation. Following removal of condyles of the femur, a tissue specimen about 1 cm in length was harvested, with the implant as a center, and fixed with 40 g/L paraformaldehyde. Specimens were then decalcified with 10% EDTA and dehydrated and embedded with paraffin following routine procedures. Slices of 5-μm-thick sections were stained with hematoxylin-eosin, Masson's trichrome, and toluidine blue and observed under the microscope (BX51, Olympus, Tokyo, Japan).

Immunohistochemical detection of type II collagen
At postoperative 8, 12, and 24 weeks, the tissue specimens were harvested as described above and then fixed, decalcified, hydrated, embedded, sliced into 5-μm-thick sections, and stained for type II collagen expression using standard immunohistochemistry. The specimens were then assessed using an inverted phase contrast microscope (BX51; Olympus).

Scanning electron microscopy observation
At postoperative 12 and 24 weeks, tissue specimens (1 × 1 × 1 cm) were fixed with 2.5% glutaraldehyde (pH 7.2–7.4), dehydrated with ethanol series, and subject to gold sputtering. The interface between the implant and the surrounding cartilage and subchondral bone was observed by scanning electron microscopy (S3400N; Hitachi, Japan).

Results

Appearance and inner structure of biomaterial composite
The cylindrical PVA/n-HA+PA66 composite was 5 mm in diameter and 5 mm in height. The upper layer of PVA was 1.5 mm high and consisted with an ivory, smooth, and tenacious surface. By comparison, the lower layer of n-HA+PA66 was 3.5 mm high, and had a rough and stiff composition. Using scanning electron microscopy, the PVA exhibited a porous structure, with a pore diameter of 5–40 μm, a porosity of 75.3% and water ratio of 71.6%. The n-HA+PA66 component of the biomaterial was also porous, with a pore diameter of 100–400 μm and porosity of 61.7%. By X-ray diffraction analysis, the PVA appeared as a semi-crystalline polymer, with strong hydrogen bonds between the hydroxyl groups. The composite n-HA+PA66 consisted of a uniform crystal structure, with firm bonds to polyamide (Fig. 1).

Biological behaviors of rabbits
Seventy-two New Zealand rabbits were included in the final analysis. After surgery, no rabbits had died or suffered wound infection/secretion. The rabbits in the PVA/n-HA +PA66 implant group and PVA implant group showed a good range of motion. In the control group, joint motion was reduced in two rabbits and this symptom developed into knee joint stiffness at 8 weeks after surgery.

Changes in the knee joint cavity
In the PVA/n-HA+PA66 implant group, the articular surface was smooth. At 4 weeks, the gap surrounding the implant was filled with fibrous tissue, which secured the implant such that it could not be pulled out. At 8, 12, and 24 weeks, the gap surrounding the implant disappeared, and the joints regained good function. No obvious cartilage degeneration was observed, and the implant bonded well with the adjacent articular cartilage and subchondral bone. As expected, the contralateral articular surface was smooth without abrasion. No hyperplastic and plump synovial membrane formations were observed (Fig. 2a). In the PVA implant group, the surface of the implant was smooth at 4 weeks, but the implant was not firmly fastened and easily prolapsed. At 8 and 12 weeks, the implant had dropped by 2.0–3.0 mm. At 24 weeks, a small amount of degenerative change was observed in the cartilage (pale color and surface layer abrasion), and the implant was not firmly fastened into the joint (Fig. 2b). In the control group, the defect region was filled with fibrous granulation tissue at 4 weeks, which gradually enclosed the articular surface. Light colored, fibrous cartilage with a roughened surface was identified. At 24 weeks, the fibrous tissue had calcified

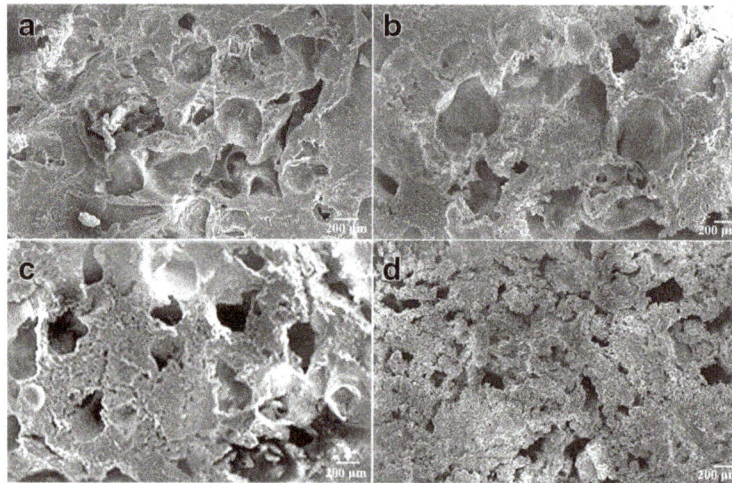

Fig. 1 Scanning electron microscopy image of the porous biomaterial nano-hydroxyapatite+polyamide 66 (×60) (**a** x80, **b** x70, **c** x60, **d** x50)

and continued to appear rough. The articular cartilage in the surrounding region presented with degenerative changes, and the articular synovium exhibited hyperplasia, swelling, and appeared plump (Fig. 2c). Severe traumatic arthritis, articular synarthrophysis, and stiffness occurred in two of the rabbits in this group.

Histomorphological observations

At 4 weeks, for rabbits in the PVA/n-HA+PA66 implant group, the fibrous tissue in the gap between the implant and adjacent tissue contained a small number of filtrated inflammatory cells, with some fibrous tissue growing into the pores of the n-HA+PA66 biomaterial. At 8 and 12 weeks, a large amount of fibrous tissues had infiltrated into the pores of the n-HA +PA66 lower layer, with the formation of some collagen and osteoid. The gap between the PVA in the upper layer and the adjacent cartilage had become filled with articular cartilage that had also started to cover the PVA surface. At 24 weeks, the lower layer

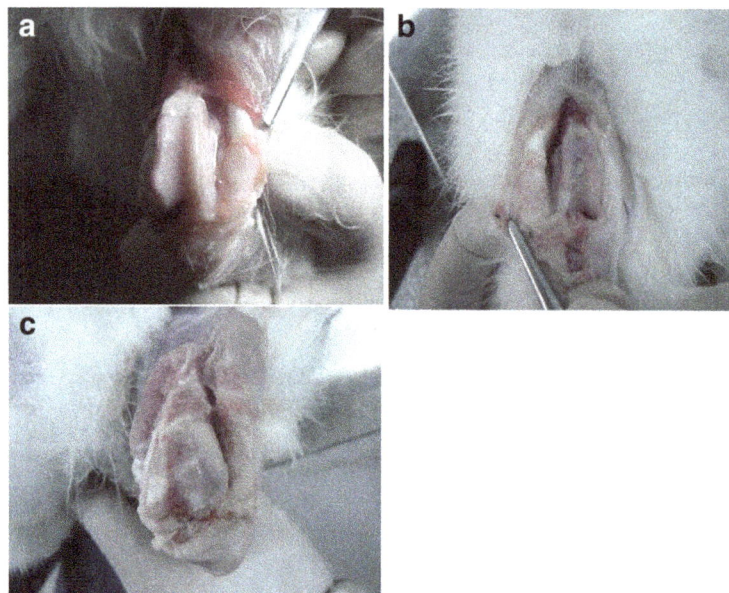

Fig. 2 At 24 weeks after implantation of polyvinyl alcohol/nano-hydroxyapatite and polyamide 66. No obvious changes were observed in the peripheral articular cartilage; the contralateral articular surface was smooth (**a**). At 24 weeks after implantation of polyvinyl alcohol, the implant had dropped and was not firmly fastened into the joint (**b**). At 24 weeks in the control group, the surface of joint appears rough and articular cartilage in the surrounding region presented with degenerative changes (**c**)

had bonded with the adjacent tissue, with much osteoid in the pores that had formed a reticular layer. No abrasion to the PVA in the upper layer was observed, and the adjacent cartilage was ordered, covering the surface of the PVA, with no obvious degeneration (Fig. 3a).

In the PVA implant group, there was a large number of infiltrated inflammatory cells at 4 weeks in the gap between the implant and the adjacent subchondral bone, with some proliferative fibrous tissue. At 8 and 12 weeks, the gap between the implant and the host tissue was filled with fibrous tissue. The biomaterial adjacent to the articular cartilage edge appeared blunted and presented with slight degenerative changes. At 24 weeks, the adjacent cartilage had thinned and continued to show degenerative changes (Fig. 3b). The fibrous tissue in the defect site of rabbits in the control group was interspersed with a large number of fibroblasts and inflammatory cells at 4 weeks. At 8 and 12 weeks, the granulation tissue had become calcified, and by 24 weeks, the majority of the defect region had formed bony trabeculae and osteoid. In the upper layer, the fibrous tissue was poorly arranged and had formed transparent cartilage; the adjacent host cartilage had thinned and begun to degenerate (Fig. 3c).

Immunohistochemical detection of type II collagen

Positive type II collagen staining was found in the PVA/n-HA+PA66 implant group at 12 weeks in the gaps between the PVA and adjacent articular cartilage and on the surface of PVA biomaterial. At 24 weeks, type II collagen staining had increased at the cartilaginous margin and on the surface of the PVA biomaterial (Fig. 4a). For rabbits in the PVA implant group, weak type II collagen staining was observed in the gap between the PVA biomaterial and the adjacent tissue, with positive staining on the surface of the PVA and in the adjacent cartilage. There was a slight increase in this staining at 24 weeks, but the staining on the surface of PVA biomaterial and in the adjacent cartilage was attenuated (Fig. 4b). In the control group, a small amount of type II collagen was present at 12 weeks, presenting as weak positive staining on the surface of the defect and in the adjacent articular cartilage. At 24 weeks, type II collagen staining was attenuated on the surface of the defect and in the adjacent articular cartilage (Fig. 4c).

Scanning electron microscopy observation

In the PVA/n-HA+PA66 implant group, a large number of fibroblasts were found in the pores of n-HA+PA66 biomaterial in the lower layer at 12 weeks, along with substantial osteoid. The osteoid was arranged in strips, and the gap between the n-HA+PA66 biomaterial and adjacent tissues contained numerous fibroblasts and collagen, with some calcified fibrous tissue surrounding the PVA in the upper layer. At 24 weeks, the n-HA+PA66 biomaterial pores in the lower layer contained osteoid that made connections with the adjacent tissue, and the PVA in the upper layer was tightly connected with the n-HA+PA66 biomaterial in the lower layer (Fig. 5a). By comparison, in the PVA implant group, a poor connection with the adjacent tissue was observed at 12 weeks,

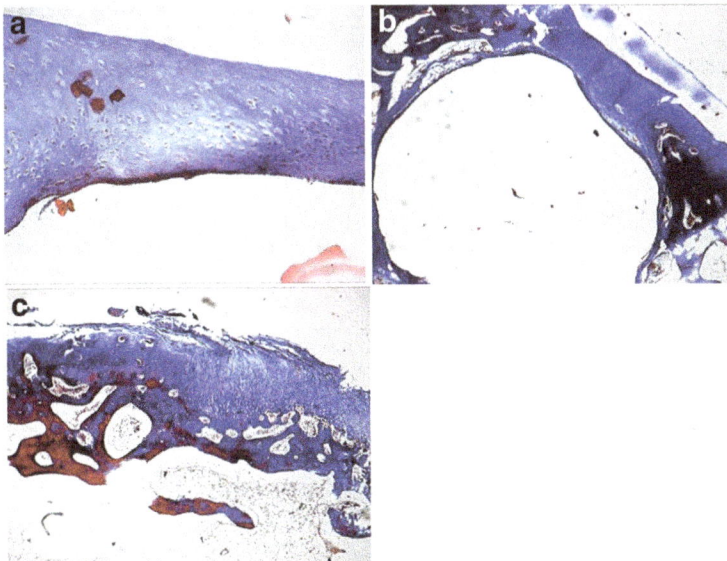

Fig. 3 At 24 weeks after implantation of polyvinyl alcohol/nano-hydroxyapatite and polyamide 66, part of the polyvinyl alcohol surface was covered by collagen (×40) (**a**). At 24 weeks in the PVA implant group, the adjacent cartilage had thinned and continued to show degenerative changes (×40) (**b**). At 24 weeks in the control group, the fibrous tissue was poorly arranged and had formed transparent cartilage (×40) (**c**)

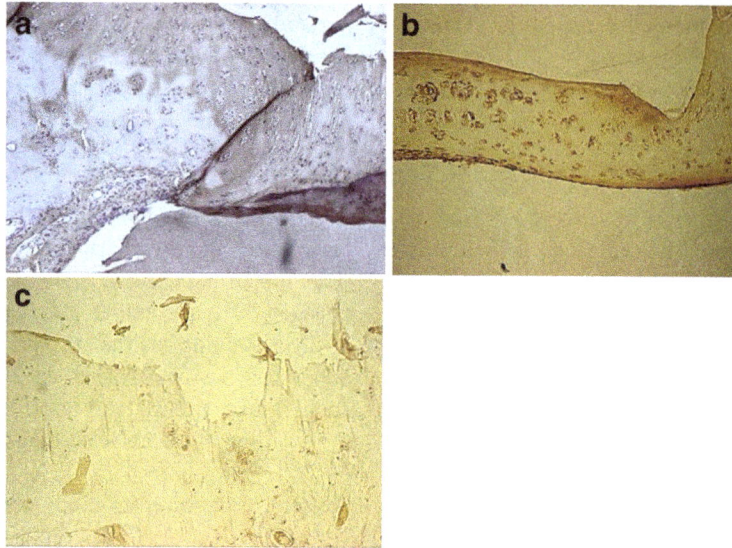

Fig. 4 At 24 weeks in PVA/n-HA+PA66 implant group, immunohistochemical detection of type II collagen showed positive staining on the surface and in the peripheral region of the polyvinyl alcohol implant (×100) (**a**). At 24 weeks in the PVA implant group, weak type II collagen staining was observed in the gap between the PVA biomaterial and the adjacent tissue(×100) (**b**). At 24 weeks in the control group, a small amount of type II collagen was present, presenting as weak positive staining on the surface of the defect (×100) (**c**)

with an obvious margin. Part of the PVA in the upper layer was covered by fibrous strips. At 24 weeks, part of the adjacent sclerotin had pulled away, enlarging the gap (Fig. 5b). In the control group, the lower part of defect region was filled with solid sclerotin and the surface was covered by a layer of fibrous tissue at 12 weeks. At 24 weeks, the lower part of the defect was filled with

sclerotin, and the upper part contained a disordered, scar-like fibrous tissue (Fig. 5c).

Discussion

Articular cartilage is a tissue without blood vessels, lymphatic vessels, and nerves. As such, chondrocytes

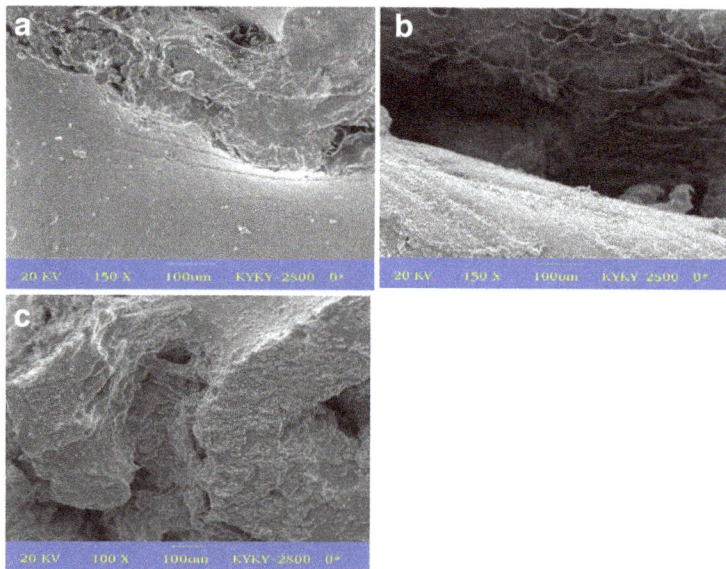

Fig. 5 At 24 weeks postoperatively, the n-HA+PA66 biomaterial in the lower layer was tightly connected with adjacent tissue and the PVA biomaterial in the *upper* layer was tightly connected with the n-HA+PA66 biomaterial in the *lower* layer (SEM × 150) (**a**). In the PVA implant group, a poor connection and gap with the adjacent tissue were observed (SEM × 150) (**b**). In the control group, the *lower* part of defect was filled with sclerotin and the *upper* part contained a disordered, scar-like fibrous tissue (SEM × 150) (**c**)

under general circumstances have limited capacity to undergo mitosis or regenerate the cartilage in response to damage or deterioration. According to the structure and characteristics of cartilage, a substitute material used as artificial cartilage should meet the following requirements: good biomechanical property, excellent lubricity and wear resistance, ability to induce chondrocyte growth, firm connection with bone base, and biocompatibility.

Histocompatibility of composite biomaterial PVA/n-HA +PA66

PVA hydrogel exhibits physical properties that are more similar to in vivo tissue than many other artificial composites. First, its expansive capability and water permeability contribute to its overall satisfactory biocompatibility [19]. Second, its flexibility and elasticity can reduce the load experienced by surrounding cells and tissue. Third, PVA exhibits a good biomechanical property, which is similar to the elastic modulus of cartilage, and has a small surface friction coefficient [20]. Therefore, PVA hydrogel is currently considered a good substitute biomaterial for articular cartilage [21–23].

Some scholars have performed studies to assess the cellular toxicity, safety, and excretion of PVA. Strong evidence exists that PVA does not cause hemolysis, allergic response, or skin irritations [24]. Our results demonstrate that PVA exhibited good compatibility with the adjacent articular cartilage; after the PVA implantation, the adjacent articular cartilage did not present with any degenerative changes, type II collagen was secreted, and chondrocytes were arranged in order. After 4 weeks, some chondrocytes were observed on the PVA surface and filled the gap between the PVA and the adjacent articular cartilage. At 24 weeks, the articular cartilage surrounding the PVA grew well and did not present with any obvious degenerative changes, showing positive type II collagen staining on the surface and at the biomaterial edge, suggestive of cartilage growth. These findings indicate that PVA exhibits good biocompatibility with adjacent host articular cartilage.

HA has a good osteoconductivity and has been well accepted as a bone repair substitute [25]. PA66 is a polymer with strong intensity, high flexibility, and good stability. Previous studies have shown that the combination of these two materials yields a high molecular weight polymer, n-HA+PA66, that was initially prepared under international advanced standards using Chinese intellectual property. In this study, according to human bone tissue compositions, we found that our novel biomaterial exhibited the strong rigidity of n-HA and the highly flexible nature of PA66, thereby generating a structure with similar properties to the bone and articular cartilage that was appropriate for presenting the PVA

biomaterial [26–28]. Zhang et al. [29] also evaluated the biological characteristics of the n-HA/PA66 composite biomaterial in vivo and in vitro, showing that the n-HA/PA66 composite biomaterial did not dissolve in the blood and induced no cell toxicity, skin irritation or allergic response, and no pyrogen reaction or other adverse reactions after intramuscular implantation for 90 days or bony implantation for 180 days. Using this composite to repair dog mandibular cortical defects, Zheng et al. [30] found that, after surgery, the wound healed well, there were no rejections, the implant made strong connections with the bone tissue, and displayed good osteoconductivity, suggesting good biocompatibility and biological activity of the material.

Integrated composite material formation by firm connection of upper and lower layers of interfaces

The PVA/n-HA+PA66 composite consisted of a uniform crystal structure, with firm bonds to polyamide, as evidenced by electron microscopy (Fig. 1). PVA and n-HA+PA66 can be integrated by freeze-thaw cycles and casting because of the porosity of the n-HA +PA66 compound, which is suitable for permeation of liquid compositions. Part of the dissolved PVA compositions casted onto the n-HA+PA66 can directly permeate into the pores of n-HA+PA66. PVA and n-HA+PA66 form a steady connection after repeated freeze-thaw cycles.

Stability and advantages of integrated composite material after implantation

Under normal conditions, subchondral and cancellous bones below the articular cartilage play an important role in protecting the articular cartilage from high stress. When the joints are exposed to high loads, the subchondral bone assigns the majority of this stress to the cancellous bone, which is arranged in a radial manner to greatly decrease the stress to articular cartilage. Brittberg et al. [31] reported that cartilage defects often involve the subchondral bone; they result in destruction of the normal cartilage and induce subsequent changes to the mechanical properties of the joint, leading to a decreased healing rate and degenerative changes. For this reason, the PVA hydrogel used as a substitute of articular cartilage should provide sufficient support to the subchondral and cancellous bones. However, a good connection between the PVA hydrogel and the bone has, until now, remained problematic. Recently, Gu et al. [32] used mechanical-chemical methods to investigate a firm connection between PVA hydrogel and metal (as a bottom layer for bone). In addition, Oka et al. [33] implanted PVA-H into the cartilage defect region and fixed it using tissue grown in titanium mesh pores. Some therapeutic effects were acquired, but the long-term bio-mechanical properties of these composites deserve further investigation.

In this study, we designed a novel artificial cartilage substitute biomaterial to solve this problem with PVA presentation for joint repair. The upper layer was made of PVA and the lower layer of n-HA+PA66, integrated by freeze-thaw cycles and casting. The upper layer functioned to substitute for articular cartilage while the lower layer substituted as a subchondral bone. The lower layer exhibited a porous structure to facilitate the ingrowth of fibrous and bony tissue. The formation of biological self-locking fixation of the n-HA+PA66 after implantation can effectively prevent displacement of the implant and greatly improve the stability and function of the artificial cartilage upper layer of the biomaterial. PVA exhibits a good stability throughout the entire lifespan, which plays a positive role in its functioning as articular cartilage.

Our results confirmed that the composite PVA/n-HA+PA66 immediately fixed into the defect, becoming integrated with the adjacent subchondral bone. At 4 weeks after implantation, the lower part of the biomaterial showed preliminary connections with the adjacent tissue. After 8 weeks, n-HA+PA66 in the lower layer attained good connections with the adjacent tissue, that gradually calcified into bone tissue. Thus, the n-HA+PA66 in the lower layer offers a strong support to the upper PVA and contributes to PVA functioning as a substitute articular cartilage.

Our results showed that the PVA alone lacked the necessary support to subchondral bone, being extremely unstable and easily deformable under the influences of external forces owing to lacking of good fixation. Electron microscopy results showed an obvious boundary between the entire PVA and the adjacent tissue that likely arose because the bone tissue and fibrous tissue cannot grow into the inner portion of the PVA. This leads to poor interconnectivity, displacement of PVA biomaterial, increased PVA abrasion, a non-uniform stress distribution, and finally degeneration of adjacent cartilage. It may even lead to osteophyma.

Conclusion

Taken together, the composite biomaterial PVA/n-HA+PA66 serves as a good integrated biomaterial substitute for articular cartilage and subchondral bone. The implanted PVA/n-HA+PA66 can reconstruct the smooth cartilage surface, reduce abrasion, postpone or prevent the occurrence of osteoarthritis, and provide an alternative biomaterial for repair of articular cartilage defects. However, the problem of abrasion in long-term application of PVA biomaterial deserves further investigation.

Abbreviations
n-HA+PA66: nano-hydroxyapatite (n-HA) and polyamide 66 (PA66); PVA: Polyvinyl alcohol hydrogel

Acknowledgments
Not applicable

Funding
No funding was received.

Authors' contributions
TG conceived and designed the experiments. TG, XT, and BL performed the experiments. TY and YL analyzed the data. TG contributed reagents/materials/analysis tools. TG wrote the paper. All authors read and approved the final manuscript.

Competing interests
The authors declare that they have no competing interests.

Author details
[1]Department of Orthopedics, Guizhou Province People's Hospital, Guiyang, Guizhou province 550002, China. [2]Department of Orthopedics, West China Hospital, Sichuan University, Chengdu, Sichuan province 610041, China. [3]Nanometer Analytical and Testing Center, Sichuan University, Chengdu, Sichuan province 610041, China.

References
1. Zhang HB, Zhang BC, Zhang HJ, Zheng SM. Experimental study of hepatocyte growth factor in repairing articular cartilage defects. Zhonghua Guke Zazhi. 2000;20:181–4.
2. Yamasaki S, Mera H, Itokazu M, et al. Cartilage Repair With Autologous Bone Marrow Mesenchymal Stem Cell Transplantation: Review of Preclinical and Clinical Studies. Cartilage. 2014;5(4):196-202.
3. Shapiro F, Koide S, Glimcher MJ. Cell origin and differentiation in the repair of full-thickness defects of articular cartilage. J Bone Joint Surg Am. 1993;75(4):532–53.
4. Madsen BL, Noer HH, Carstensen JP, Nørmark F. Long-term results of periosteal transplantation in osteochondritis dissecans of the knee. Orthopedics. 2000;23(3):223–6.
5. van der Kraan PM, Buma P, van Kuppevelt T, van den Berg WB. Interaction of chondrocytes, extracellular matrix and growth factors: relevance for articular cartilage tissue engineering. Osteoarthr Cartil. 2002;10(8):631–7.
6. Wang CY, Guo XM, Fang ZQ, Duan CM, Zhao Q, Wang YH, Chen JH, Bo B, Fan M, Lu JX. Repair of sheep articular cartilage defects by tissue engineered cartilage: an experimental study. Junshi Yixue. 2002;26:81–5.
7. Li SP. Introduction of biomedical materials. Wuhan: Wuhan Gongye Daxue Chubanshe; 2000.
8. Ząbek A, Małecka B, Kołodzińska A, Maziarz A, Lelakowski J, Kutarski A. Early abrasion of outer silicone insulation after intracardiac lead friction in a patient with cardiac device-related infective endocarditis. Pacing Clin Electrophysiol. 2012;35(6):e156–8.
9. Tsui YK, Gogolewski S. Microporous biodegradable polyurethane membranes for tissue engineering. J Mater Sci Mater Med. 2009;20(8):1729–41.
10. Buckwalter JA, Mankin HJ. Articular cartilage: tissue design and chondrocyte-matrix interactions. Instr Course Lect. 1998;47:477–86.
11. Chen G, Hoffman AS. Graft copolymers that exhibit temperature-induced phase transitions over a wide range of pH. Nature. 1995;373(6509):49–52.
12. Alhalafi AM. Applications of polymers in intraocular drug delivery systems. Oman J Ophthalmol. 2017;10(1):3–8.
13. Rafique A, Mahmood Zia K, Zuber M, Tabasum S, Rehman S. Chitosan functionalized poly(vinyl alcohol) for prospects biomedical and industrial applications: a review. Int J Biol Macromol. 2016;87:141–54.
14. Vellayappan MV, Balaji A, Subramanian AP, John AA, Jaganathan SK,

Repair of articular cartilage and subchondral defects in rabbit knee joints with a polyvinyl...

141

Murugesan S, Mohandas H, Supriyanto E, Yusof M. Tangible nanocomposites with diverse properties for heart valve application. Sci Technol Adv Mater. 2015;16(3):033504.

15. Guo D, Xu K. Application of polyvinyl alcohol in biomedical engineering. Sheng Wu Yi Xue Gong Cheng Xue Za Zhi. 2005;22(3):602–5.

16. Alexandre N, Costa E, Coimbra S, Silva A, Lopes A, Rodrigues M, Santos M, Maurício AC, Santos JD, Luís AL. In vitro and in vivo evaluation of blood coagulation activation of polyvinyl alcohol hydrogel plus dextran-based vascular grafts. J Biomed Mater Res A. 2015;103(4):1366–79.

17. Kobayashi M, Oka M. Composite device for attachment of polyvinyl alcohol-hydrogel to underlying bone. Artif Organs. 2004;28(8):734–8.

18. Ushio K, Oka M, Hyon SH, Hayami T, Yura S, Matsumura K, Toguchida J, Nakamura T. Attachment of artificial cartilage to underlying bone. J Biomed Mater Res B Appl Biomater. 2004;68(1):59–68.

19. Xu FL, Li YB, Li JD, Mu YH. Swelling properties of nano-hydroxyaptite/polyvinyl alcohol hydrogel composite. Cailiao Gongcheng. 2005;50:15–18,22.

20. Williams S. Mechanical testing of a new biomaterial for potential use as a vascular graft and articular cartilage replacement [dissertation]. Atlanta: Georgia Institute of Technology; 2006.

21. Katta JK, Marcolongo MS, Lowman AM, Mansmann KA. Friction and wear characteristics of PVA/PVP hydrogels as synthetic articular cartilage. IEEE. 2004;4:142–3.

22. Li Y, Gao J, Liu G, Gu Z, Ma Y, Xue H. Swelling characterization of poly (vinyl alcohol) hydrogel for prosthetic intervertebral disc nucleus. Sheng Wu Yi Xue Gong Cheng Xue Za Zhi. 2005;22(5):995–8.

23. Kobayashi M, Toguchida J, Oka M. Development of an artificial meniscus using polyvinyl alcohol-hydrogel for early return to, and continuance of, athletic life in sportspersons with severe meniscus injury. II: animal experiments. Knee. 2003;10:53.

24. Baker MI, Walsh SP, Schwartz Z, Boyan BD. A review of polyvinyl alcohol and its uses in cartilage and orthopedic applications. J Biomed Mater Res B Appl Biomater. 2012;100:1451–7.

25. Du C, Cui FZ, Feng QL, Zhu XD, de Groot K. Tissue response to nano-hydroxyapatite/collagen composite implants in marrow cavity. J Biomed Mater Res. 1998;42:540–8.

26. Xu YH, Li SQ, Li ZA. Development of nanometer hydroxyapatite complex materials-cytotoxicity test of nano-hydroxyapatite by MTT-assay. Shiyong Kouqiang Yixue Zazhi. 2004;20:147–50.

27. Yang X, Song Y, Liu L, et al. Anterior reconstruction with nano-hydroxyapatite/polyamide-66 cage after thoracic and lumbar corpectomy. Orthopedics. 2012;35(1):e66-73.

28. Meng CY, An H, Jiang DM, Li YB, Wei J. Biocompatibility and security of new type nano hydroapatite crystals and polyamide for bone reconstruction and repair after implanting in vivo. Zhongguo Linchuang Kangfu. 2004;8:6330–545.

29. Zhang L, Li YB, Wang XJ, Wei J, Peng XL. Studies on porous scaffold made of the nano-HA/PA66 composite. J Mater Sci. 2005;40:107–10.

30. Zheng Q, Zhou LW, Wei SC, Li YB, Wei J. Experimental study on the reconstruction of mandibular defects with a new bioactive artificial bone nano-hydroxyapatite/polyamide-66 in dogs. Zhonghua Kou Qiang Yi Xue Za Zhi. 2004;39(1):60–2.

31. Brittberg M, Nilsson A, Lindahl A, Ohlsson C, Peterson L. Rabbit articular cartilage defects treated with autologous cultured chondrocytes. Clin Orthop Relat Res. 1996;326:270–83.

32. Gu ZQ, Xiao JM, Lou SQ. The mechanical-chemical attachment between the artificial articular cartilage (PVA-hydrogel) and metal substrate (or underlying bone). Biomed Mater Eng. 1999;9(5–6):347–51.

33. Oka M. Biomechanics and repair of articular cartilage. J Orthop Sci. 2001;6(5):448–56.

20

A randomized controlled trial on the effects of collagen sponge and topical tranexamic acid in posterior spinal fusion surgeries

Derong Xu, Qianyu Zhuang, Zheng Li, Zhinan Ren, Xin Chen and Shugang Li[*]

Abstract

Background: This is a randomized controlled trial research to assess the hemostatic efficacy of gelatin sponge, collagen sponge, and topical use of tranexamic acid (TXA) on postoperative blood loss in posterior spinal fusion surgeries.

Methods: We recruited patients with spinal degenerative diseases into the study from November 2013 to October 2016. All the participants were assigned to 3 groups using a simple, equal-probability randomization scheme: group A is a control group utilizing gelatin sponge, while groups B and C are experimental groups, applying collagen hemostatic sponge and topical TXA respectively. Postoperative blood loss, rates of transfusion, and hospitalization were compared among the 3 groups.

Results: In our study, the volume of drainage and blood content in drainage on the first postoperative day (POD 1) of patients in the experimental groups were significantly less than those in the control group, as well as rates of transfusion and postoperative hospitalization ($P < 0.05$). When compared with the control group, the volume of drainage decreased by 22.7% in group B and 56.2% in group C, while the blood content in drainage decreased by 28.8 and 75% respectively.

Conclusions: In this study, collagen and topical use of TXA have both proven to be effective and safe for patients undergoing posterior spinal fusion surgeries, while TXA has exhibited better efficacy. The total amount of perioperative blood loss reduced significantly without increasing incidence of related complications.

Trial registration: A randomized controlled trial for effects of collagen sponge and topical tranexamic acid in posterior lumbar fusion surgeries. ChiCTR-IIR-17010785.

Keywords: Spinal fusion surgery, Collagen sponge, Topical TXA, Blood loss

Background

Effective measures to control perioperative bleedings is a common issue that should be taken seriously, especially in complex and high-risk multilevel spinal fusion surgeries. Excessive blood loss may result in diverse undesirable consequences, such as severe anemia, massive transfusions, prolonged hospitalization, increased incidence of wound infections, and medical expenses [1, 2]. Therefore, many blood protection measures have been implemented to control bleeding in spinal surgeries, including hypotensive anesthesia, intra-operative cell salvage systems, and application of hemostatic agents [3].

The gelatin sponge has been used in surgical procedures for several decades; it has no bioactivity and controls bleeding mainly by volume expansion and mechanical compression. In contrast to gelatin sponge, collagen sponge contains hemostatic agents that are purified from original type I collagen. So besides physical compression, the biological components in collagen sponge possess hemostatic function by activating the platelets and intrinsic coagulation pathway. In addition, Lan [4] pointed out that the excellent hemostatic effect of collagen sponge may lead to a higher platelet ratio resulting from the blood adsorption.

As an antifibrinolytic agent, tranexamic acid (TXA) can block the interaction of plasminogen and plasmin by competing with the lysine residues on the surface of fibrin to inhibit the fibrinolysis and consequently stabilize

* Correspondence: lishugangpumc@163.com
Department of Orthopedic Surgery, Peking Union Medical College Hospital, No.1 Shuai Fu Yuan, Wang Fu Jing Street, Beijing 100730, China

clot [5]. It could be applied intravenously or topically [6]. Lots of researches have demonstrated that intravenous TXA (IV TXA) can reduce blood loss and transfusion requirements in total knee arthroplasty (TKA), total hip arthroplasty (THA), and spinal fusion surgeries [7–9]. However, IV TXA might be accompanied with serious side effects, which are quite rare but do exist, especially in patients with hypercoagulability, severe ischemic heart diseases, and renal failure [10]. On the other hand, there are relatively fewer reports about the safety and efficacy of topical use of TXA in spinal surgeries.

The goal of this study was to evaluate the efficacy of three different methods—gelatin sponge, collagen sponge, and topical TXA in reducing blood loss in patients undergoing posterior spinal fusion surgeries. Additionally, we observed the incidence of perioperative complications, rates of transfusion, and hospitalization as well.

Methods

This is a randomized controlled clinical study. Patients diagnosed with spinal degenerative diseases at Peking Union Medical Hospital were recruited into research from November 2013 to October 2016. The inclusion criteria were spinal degenerative diseases, such as spinal stenosis, disc diseases, and instability (e.g., grade I–II spondylolisthesis, spondylolisthesis/spondylolysis) indicated for surgical treatments. The exclusion criteria were as follows: (1) patients with comorbid severe medical diseases such as osteoporosis, anemia, renal failure, and cardiovascular diseases; (2) patients with abnormal coagulation function; (3) patients who have taken anti-platelet aggregates such as aspirin or anticoagulants in the last month; and (4) patients who had a history of thromboembolisms.

All the participants were assigned to 3 groups using a simple, equal-probability randomization scheme: because of limited hemostatic effect as explained before, patients utilizing gelatin sponge in group A were referred as control group, patients in group B were applied with collagen hemostatic sponge group, and patients in group C were applied with topical TXA. The participants were presented in a flow diagram in Fig. 1.

All the surgeries were performed by the same surgeons. After general anesthesia, patients were performed total laminectomy with pedicle screw instrumentation by free-hand technique. In addition to posterior bony structure decompression, patients underwent discectomy if diagnosed with disc herniation. After articular process fusion with bone grafting, we took different hemostatic measures according to group allocation. For patients in group A and group B, we applied gelatin sponges and collagen hemostatic sponges separately. According to the size of exposed spinal dura, we cut the hemostatic materials into proper shape to ensure the entire dura was covered. For patients in group C, we soaked the surgical field with TXA (1 g in 100 ml saline solution) for 5 min and then aspirated the TXA solution before stitching the wound. All the operations were accomplished by the same surgeons.

We estimated intraoperative blood loss based on weight of soaked surgical sponges and volume in suction canisters subtracting irrigation fluid added to the surgical field. At the end of the operation, we placed deep drainage below the fascia. The amount of drainage on

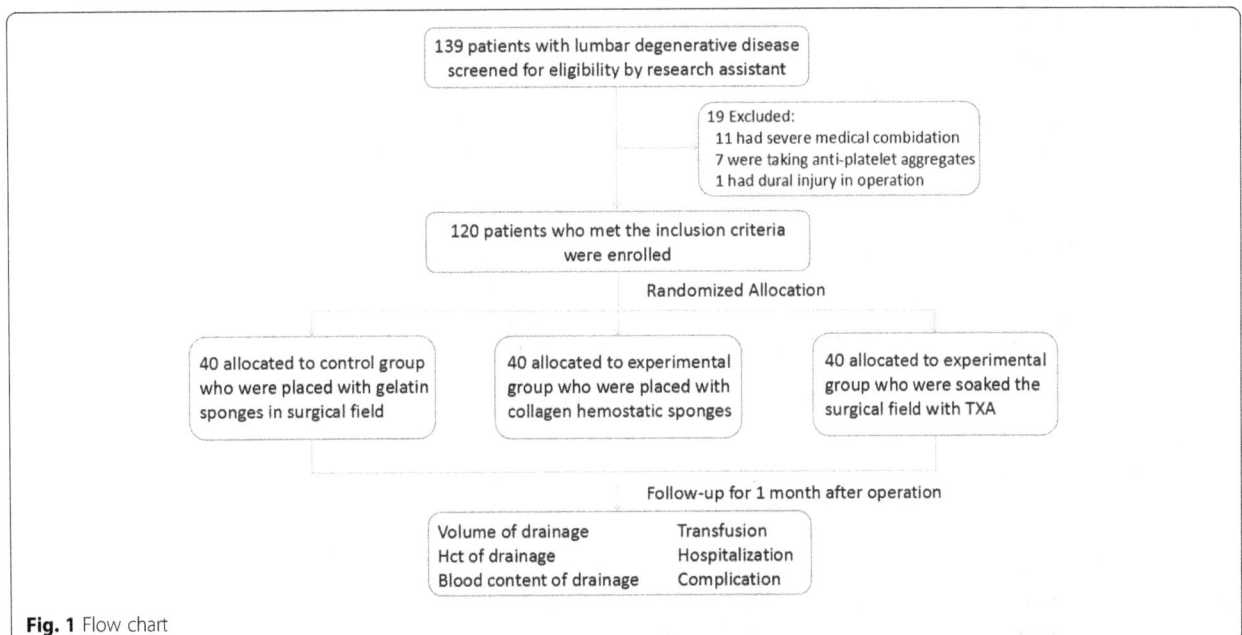

Fig. 1 Flow chart

postoperative day 1, postoperative day 2, and the total drainage volume were recorded.

The drainage was routinely removed when the drain output was less than 50 ml per 24 h. Recorded clinical data includes age, height, weight, body mass index (BMI), operative durations, surgical levels, intraoperative blood loss, related complications, and length of hospital stays.

Transfusion

No patients received CellSaver autologous blood transfusions during operation in our study. Routine blood tests including hematocrit (HCT), hemoglobin (HGB), and coagulation index were examined on the preoperative day and at 8, 24, 48, and 72 h post-operation. Transfusion was carried out for patients with hemoglobin level less than 8 g/dL and for symptomatic patients with hemoglobin level between 8 and 10 g/dL, such as persistent tachycardia (heart rate N100 for at least 4 h), chest pain, dyspnea, and hypotension (a drop in blood pressure N20 mmHg).

Complications

Venous Doppler ultrasonography was performed before patients discharge, and 1 month after operation, complications such as deep venous thrombosis (DVT)/pulmonary embolism (PE), spinal hematomas/seromas, and wound infections were investigated.

Statistics

The Pearson chi-square test was used to analyze categorical variables. The differences in perioperative data among 3 groups were analyzed using the one-way ANOVA. In all analyses, the level of statistical significance was set at $P < 0.05$. All data analyses were performed with the SPSS 19.0 software package. Four parameters were compared within 3 groups: (1) volume of drainage in postoperative day (POD) 1, POD 2, and patient's total drain output; (2) HCT of drainage in POD 1, POD 2, and POD 3; (3) blood content in drainage at different time points; and (4) transfusion rates and hospitalization durations.

This RCT study was approved by the ethical committee at Peking Union Medical College Hospital; the reference number is ZS-1000. All participants provided written informed consents for the study and surgery.

Results

Baseline characteristics

One hundred twenty patients who met the inclusion criteria participated in this study. According to the randomization scheme, there were 40 patients assigned to each group. The basic information of patients in these 3 groups is listed in Table 1. No significant differences in sex, age, BMI, preoperative HGB, surgical level, intra-

Table 1 Demographic date

Variable	Group A	Group B	Group C	P
N	40	40	40	
Age (year)	57.4 ± 10.7	58 ± 12.3	53.1 ± 12	P > 0.05
Sex				
Males	13	18	19	P > 0.05
Females	27	22	21	P > 0.05
BMI (kg/cm²)	24.9 ± 3.9	25 ± 3.3	25.6 ± 2.8	P > 0.05
Preoperative HGB (g/l)	126.8 ± 8.6	123.4 ± 10.3	139.4 ± 13.6	P > 0.05
Surgical level	2.31 ± 0.09	2.76 ± 0.12	2.40 ± 0.10	P > 0.05
Operative time (min)	144.5 ± 40.2	128 ± 40.9	121 ± 19.1	P > 0.05
Intra-operative blood loss (ml)	190 ± 123.2	223.8 ± 163	176 ± 100.5	P > 0.05
Mean duration of hospital stay (days)	7.82 ± 1.2	6.09 ± 1.3	6.13 ± 1.3	P = 0.001
Number of transfusion	12	3	3	P = 0.001

operative blood loss, or operative time were detected in 3 groups ($P > 0.05$).

Drainage

Our results showed that postoperative drainages were significantly different among the 3 groups (Table 2). Drainages in experimental groups were less than control group. In addition, patients with topical TXA in group C exhibited the least volume on POD 1 and of total postoperative drainage ($P < 0.05$).

Most of previous studies treated volume of drainage as postoperative blood loss; however, the volume of drainage is not equal to the postoperative blood loss according to the Gross formula. Because the component of drainage varied with time varying, so postoperative blood loss does not depend on the amount of fluid loss but the pure blood contained in drainage [11, 12]. In our study, we also examined complete blood count (CBC) for every drainage sample to obtain data of HCT and hemoglobin (HGB), which were used to calculate the precise blood contained in drainage. The pure blood loss in drainage = volume of drainage × $HCT/HCT_{average}(HCT_{average} = HCT_{pre} + HCT_{post})$.

According to the results detailed in Table 3, the average HCT of drainage in group C was lower than the other two groups (group A > group B > group C) in the postoperative 24 h; the difference showed statistical

Table 2 The information of postoperative drainage

Variable	Group A	Group B	Group C	P
Volume of drainage in POD 1 (ml)	232.8 ± 75.9	175.6 ± 76.8	90.9 ± 49.8	P = 0.001
Volume of drainage in POD 2 (ml)	74.1 ± 32.8	57.3 ± 34.5	41.1 ± 23	P = 0.001
Total volume of drainage (ml)	301.3 ± 110.9	232.8 ± 98	131.9 ± 78	P = 0.001

Table 3 The actual blood contain of postoperative drainage

Variable	Group A	Group B	Group C	P
HCT of drainage in POD 1 (%)	21.2 ± 6.1	19.3 ± 6.3	14.2 ± 5.3	P = 0.001
HCT of drainage in POD 2 (%)	11.7 ± 4.5	13.3 ± 4.7	9.6 ± 3.9	P > 0.05
HCT of drainage in POD 3 (%)	6.3 ± 2.1	5.2 ± 1.2	4.9 ± 1.3	P > 0.05
Drainage blood in POD 1 (ml)	137.1 ± 68.6	94.1 ± 52.2	34.8 ± 25.4	P = 0.001
Drainage blood in POD 2 (ml)	23 ± 18	20.6 ± 16.5	15.2 ± 4.5	P > 0.05
Total volume of drainage blood (ml)	160.2 ± 82.8	114.4 ± 60.7	39.9 ± 28.5	P = 0.001

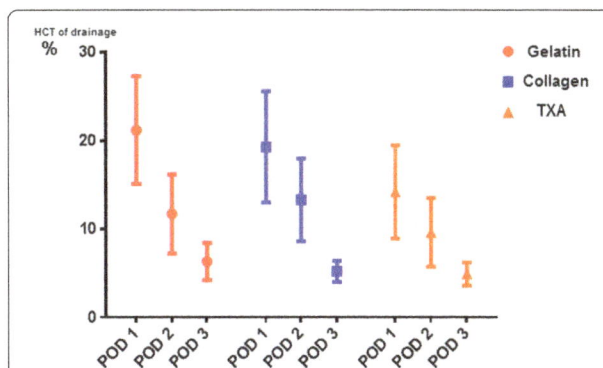

Fig. 3 Time variation of HCT of drainage. The HCT of drainage declined gradually over time

significance. While in the next 24 h, the HCT of drainage declined and no noticeable difference was observed in among groups. With the volume and HCT of drainage every day, we got accurate postoperative blood loss that is showed in Table 3 and Figs. 2 and 3. It is clear that total amount of postoperative blood loss in experimental groups was less than control group (group A > group B > group C), especially on the first day ($P < 0.05$).

Transfusion and hospitalization

There were 12 cases (30%) received transfusion in group A, which were in contrast to 3 cases (7.5%) in group B and 3 cases (7.5%) in group C. The hospitalization in experimental groups was less than that in control group as well (7.82 ± 1.2 vs 6.09 ± 1.3 vs 6.13 ± 1.3); these two indices have significant difference between experimental groups and control group ($P = 0.001$).

Complication

There were no perioperative complications, such as DVT/PE, postoperative hematomas or seromas, and postoperative infections in the 3 groups.

Discussion

Gelatin sponge, collagen sponge, and TXA have been introduced to reduce surgical bleedings as hemostatic agents for many years. In our study, the intraoperative blood loss in 3 groups had no statistical difference because the intervention happened at the end of surgery. However, the postoperative blood loss in experimental groups was much less than control group via measurement of drainage and its blood content (Fig. 4). The drainage decreased by 22.7 and 56.2% in group B and group C when compared with control group, respectively. The result is similar to many previous studies which have proven that collagen hemostatic sponge and TXA can effectively reduce postoperative blood loss in orthopedic operations [13–15]. Cho [13] soaked the absorbable gelatin sponge in thrombin and applied over the exposed spine before wound closure; the result demonstrated that patients' postoperative drain output (93 vs 204 ml, $P < 0.001$) and consequent hospital stays (1.3 days vs 2.2 days) could be further reduced. A meta-analysis of randomized controlled trials performed by Shangquan Wang has revealed that both topical TXA and intravenous TXA have been effective in reducing blood loss and

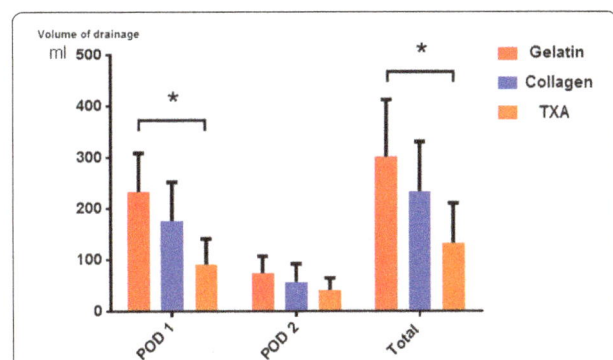

Fig. 2 Postoperative drainage in 3 groups. The postoperative drainage in experimental groups is much less than control group in POD 1 as well as total volume, and TXA group shows the best effect. There was no significant difference in 3 groups in POD 2

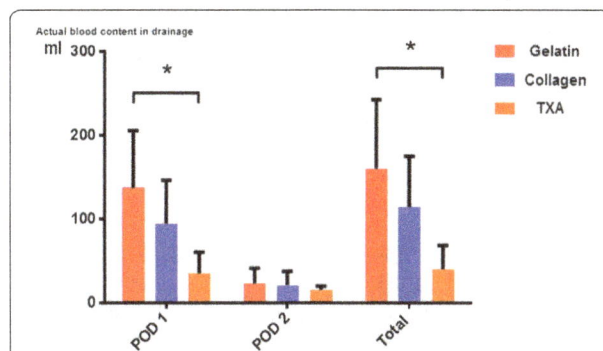

Fig. 4 Postoperative blood content in drainage. The calculated actual postoperative blood loss in experimental groups is also less than control group in POD 1 as well as total volume, and TXA group shows the best effect. There was no significant difference in 3 groups in POD 2

transfusion rates in patients who underwent TKA [10]. However, the used methods were completely different and there remains no consensus regarding to the relative efficacy of these two treatments. The aim of our study was to compare hemostatic effects of collagen sponge and topical TXA in a prospective randomized clinical trial for patients who undergo spinal fusion surgeries.

As mentioned before, it is more accurate to take blood content as an indicator of postoperative blood loss. According to our calculation, the blood content in drainage decreased respectively by 28.8 and 75% in collagen hemostatic sponge group and TXA group compared with gelatin sponge group. Based on results of drainage and blood content, TXA showed more effective hemostasis than collagen sponge. The reasons for this difference require further exploration, and it might relate to the fact that soaked TXA has a larger influential area than collagen's partial coverage.

Additionally, the rate of transfusion is an important indicator to evaluate efficacy of blood conservations. Hossein Elgafy' systematic review shows that for adult spine fusion surgery patients, the mean blood loss ranged from 650 to 2839 ml per patient and the proportion requiring transfusion ranged from 50 to 81% without plotting any strategy to reduce hemorrhage [1]. Jian Wu [16] reported that application of absorbable gelatin sponge in multilevel posterior spinal fusion surgery can decrease allogeneic blood transfusion rates (34.1 vs 58.5%, $P = 00.046$). As for TXA, Shi performed a prospective, randomized, double-blind, placebo-controlled study, in which the eligible patients were randomized to receive either a bolus dose of 30 mg/kg intravenous TXA, a maintenance dosage of 2 mg/kg/h TXA, or an equivalent volume of normal saline. The result showed that the blood transfusion rates did not vary significantly [17]. In our study, the amount of allogeneic blood transfusion of experimental groups was only 1/4 of the control group; meanwhile, there were no differences between collagen sponge group and topical TXA group. Compared with Shi's study, topical TXA showed better effect than intravenous TXA in reducing postoperative blood transfusion.

The decreased perioperative blood loss and transfusion rate contribute to not only a lower risks of anemia and infections but also better recovery and shorter hospitalization. In our study, there was an obvious shortened time for postoperative hospitalization in experimental groups. The average postoperative stay time of collagen sponge group was 6.09 days and topical TXA group was 6.13 days, which were much shorter than 7.82 days in control group. Reasons for the improvement are probably multifactorial, including less postoperative bleeding in wound, lower incidence of anemia, and better spirits and condition that all lead to earlier functional exercises.

Furthermore, each method has its own advantages and proper scope. It is convenient for collagen hemostasis sponge to cover hemorrhagic sites whenever needed during the operation. Especially for emergency bleeding, collagen sponge also has compression function which is more effective for bleeding resulted from large vessels lacerated. For TXA, because of its liquid characteristics, it can be used for particular spinal anatomical structures and is more effective for capillary hemorrhage.

Some limitations in our study must be pointed out. The sample size was small as only 40 cases were included in each group. As many cases with severe contraindications had been excluded from our trial, it is not enough to declare that all the hemostatic measures were safe under all clinical circumstances. In the future, we will perform a further validation on a larger sample size.

Conclusion

In this study, collagen sponge and topical TXA for patients undergoing spinal fusion surgeries were found to be effective, both of them can significantly decrease the total amount of postoperative blood loss, rates of allogeneic transfusion and hospital stays. In the meanwhile, no difference in the complication rates has been found. In comparison with collagen sponge, topical TXA is more effective in reducing postoperative drainage and bleeding, while no significant difference in transfusion rates and postoperative hospitalization.

Abbreviations
BMI: Body mass index; DVT: Deep venous thrombosis; HCT: Hematocrit; HGB: Hemoglobin; IV TXA: Intravenous TXA; PE: Pulmonary embolism; POD 1: Postoperative day 1; POD 2: Postoperative day 2; POD 3: Postoperative day 3; THA: Total hip arthroplasty; TKA: Total knee arthroplasty; TXA: Tranexamic acid

Acknowledgements
None

Funding
We get funding from Peking Union Medical College Hospital in the clinical collection, analysis, and interpretation of data.

Authors' contributions
In our study, SGL and DRX participated in the design of the study and ZNR and XC performed the statistical analysis. DRX and QYZ drafted the manuscript, and ZL helped to draft the manuscript. All authors read and approved the final manuscript.

Competing interests
The authors declare that they have no competing interests.

References
1. Elgafy H, Bransford RJ, McGuire RA, et al. Blood loss in major spine surgery. Spine (Phila Pa 1976). 2010;35(9 Suppl):S47-56.
2. Smorgick Y, Baker KC, Bachison CC, et al. Hidden blood loss during posterior spine fusion surgery. Spine J. 2013;13(8):877–81.

3. Huang YH, Ou CY. Significant blood loss in lumbar fusion surgery for degenerative spine. World Neurosurg. 2015;84(3):780–5.

4. Lan G, Lu B, Wang T, et al. Chitosan/gelatin composite sponge is an absorbable surgical hemostatic agent. Colloids Surf B Biointerfaces. 2015; 136:1026–34.

5. Cheriyan T, Maier SP 2nd, Bianco K, et al. Efficacy of tranexamic acid on surgical bleeding in spine surgery: a meta-analysis. Spine J. 2015;15(4):752–61.

6. Huang G-P, Jia X-F, Xiang Z, et al. Tranexamic acid reduces hidden blood loss in patients undergoing total knee arthroplasty: a comparative study and meta-analysis. Med Sci Monit. 2016;22:797–802.

7. DiBlasi JF, Smith RP, Garavaglia J, et al. Comparing cost, efficacy, and safety of intravenous and topical tranexamic acid in total hip and knee arthroplasty. Am J Orthop (Belle Mead NJ). 2016;45(7):E439–e443.

8. Xie J, Ma J, Yao H, et al. Multiple boluses of intravenous tranexamic acid to reduce hidden blood loss after primary total knee arthroplasty without tourniquet: a randomized clinical trial. J Arthroplast. 2016;31(11):2458–64.

9. Choi HY, Hyun SJ, Kim KJ, et al. Effectiveness and safety of tranexamic acid in spinal deformity surgery. J Korean Neurosurg Soc. 2017;60(1):75–81.

10. Wang S, Gao X, An Y. Topical versus intravenous tranexamic acid in total knee arthroplasty: a meta-analysis of randomized controlled trials. Int Orthop. 2017;41(4):739–48.

11. Gross JB. Estimating allowable blood loss: corrected for dilution. Anesthesiology, 1983;58(3): 277–80.

12. Xu D, Ren Z, Chen X, et al. A randomized controlled trial on effects of different hemostatic sponges in posterior spinal fusion surgeries. BMC Surg. 2016;16(1):80.

13. Cho SK, Yi J-S, Park MS, et al. Hemostatic techniques reduce hospital stay following multilevel posterior cervical spine surgery. The Journal of Bone and Joint Surgery-American Volume. 2012;94(21):1952–8.

14. Hu H-M, Chen L, Frary CE, et al. The beneficial effect of Batroxobin on blood loss reduction in spinal fusion surgery: a prospective, randomized, double-blind, placebo-controlled study. Arch Orthop Trauma Surg. 2015;135(4):491–7.

15. Lin C, Qi Y, Jie L, et al. Is combined topical with intravenous tranexamic acid superior than topical, intravenous tranexamic acid alone and control groups for blood loss controlling after total knee arthroplasty: a meta-analysis. Medicine (Baltimore). 2016;95(51):e5344.

16. Wu J, Jin Y, Zhang J, Shao H, Yang D, Chen J. Hemostatic techniques following multilevel posterior lumbar spine surgery. J Spinal Disord Tech. 2014;27(8):442–6.

17. Shi H, Ou Y, Jiang D, et al. Tranexamic acid reduces perioperative blood loss of posterior lumbar surgery for stenosis or spondylolisthesis: a randomized trial. Medicine (Baltimore). 2017;96(1):e5718.

21

Trajectory of instantaneous axis of rotation in fixed lumbar spine with instrumentation

Masataka Inoue[1†], Tetsutaro Mizuno[2†], Toshihiko Sakakibara[2], Takaya Kato[3], Takamasa Yoshikawa[1], Tadashi Inaba[1] and Yuichi Kasai[2*]

Abstract

Background: Several studies showed instantaneous axis of rotation (IAR) in the intact spine. However, there has been no report on the trajectory of the IAR of a damaged spine or that of a fixed spine with instrumentation. It is the aim of this study to investigate the trajectory of the IAR of the lumbar spine using the vertebra of deer.

Methods: Functional spinal units (L5–6) from five deer were evaluated with six-axis material testing machine. As specimen models, we prepared a normal model, a damaged model, and a pedicle screw (PS) model. We measured the IAR during bending in the coronal and sagittal planes and axial rotation. In the bending test, four directions were measured: anterior, posterior, right, and left. In the rotation test, two directions were measured: right and left.

Results: The IAR of the normal model during bending moved in the bending direction. The IAR of the damaged model during bending moved in the bending direction, but the magnitude of displacement was bigger compared to that of the normal model. In the PS model, the IAR during bending test hardly moved. During rotation test, the IAR of the normal model and PS model located in the spinal canal, but the IAR of the damaged model located in the posterior part of the vertebral body.

Conclusions: In this study, the IAR of damaged model was scattering and that of PS model was concentrating. This suggests that higher mechanical load applied to the dura tube and nerve roots in the damaged model and less mechanical load applied to that in the PS model.

Keywords: Biomechanics, Lumbar spine, Animal experiment, Spinal instrumentation, Instantaneous axis of rotation, Trajectory

Background

The instantaneous axis of rotation (IAR) is one of the evaluation metrics used in spinal biomechanics. Usually, the motion of a rigid body comprises translational motion and rotational motion. By regarding translational motion as rotational motion having a rotation radius of infinite length, the motion of a rigid body can be represented by the rotation around a certain point. Applying this principle to the spine, the motion of a functional spinal unit can be represented by the rotation around a point. The magnitude of the displacement of the rotating object is proportional to the horizontal distance from

the axis of rotation, and the displacement is larger in positions farther from the IAR. By examining the IAR, it is possible to know the deformation behavior of the spine. Moreover, we can evaluate spinal motion characteristics in detail to investigate the trajectory of the IAR (t-IAR).

There have been numerous studies on the IAR of the lumbar spine. White et al. reported the position of the IAR during bending and rotation of an intact spine [1]. Sakamaki et al., Sengupta et al., and Haher et al. examined the IAR of the lumbar spine with damaged intervertebral disc and facet joint [2–4]. Alapan et al. investigated the effect of ligament failure on the IAR in the lower lumbar spine [5]. Orribo et al. and Huang et al. examined the IAR of a fixed spine and a spine with a replaced disc [6, 7]. Collectively, the results from these studies show that the IAR of the lumbar spine is located in stable direction.

* Correspondence: ykasai@clin.medic.mie-u.ac.jp
†Equal contributors
2Department of Spinal Surgery and Medical Engineering, Mie University Graduate School of Medicine, 2-174 Edobashi, Tsu City 514-8507, Mie prefecture, Japan
Full list of author information is available at the end of the article

Although the IAR seems to remain stationary during exercise load, Wachowski et al. and Mansour et al. reported that the IAR moves constantly during bending and rotation of an intact spine [8, 9]. However, there have been few reports on the t-IAR of a damaged spine or that of a fixed spine with instrumentation [10]. This study was conducted for the purpose of discussing the clinical problems of the unstable spine or the spine fixed by instrumentation by determining the t-IAR.

In this study, we used deer spine as a specimen. Since it cannot be said that the autopsy of the spine is approximate between deer and human, it is impossible to compare the biomechanics data simply by range of motion (ROM). As described by Wasinpongwanich et al., however, when the ROM change rate, an index to evaluate how the intervertebral stability will change when the normal spine of deer is injured or fixed by instrumentation, is examined, the ROM change rate in the normal, damaged, and PS fixation models in deer approximates very much to that of humans [11]. In the experiment to explore the biomechanical tendency like this study, the spine of culled deer is therefore considered available as an alternative of humans [12–14].

Methods

Functional spinal units (L5–6) from five deer were used as specimens. Because L5–6 is the biggest in deer lumbar spine, damaged models or PS fixation models may be made easily. The deer were culled as part of a wildlife management program. After thawing each of the frozen lumbar spines at room temperature, the muscles and fat were removed while retaining the internal stabilizing elements. The cranial and caudal portions of each specimen were fixed to the jig with dental resin. As specimen models, we stepwisely prepared a normal model, a damaged model, and a pedicle screw (PS) model. Internal stabilizing elements were retained in the normal model. The damaged model was made by drilling through holes (diameter: 3 mm) at sites 1/4, 1/2, and 3/4 of the distance from the anterior surface on the L5/6 vertebral disc and removing its supraspinous ligament, interspinous ligament, and both facet joints (Fig. 1). The PS model was similar to the damaged model but fixed

with 6.5×40 mm PSs and rods (KiSCO: S-LineII, Saint-Priest, France) (Fig. 2).

For the tests, a six-axis material testing machine developed in our laboratory was used (Fig. 3) [15]. This testing machine adopts a parallel mechanism. A set of two actuators is located parallel at 120° to the object, and each of the six actuators is independently controlled. At the lower end of six actuators, a six-axis kinesthetic sensor is equipped to detect forces in the x-, y-, and z-axes and the torque around each axis. Furthermore, this kinesthetic sensor enables force control by feeding back the detected values to the control system and enables motion with multiple degrees of freedom.

Bending in the coronal and sagittal planes (bending test) and axial rotation (rotation test) were conducted for each model using this testing machine. In the bending test, linear and angular displacements were measured: anterior, posterior, right, and left. In the rotation test, two directions were measured: right and left. The torque was set at 3.0 Nm for the bending test and 4.0 Nm for the rotation test. Each test was repeated twice. And 100 N axial preloads are provided in all tests. The number of degrees of freedom in the bending test was set to three to allow genuine bending in one plane. The number of degrees of freedom in the rotation test was set to four to allow displacement along the x-, y-, and z-axes and rotation around the z-axis.

Linear and angular displacements from the time of no load to the time of maximum torque during the bending and rotation tests were measured. The IAR was calculated for every 0.2-degree increment of angular displacement. To calculate the IAR, the angular displacement and position coordinates for before and after motion in a corresponding section were used. An example of calculating the IAR (point C) when the position coordinates change from point A to point B is shown in Fig. 4. The position coordinates of point A, point B, and the angle β are obtained from the testing machine. First, the length L and the angle θ formed by the line segment AB and the horizontal plane are determined using Eqs. (1) and (2).

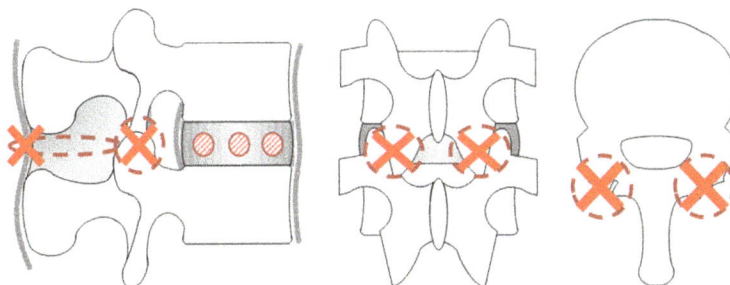

Fig. 1 Damaged model

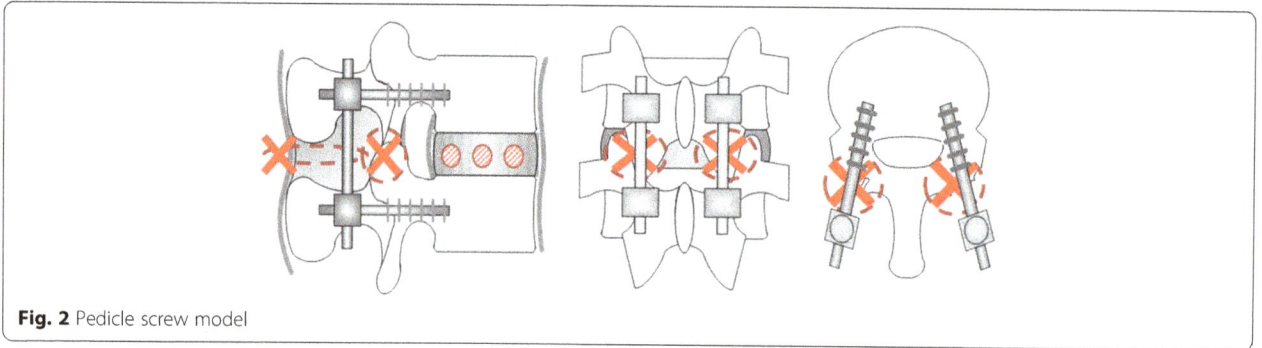

Fig. 2 Pedicle screw model

$$L = \sqrt{(y_b - y_a)^2 + (z_b - z_a)^2} \tag{1}$$

$$\theta = \tan^{-1}(y_b - y_a / z_b - z_a) \tag{2}$$

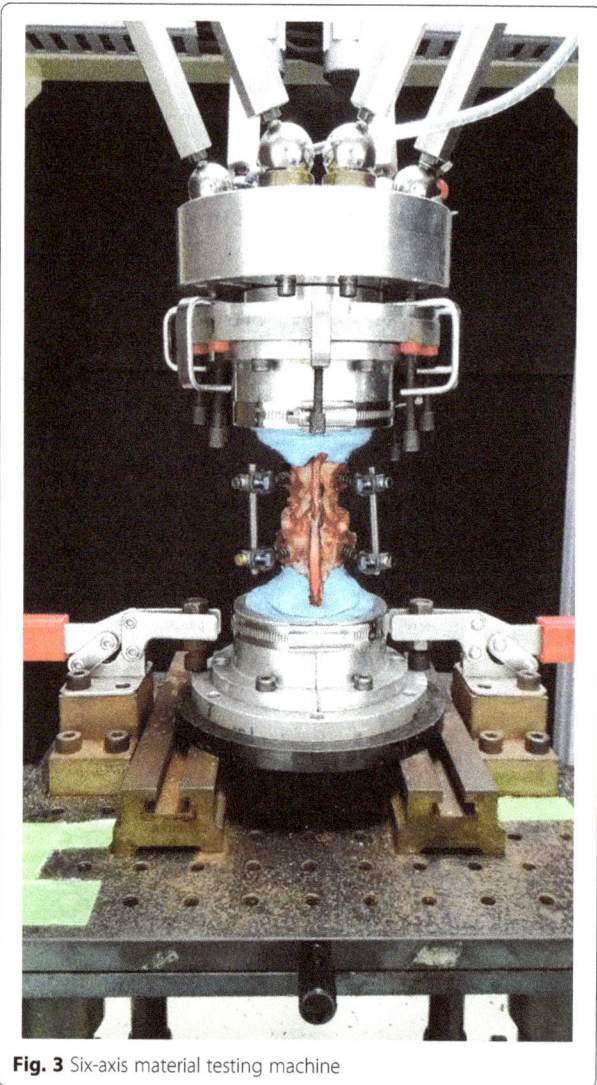

Fig. 3 Six-axis material testing machine

Next, consider the triangle ACD comprising point A, point C shown in Fig. 4, the line segment AB, and point D, which is a point of intersection of the line segment AB and its vertical bisector. The angle α is obtained from the sum of the interior angles of the triangle. The length R is calculated from the trigonometric ratio (Eq. (3)).

$$R = \frac{L}{2 \sin \frac{\beta}{2}} \tag{3}$$

The position coordinates of point C are obtained from Eq. (4). Point C is distance R away from point A. The angle of point C is $\theta + \alpha$ to the x-axis.

$$y = y_a + R \cos(\theta + \alpha)$$

$$z = z_a - R \sin(\theta + \alpha) \tag{4}$$

We calculate the IAR from data of second reciprocating motion of the bending and rotation. In the anterior–posterior bending test, β represents the angular displacement around the x-axis of the upper vertebral body compared to the angular displacement of the lower vertebral body, and $(y_b - y_a)$ and $(z_b - z_a)$ represent the magnitude of translation in the y- and z-axis directions of the upper vertebral body compared to the magnitude of translation of the lower vertebral body, respectively. The IAR during the bending and rotation tests can also be calculated using the magnitudes of angular displacement and translation from the upper vertebral body compared to the magnitudes of angular displacement and translation of the lower vertebral body.

The t-IAR in the anterior–posterior bending test was overlaid on the coordinate system, in which the caudal posterior end of the intervertebral disc is the origin O, the anterior–posterior direction of the vertebra is the y-axis (anterior is positive), and the cranial-to-caudal side direction is the z-axis (cranial side is positive). The t-IAR in the left–right bending test was overlaid on the coordinate system, in which the midpoint of the left and right horizontal diameters of the intervertebral disc on the caudal posterior

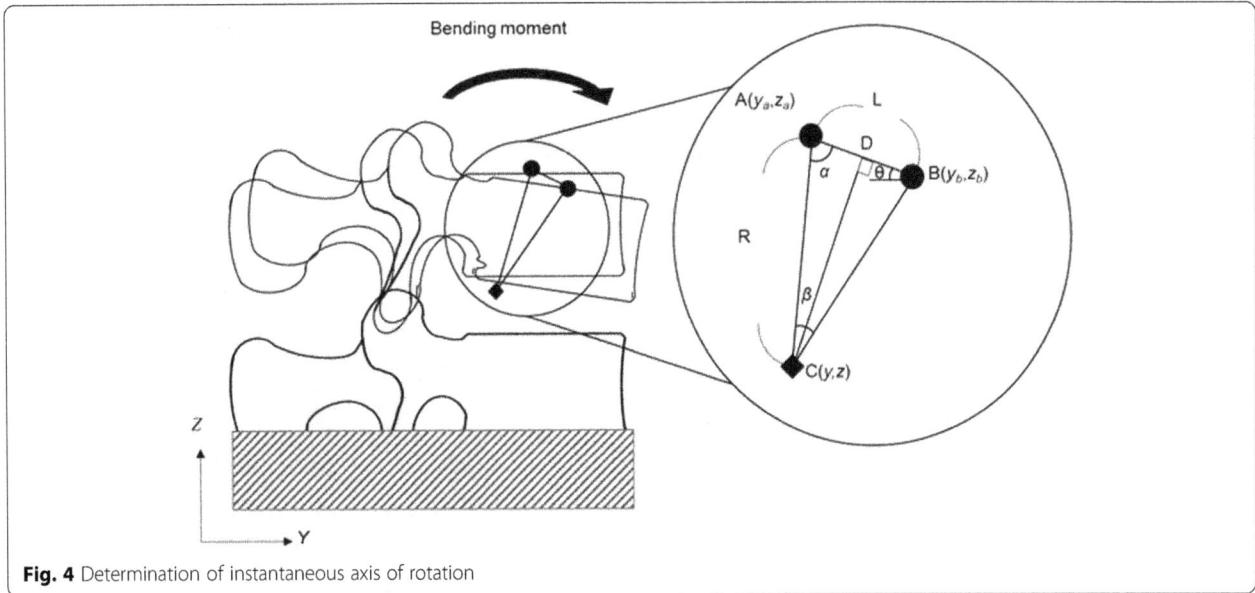

Fig. 4 Determination of instantaneous axis of rotation

edge is the origin O, the left–right direction of the vertebra is the x-axis (right side is positive), and the cranial-to-caudal direction is the z-axis (cranial side is positive). Further, the t-IAR in the rotation test was overlaid on the coordinate system, in which the midpoint of the left and right horizontal diameters of the vertebral body on the posterior edge is the origin O, the left–right direction of the spine is the x-axis (right side is positive), and the anterior–posterior direction is the y-axis (anterior is positive) (Fig. 5). The means of the t-IAR of five specimens are plotted in Figs. 6, 7, and 8.

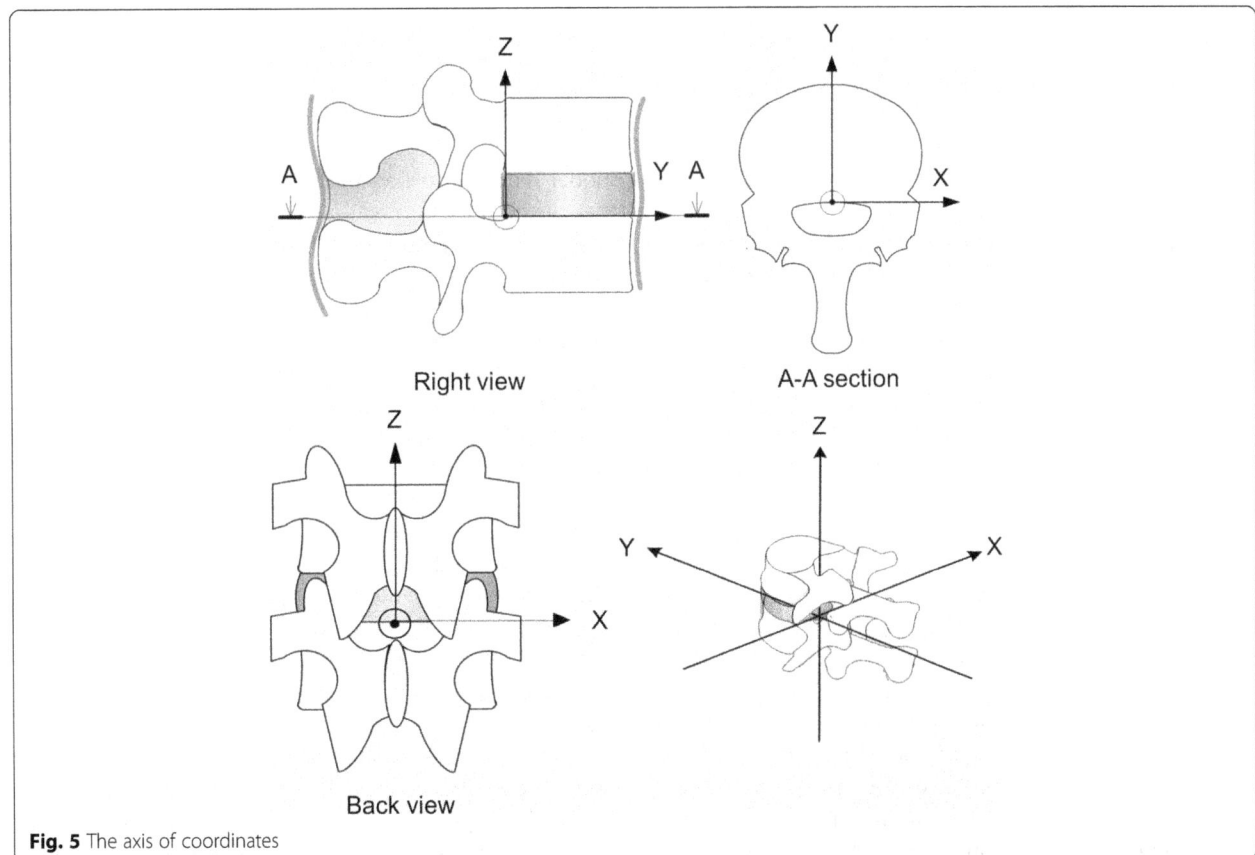

Fig. 5 The axis of coordinates

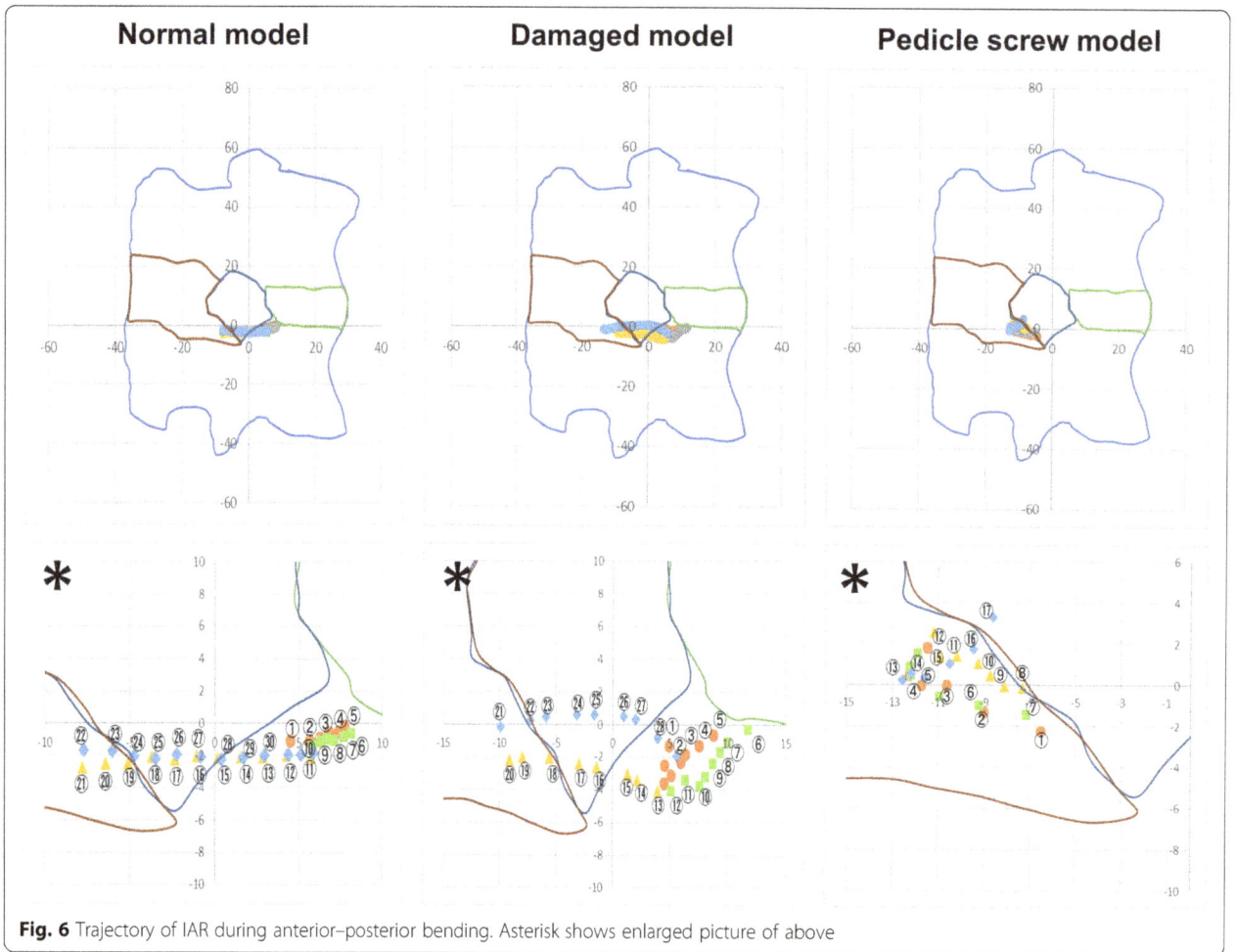

Fig. 6 Trajectory of IAR during anterior–posterior bending. Asterisk shows enlarged picture of above

Results

Anterior–posterior bending

Figure 6 shows the IAR during anterior–posterior bending. In this figure, the trace plotted with circles represents the t-IAR during anterior bending, the trace plotted with squares represents the t-IAR when returning to the midline after anterior bending, the trace plotted with triangles represents the t-IAR during posterior bending, and the trace plotted with rhomboids represents the t-IAR when returning to midline after posterior bending. The numbers in Fig. 1 indicate the order of movement of the t-IAR. Each of the five specimens tended to exhibit the same shift of the t-IAR during anterior–posterior bending.

The IAR of the normal and damaged models tends to be located in the anterior region of the vertebral body during anterior bending and in the posterior region of the vertebral body during posterior bending. On the other hand, the IAR of the PS model is in the posterior region of the spine. Particularly, the IAR during posterior bending is in a cranial position compared with the IAR during anterior bending. The t-IAR of the damaged

model during anterior–posterior bending is longer than that of the normal model. On the other hand, the t-IAR of the PS model is shorter than that of the normal and damaged models.

Left–right bending

Figure 7 shows the IAR during left–right bending. In this figure, the trace plotted with circles represents the t-IAR during bending to the left, the trace plotted with squares represents the t-IAR when returning to midline after bending to the left, the trace plotted with triangles represents the t-IAR during bending to the right, and the trace plotted with rhomboids represents the t-IAR when returning to midline after bending to the right. The numbers in Fig. 2 indicate the order of movement of the t-IAR. Each of the five specimens tended to exhibit the same shift of the t-IAR during left–right bending.

The IAR of the normal and damaged models during left–right bending is located on the left side of the vertebral body during bending to the left and on the right side of the vertebral body during bending to the right.

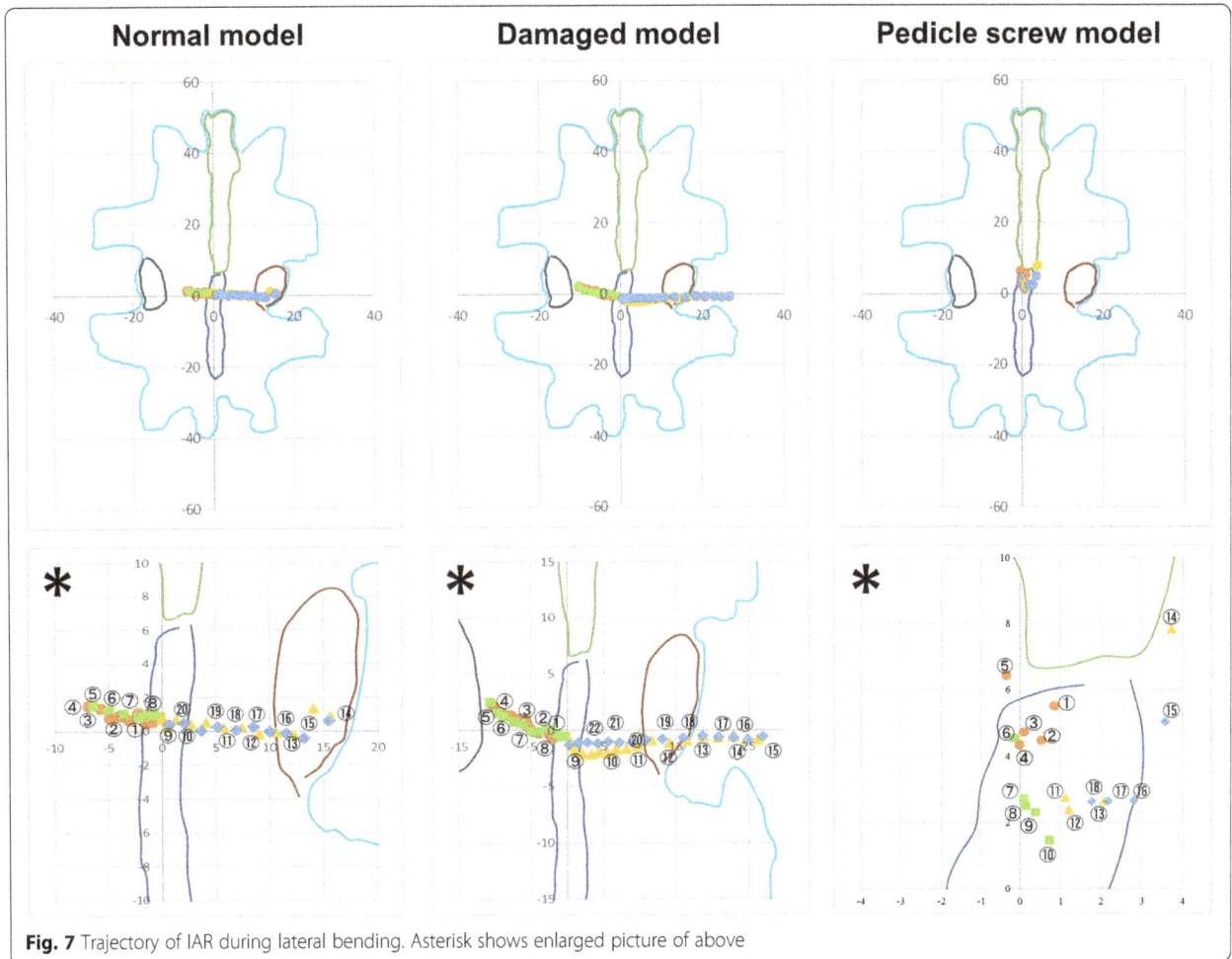

Fig. 7 Trajectory of IAR during lateral bending. Asterisk shows enlarged picture of above

On the other hand, the IAR of the PS model is primarily located in the center of the vertebral body. While the t-IAR of the normal and damaged models during left–right bending is in the intervertebral disc, the t-IAR of the PS model is in a cranial position. The t-IAR of the damaged model is longer than that of the normal model. In contrast, the t-IAR of the PS model is shorter than that of the normal and damaged models.

Rotation

Figure 8 shows the IAR during rotation. In this figure, the trace plotted with circles represents the t-IAR during rotation to the left, the trace plotted with squares represents the t-IAR when returning to midline after rotation to the left, the trace plotted with triangles represents the t-IAR during rotation to the right, and the trace plotted with rhomboids represents the t-IAR when returning to midline after rotation to the right. Each of the five specimens tended to exhibit the same shift of the t-IAR during rotation.

Now, t-IAR always exists in the spinal canal in the normal model and PS model in axial rotation, but it transfers anteriorly into the vertebral body in the damaged model. In the damaged model, moreover, t-IAR does not move so much in comparison with the other models. From the above, it is considered that the normal model and PS model have a small dynamic load onto the dural tube in the spinal canal, but in the damaged model, a load is always put on the dural tube. It is therefore presumed that persistent dynamic stress is placed on the dural tube when intervertebral instability is observed.

Discussion

This study is the first to examine the t-IAR of a damaged lumbar spine and instrumented spine during bending in the coronal and sagittal planes and axial rotation.

According to the results of the present study, the IAR of the normal model during bending moves in the bending direction, but remains in the spinal canal during rotation. These results agree with that from a study by Wachowski et al., who studied the kinematics of spinal segment [8]. Further, since the t-IAR of the normal model during bending and rotation remains in the spinal

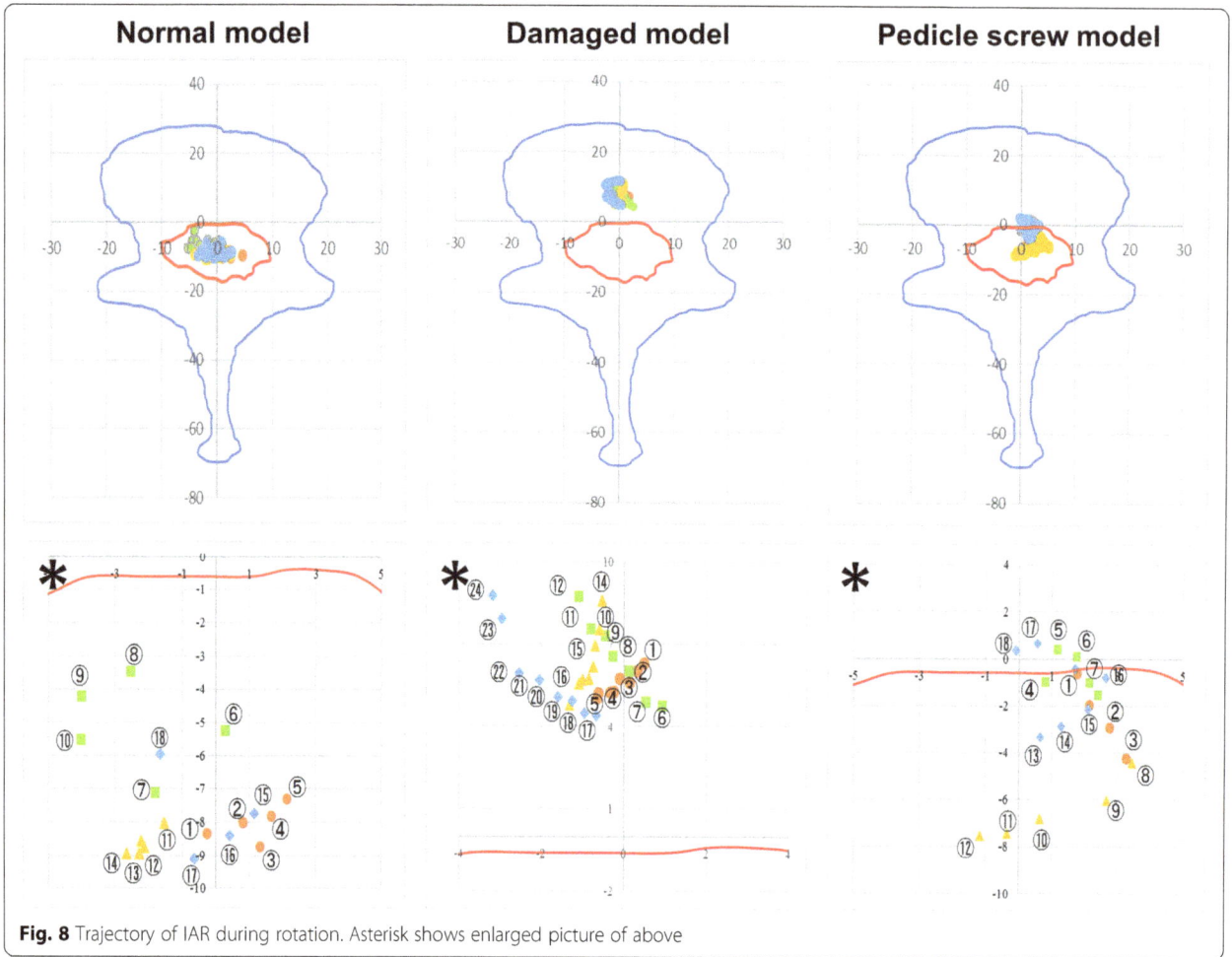

Fig. 8 Trajectory of IAR during rotation. Asterisk shows enlarged picture of above

canal, the displacement and shear load occurring in the dura mater tube and nerve roots in the spinal canal are considered small.

Similar to the normal model, the IAR of the damaged model during bending moved in the bending direction. However, the magnitude of displacement of the IAR of the damaged model is bigger compared to that of the normal model, and the IAR is away from the spinal canal. Thus, the shear load occurring in the dura mater tube and nerve roots of the damaged model is higher than that of the normal model. Ahmadi et al. also reported that arc length of instantaneous center of rotation was significantly higher in patients with low back pain, and this might be one of the causes of low back pain or nervous symptoms [16]. The t-IAR during rotation is primarily located in the vertebral body. This suggests that the rigidity in the posterior region of the spine is decreased because of the damage to both facet joints, and the rigidity in the anterior region of the spine is relatively increased. The IAR was primarily located in the spinal canal in the normal model, but shifted to the vertebral body in the damaged model. Higher shear load

is applied to the dura mater tube or nerve roots in the spinal canal and may worsen neurological symptoms. Therefore, IAR analysis reconfirms that fusion surgery is necessary for trauma with facet joint injury or patients with degenerative disease.

In the PS model, the IAR during anterior–posterior bending is primarily located in the posterior region of the spine. This is likely caused by the PS instrumentation increasing the rigidity in this region. During anterior–posterior bending of the spine, a high load might have been applied to the front of the vertebra and intervertebral disc, as well as the anterior tip of the PS. Further, the t-IAR during posterior bending shifts to a cranial position compared with the t-IAR during anterior bending. This suggests that a high load might have been applied to the cranial region of the specimen during anterior bending and to the caudal region of the specimen during posterior bending of the spine instrumented with PS. During left–right bending, the IAR is primarily located in the center of the vertebral body in the PS model, which seems to be the ideal position. Further, during rotation, the IAR is primarily located in the posterior region of the vertebral body in the vicinity of the spinal canal, and instrumentation with PS is considered to reduce the mechanical load applied to the dura tube or nerve roots.

This study has several limitations: (1) the specimens were spinal columns from deer, (2) only five samples were tested, (3) PSs for humans were used, and (4) coupling motion was not considered. In the future, we plan to conduct similar experiments using human cadavers, increase the number of samples, and perform experiments and repeated loading tests for the coupling motion.

Conclusion

We examined the t-IAR in different spine models subjected to bending and rotation. The model with damage to the intervertebral disc and facet joint exhibited increased intervertebral instability, which led to higher mechanical load on the dura tube or nerve roots. The mechanical load on the dura tube or nerve roots was reduced in the model with PS instrumentation, but this model exhibited a higher mechanical load on the front of the vertebral body and intervertebral disc and on the anterior tip of the PS during anterior–posterior bending.

Abbreviations

IAR: Instantaneous axis of rotation; PS: Pedicle screw; ROM: Range of motion; t-IAR: Trajectory of the IAR

Acknowledgements

Mr. Inoue and Dr. Mizuno contributed equally to the manuscript.

Funding

None

Authors' contributions

MI drafted the manuscript, did the first selection of articles, and assessed the quality of the papers. TM, TS, TK, and TY gave important input for the method part of this paper, assessed the quality of the papers, and performed the statistical analysis, and TM revised the manuscript critically for its content. TI and YK helped to draft and correct the manuscript. All authors read and approved the final manuscript.

Competing interest

Department of Spinal Surgery and Medical Engineering, Mie University Graduate School of Medicine, is a donated fund laboratory of KiSCO Co. Ltd., Japan.

Author details

[1]Department of Mechanical Engineering, Graduate School of Engineering, Mie University, 1577 Kurimamachiya-cho, Tsu City 514-8507, Mie prefecture, Japan. [2]Department of Spinal Surgery and Medical Engineering, Mie University Graduate School of Medicine, 2-174 Edobashi, Tsu City 514-8507, Mie prefecture, Japan. [3]Community-University Research Cooperation Center, Mie University, 1577 Kurimamachiya-cho, Tsu City 514-8507, Mie prefecture, Japan.

References

1. White AA, Panjabi MM. The basic kinematics of the human spine: a review of past and current knowledge. Spine. 1978;3(1):12–20.
2. Sakamaki T, Katoh S, Sairyo K. Normal and spondylolytic pediatric spine movements with reference to instantaneous axis of rotation. Spine(Phila Pa 1976). 2002;27(2):141–5.
3. Sengupta DK, Demetropoulos CK, Herkowitz HN. Instant axis of rotation of L4-5 motion segment—a biomechanical study on cadaver lumbar spine. J Indian Med Assoc. 2011;109(6):389. -90,392-3,395
4. Haher TR, O'Brien M, Felmly WT, et al. Instantaneous axis of rotation as a function of the three columns of the spine. Spine(Phila Pa 1976). 1992;17(6 Suppl):S149–54.
5. Alapan Y, Demir C, Kaner T, et al. Instantaneous center of rotation behavior of the lumbar spine with ligament failure. J Neurosurg Spine. 2013;18:617–26.
6. Perez-Orribo L, Zucherman J, Hsu K, et al. Biomechanics of a posterior lumbar motion stabilizing device. Spine. 2016;41(2):E55–63.
7. Huang RC, Girardi FP, Cammisa FP Jr, et al. The implications of constraint in lumbar total disc replacement. J Spinal Dsord Tech 2003;16(4):412-417.
8. Wachowski MM, Mansour M, Lee C, et al. How do spinal segments move? J Biomech. 2009;42(14):2286–93.
9. Mansour M, Spiering S, Christoph L, et al. Evidence for IHA migration during axial rotation of a lumbar spine segment by using a novel high-resolution 6D kinematic tracking system. J Biomech. 2004;37:583–92.
10. Anderst W, Baillargeon E, Donaldson MW, et al. Motion path of the instant center of rotation in the cervical spine during in vivo dynamic flexion-extension: implications for artificial disc design and evaluation of motion quality following arthrodesis. Spine. 2013;38(10):E594–601.
11. Wasinpongwanich K, Sakakibara T, Yoshikawa T, et al. Are deer and boar spine a valid biomechanical model for human spines? J Spine. 2014;3:5. https://doi.org/10.4172/2165-7939.1000187.
12. Kumar N, Kukreti S, Ishaque M, et al. Anatomy of deer spine and its comparison to the human spine. Anat Rec. 2000;260:189–203.
13. Kumar N, Kukreti S, Ishaque M, et al. Functional anatomy of the deer spine: an appropriate biomechanical model for the spine. Anat Rec. 2002;266:108–17.
14. Liu GM, Li YQ, CJ X, et al. Feasibility of vertebral internal fixation using deer and sheep as animal models. Chin Med J. 2010;123:2379–83.
15. Fujiwara M, Masuda T, Inaba T, et al. Development of 6-axis material tester for measuring mechanical spine properties. J Robot Mechatron. 2006;18(2):160–5.
16. Ahmadi A, Maroufi N, Hamid B, et al. Kinematic analysis of dynamic lumbar motion in patients with lumbar segmental instability using digital videofluoroscopy. Eur Spine J. 2009;18:1677–85.

22

Comparison of three different fixation constructs for radial neck fractures: a biomechanical study

Hongwei Chen[1], Dengying Wu[2], Tianlong Pan[2], Jun Pan[2], Rui Zhang[2] and Xuchao Shi[2*]

Abstract

Background: Fixation of radial neck fractures can be achieved with a plate and screw construct or with two screws. This study evaluated the biomechanical properties of three different fixation methods following radial neck fractures.

Methods: Twenty-four fourth-generation composite radii were sawed to simulate an unstable radial neck fracture. They were then instrumented with a plate and screw construct or two different orientations (crossed and parallel) of screw fixation. Implants were tested under bending and torsional loads via a tension torsion composite test system. Bending and torsional failure loads were added to the remaining implant-radius constructs if they did not fail during the previous tests.

Results: During the bending loading test, the crossed-screw group showed the greatest stiffness, followed by the parallel-screw group, the plate group demonstrating the weakest stiffness. There was no significant difference between the crossed- and the parallel-screw groups. However, there was a significant difference between the two screw groups and the plate group. During the bending failure test, the largest stiffness was found for the crossed-screw group, while the plate group exhibited the smallest stiffness. There was a significant difference between the three groups. During the torsion loading test, the highest stiffness was observed for the crossed-screw group, while the plate group showed the lowest stiffness. In the torsion failure test, the failure torques were 11.97 ± 2.659, 8.531 ± 1.768, and 7.079 ± 1.666 N m respectively for the crossed-screw, parallel-screw, and plate groups. There was a significant difference between the crossed-screw group and the two other groups.

Conclusions: Crossed screws and plate fixation are commonly used in clinical practice to treat simple radial neck fractures. While the present study shows that the parallel-screw method results in similar biomechanical strength as the two other techniques, it has the advantages of reaching limited wound exposure and having the implant buried. Therefore, it may be widely used in clinical practice.

Keywords: Radial neck fractures, Screw, Biomechanical comparison, Different fixation constructs

Background

Radial head and neck fractures are uncommon, their reported incidence being approximately 55.4 per 100,000 persons [1]. The injury mechanism of the radial neck is usually an axial load caused by valgus and fall [2, 3], during which the radial capitellar joint usually transfers 60% of the upper limb load [4]. In order to restore stability and alignment of the displaced radial head and neck

following a fracture and to enable then an early range of motion, open reduction with internal fixation (ORIF) is essential [5–7]. There are controversial and varied treatment choices for radial head and neck fractures. However, there is still no consensus regarding the best treatment to dispense for Mason–Johnston types II–IV fractures [8]. The Mason classification has been widely used to describe the radial head and neck fracture [9]. Broberg and Morrey [10] modified this classification with type II fractures being those having more than 2 mm of displacement and involving at least 30% of the radial head. Johnston [11] then added a type IV fracture

* Correspondence: shixuchao0577@163.com
[2]Department of Orthopaedics Surgery, The Second Affiliated Hospital and Yuying Children's Hospital of Wenzhou Medical University, NO.109, Xue Yuan West Road, Wenzhou, Zhejiang Province 325027, China
Full list of author information is available at the end of the article

to the classification, which corresponds to a radial head or neck fracture associated with an elbow dislocation. The purpose of this study was to determine the biomechanical properties of the bending and torsional stiffnesses of a plate and two different screw fixation orientations (crossed and parallel) in an unstable radial neck fracture. Only five studies evaluating the biomechanical characteristics of various radial head implants were found in the literature [12–16].

A simple radial neck fracture model was used to standardize our investigation. Although this model does not reproduce radial head and neck fractures, the results of this study can still help orthopedic surgeons to develop the most reasonable internal fixation pattern. We aimed at comparing the stiffness and strength of the plate and two different screw orientations, the plate and the crossed screw being commonly used in clinical practice, and the parallel screw being specifically designed by us for this study.

Methods

We used 24 identical (i.e., same size and density) synbone radii (SYNBONE AG, Malans, Switzerland). Each radius was cut at the mid-shaft level, leaving an approximately 10-cm long proximal segment. A transverse osteotomy was then made at the head-neck junction by using a micro-sagittal saw, this simulating a longitudinally unstable radial neck fracture.

Three different fixation devices were tested for reconstruction after the osteotomy: a radial head plate and screws (Stryker, Mahwah, NJ, USA) or two different orientations (crossed and parallel) of screw fixation (AO, Davos, Switzerland). The plate group included a plate construct involving five bicortical screws. In the crossed-screw group, the screws were placed approximately 60° apart, as described by Smith and Hotchkiss [17]. In the parallel-screw group, the screws were inserted in parallel to each other. The two screws were inserted into the radial head from the outer edge of the top at 45° of the radial head axis. The length of the two screws was uniform, and the distance between the two screws was 5 mm. The plate was placed in the safe zone of the radial head, which lies on the dorsal surface of the radius [18]. The fixations were evaluated using X-ray images. Figure 1 shows X-rays of the reconstructed radial heads with the three different fixation devices described above. The transversely cut end of the radial shaft was then potted in a metal tube by using polymethylmethacrylate (PMMA). Figure 2 displays some representative potted specimens. An Electro Force 3510 Tension torsion composite test system (Bose, MA, USA) was used to test the specimens. The testing machine features up to ± 75,000 N of axial force capacity and ± 50 N m of torque capacity.

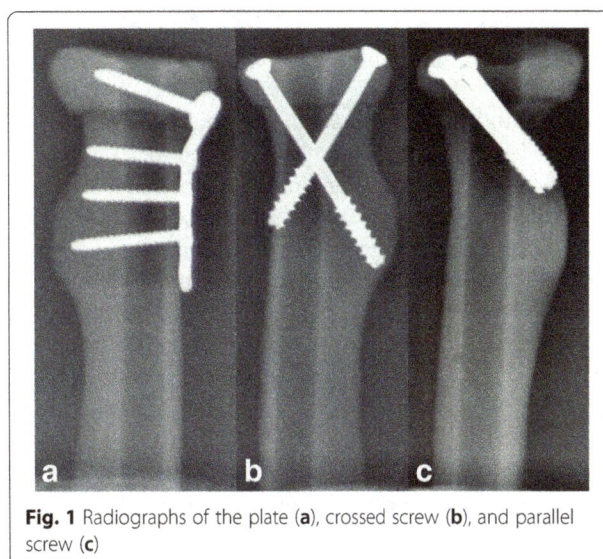

Fig. 1 Radiographs of the plate (**a**), crossed screw (**b**), and parallel screw (**c**)

Bending load test

The bending load was applied to the radial head through a custom solid cup made of PMMA. The loading orientation was posterior to anterior. Before the actual test, a preload of 10 N was applied three times at the same velocity (2 mm/min) to the radial head which had to resist to a horizontal slide. This position was regarded as the baseline to record the displacement of the head and the data were then cleared. Next, the construct was loaded in compression at a rate of 2 mm/min. The test was stopped when the displacement of the radial head reached 2 mm.

After the bending load test, if the fracture models did not fail, a failure load test was performed at a rate of 2 mm/min. Bending stiffness and bending failure loads were recorded.

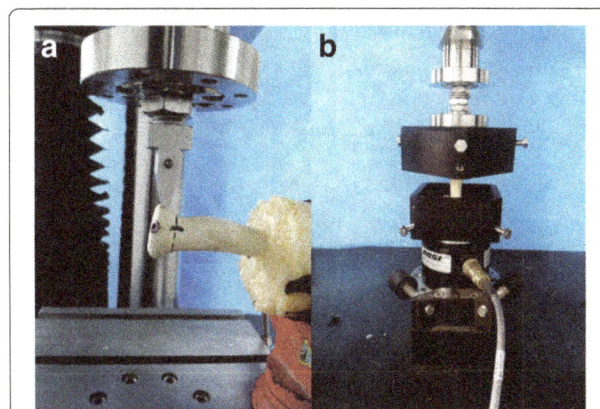

Fig. 2 The radial head model was placed in the instrument for bending (**a**) and torsional (**b**) loading

Torsional load test

First, the head of the radial was coupled with the actuator of the Electro Force 3510 Tension torsion composite test system with the use of an additional double gimbal fixture (Bose, MA, USA). Radii were then loaded for 10 cycles at 1 Hz in both the anterior and posterior torsional direction at five levels: $-0.5°$, $-1.0°$, $-1.5°$, $-2.0°$, and $-2.5°$. The torsional stiffness obtained was then used to evaluate the ability of the fixed structure to resist rotation.

Similarly to the bending load test procedure presented above, the fracture models underwent a failure load test at a rate of 5°/min if they did not fail after the torsional load test. Torsional stiffness and torsional failure loads were recorded.

Failure of the model was defined as (1) a new fracture line appearing in the model in addition to the original fracture line; (2) an internal fixation failure, such as plate or screw bending, cutting, or fracture; (3) a lateral displacement of the radial head superior to 5 mm or a torsion displacement of the radial head that exceeded 14.5°; and (4) a flat load-displacement curve in the data acquisition image or an absence of change in the displacement of the model while the load still increased.

The stiffness was defined as the slope of the regression line fitted to the loading segment of the cyclic load displacement curves. Data of each group are presented as mean ± standard deviation (SD). For statistical analysis, SPSS 21.0 (IBM Corporation, Armonk, NY, USA) was used. Mechanical parameters were compared by using one-way analyses of variance. The level of statistical significance was set at $p < 0.05$.

Results

We compared the stiffness of the three structures from the five bending load levels (Table 1). The stiffness of the crossed-screw group was the largest compared with the two other structures. Although the stiffness of the parallel-screw group appeared smaller than the crossed-screw group, our results revealed no statistical difference for all levels (Table 2). The stiffness of the plate group was smaller than that of the parallel-screw ($p = 0.003$) and crossed-screw groups ($p < 0.001$). All bending load data were processed as a displacement-load curve, as

Table 1 Bending stiffness of plate, crossed-screw, and parallel-screw constructs

Load (mm)	Mean ± SD (N/mm)		
	Plate group	Crossed-screw group	Parallel-screw group
0.4	45.56 ± 7.23	68.86 ± 10.07	68.24 ± 19.82
0.8	46.69 ± 5.31	65.11 ± 10.60	66.01 ± 10.61
1.2	49.68 ± 6.98	69.53 ± 10.46	68.57 ± 9.87
1.6	47.98 ± 7.46	73.37 ± 11.16	67.29 ± 9.26
2.0	48.44 ± 6.29	69.66 ± 10.65	66.82 ± 9.30

Table 2 Comparison of three constructs during bending

Constructs' type (average N)	P		
	Plate group	Crossed-screw group	Parallel-screw group
Plate group		0.000	0.003
Crossed-screw group	0.000		0.427
Parallel-screw group	0.003	0.427	

depicted in Fig. 3. The three curves in the figure represent the three different load-displacement variations. It can be observed that the load-displacement variation was approximately linear in the range of 0–2 mm for the three groups. A first analysis revealed that the three sets of data met the homogeneity of variance criterion. The average stiffness of the plate group was 48.73 ± 6.801 N/mm. The parallel-screw group was 25.28% stiffer than the plate group while the crossed-screw group was 46.21% stiffer than the plate group (Table 3). A stiffness comparison between the three groups is presented in Fig. 4. The bending failure load test revealed that the failure load was the largest for the crossed-screw group (418.51 ± 70.68 N), whereas the minimum failure load was observed for the plate group with only 279.22 ± 75.36 N, the parallel-screw group standing between the two groups with 399.73 ± 81.60 N (Fig. 5). There was no statistical difference between the two screw groups. However, the plate group was statistically different from the two other groups.

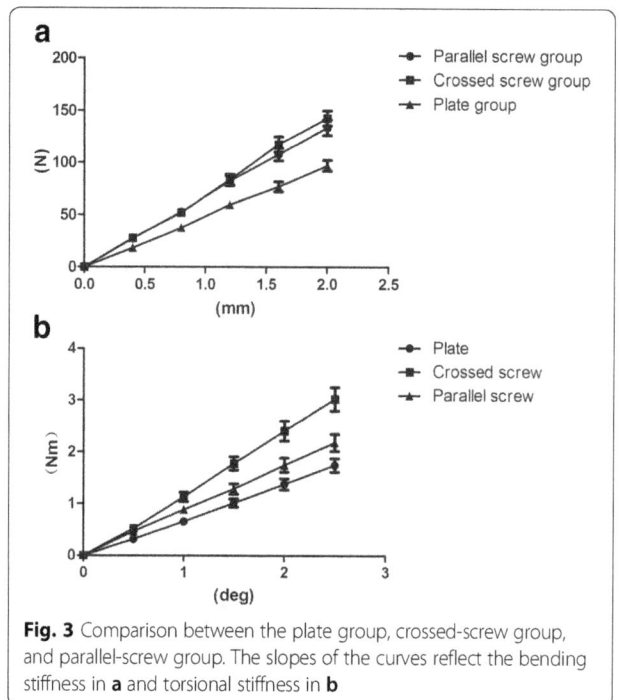

Fig. 3 Comparison between the plate group, crossed-screw group, and parallel-screw group. The slopes of the curves reflect the bending stiffness in **a** and torsional stiffness in **b**

Table 3 Average stiffness on bending and torsion of plate, crossed-screw, and parallel screw constructs

	Plate group	Crossed-screw group	Parallel-screw group
Bending average (N/mm)	48.73 ± 6.80	71.25 ± 10.88	67.05 ± 8.54
Torsion average (Nm/°)	0.69 ± 0.12	1.22 ± 0.22	0.95 ± 0.17

We also compared the behavior of the three structures at the five different levels during the torsion loading test (Table 4 and Fig. 3). Average torsional stiffness is presented in Table 3 and Fig. 4 for the three structures. The crossed-screw group demonstrated the greatest stiffness, followed by the parallel-screw group and then the plate group. As presented in Table 5, statistical results

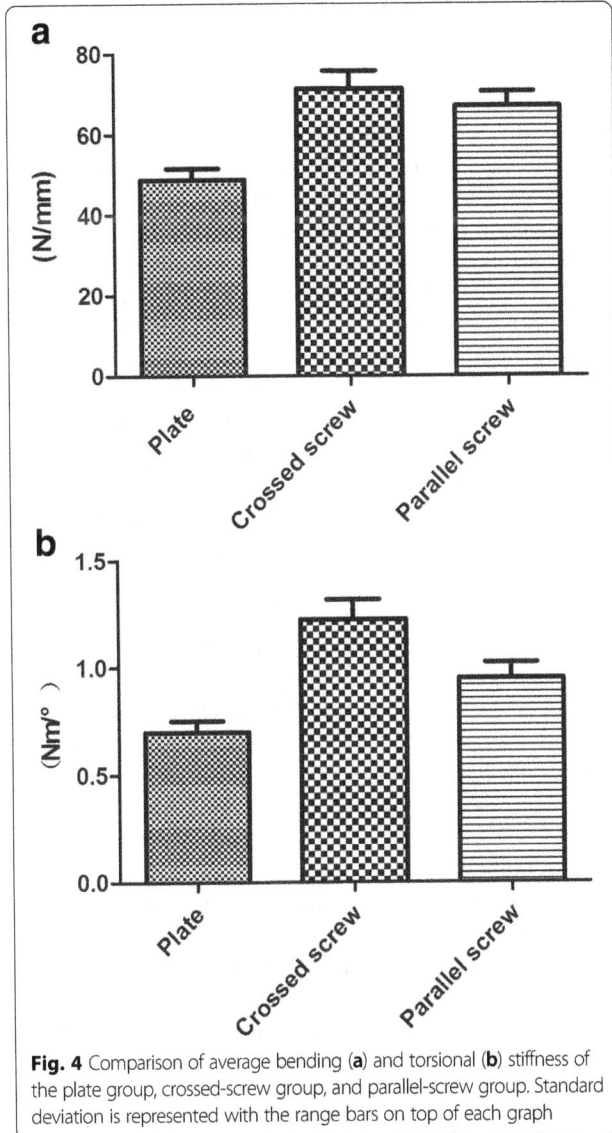

Fig. 4 Comparison of average bending (**a**) and torsional (**b**) stiffness of the plate group, crossed-screw group, and parallel-screw group. Standard deviation is represented with the range bars on top of each graph

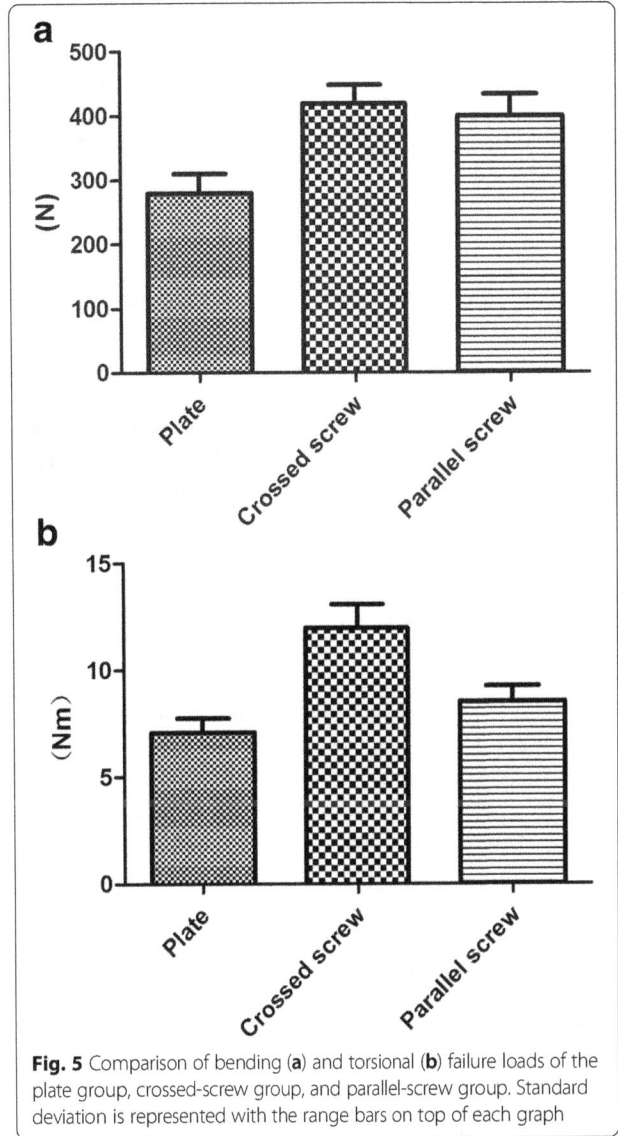

Fig. 5 Comparison of bending (**a**) and torsional (**b**) failure loads of the plate group, crossed-screw group, and parallel-screw group. Standard deviation is represented with the range bars on top of each graph

revealed that the average stiffnesses of the three groups were significantly different from each other ($p < 0.05$). Results of the torsion failure test showed that stiffness was significantly higher for the crossed-screw group than for the parallel-screw and plate groups, with no

Table 4 Rotation stiffness of plate, crossed-screw, and parallel-screw constructs

Rotation degree (°)	Mean ± SD (Nm/°)		
	Plate group	Crossed-screw group	Parallel-screw group
0.5	0.31 ± 0.08	0.51 ± 0.13	0.46 ± 0.09
1.0	0.65 ± 0.09	1.12 ± 0.22	0.88 ± 0.18
1.5	1.01 ± 0.19	1.77 ± 0.31	1.28 ± 0.24
2.0	1.37 ± 0.26	2.4 ± 0.46	1.74 ± 0.33
2.5	1.74 ± 0.31	3.02 ± 0.55	2.17 ± 0.40

Table 5 Comparison of three constructs during torsion

Constructs' type (average Nm)	P		
	Plate group	Crossed-screw group	Parallel-screw group
Plate group		0.000	0.029
Crossed-screw group	0.000		0.019
Parallel-screw group	0.029	0.019	

significant difference between the parallel-screw group and the plate group (Fig. 5).

Discussion

The surgical management of radial head and neck fractures has evolved over the last decades. For radial head and neck fractures of type II, there is no general agreement in the literature on the superiority of any surgical or conservative treatment over the other. Radial head fractures of type III are commonly treated with surgery. Several surgical treatment options can be performed: ORIF by screws, plates, k-wires or biodegradable pins, implantation of a prosthesis [19, 20], or resection of the radial neck [21–23]. Regarding the initial stability of the forearm and elbow, and the later development of arthritis, ORIF is believed to be a superior technique compared with the radial head resection for the treatment of unstable, displaced radial head fractures [5, 24, 25]. Ikeda et al. [25] compared the clinical results obtained after either resection or ORIF of Mason type III fractures. They reported a better outcome with better function for patients in whom the radial head was reconstructed than for patients whose radial head was resected.

Most studies have reported ORIF results for fractures of both the radial head and neck. However, only few studies have published results on adult-only radial neck fractures. Esser et al. [5] followed up for 7 years 26 patients who were treated with ORIF via a plate fixation. None of them presented with bad outcomes. Nevertheless, many articles pointed out that the treatment of radial neck fracture with plate fixation may produce a variety of complications. In 2007, Smith et al. [16] reported that 6 out of 10 patients were not satisfied after being treated with a plate. In a study by Li et al. [26], 58 patients were reviewed for 1 year. The mean range of forearm rotation in the screw group was significantly better than that in the plate group, and the screw group had a lower incidence of heterotopic ossification than the plate group. Based on these studies, we asked ourselves whether screw fixation was a better technique than using a plate to treat radial head and neck fractures. A simple biomechanical study of the fracture of the radial neck was made by Gutowski et al. [15]. They compared two oblique headless compression screws and a radial neck plate. They concluded that the two

strategies provide similar strength and stiffness for the fixation of transverse radial neck fractures. However, the two oblique screws might be preferred for simple transverse neck fractures since this strategy requires limited wound exposure and the implant is buried. The above two studies seem to indicate that the use of screws is better than the use of plate for treating radial neck fractures.

In our study, the stiffness of the radial neck fractures was compared between the three fixation methods in order to evaluate the effect of these structures on fracture stability. These structures can enable the injured patients to perform postoperative functional exercise earlier. Since bending and torsion are the main forces applied to the radial head and neck during normal elbow movements, we used these two force types as our loading parameters. During the bending test, the crossed-screw group and the parallel-screw group had similar stiffness whereas the smallest stiffness was observed for the plate group. We believe that the screw groups were directly connected through the internal ends of the fracture. In the plate group, the plate was fixed with screws in one end of the fracture, and there was no rigid connection within the fracture site. Also, only the lateral side of the fracture end was connected by the plate, and the fixed force was in the lateral fracture side. The load of the crossed-screw group was larger than that of the plate group in the bending failure load test, which is consistent with the results reported in Gutowski's study.

The stiffness of the crossed-screw group was the largest in the torsion test, whereas the stiffness of the plate group was the smallest. This suggests that the crossed screws have a good anti-torsion effect, can provide good fracture stability, and promote early functional exercise without any displacement of the fracture ends. During the failure test, the crossed-screw group shows a significantly larger stiffness than the parallel-screw group and the plate group. We believe that at the proximal end of the fracture, the fixation of the parallel screws and the plate were eccentric, whereas it was in the center distribution of the radial axis for the crossed-screw group. During the torsion process, only one side was forced on the fracture ends of the plate and parallel-screw groups, while the two sides of the fracture were stressed in the crossed-screw group. Therefore, the stiffness of the crossed-screw group was larger than the two other groups.

As shown in Fig. 6, the failure modes were different among the three groups. In the plate group, the plate was deformed at the fracture site, but the screws on the plate did not shift. In the parallel-screw group, a new fracture was noticed in the proximal part of the fracture, but no change was observed in the distal part of the fracture. In the crossed-screw group, one or two screws at the distal end of the fracture were cut out.

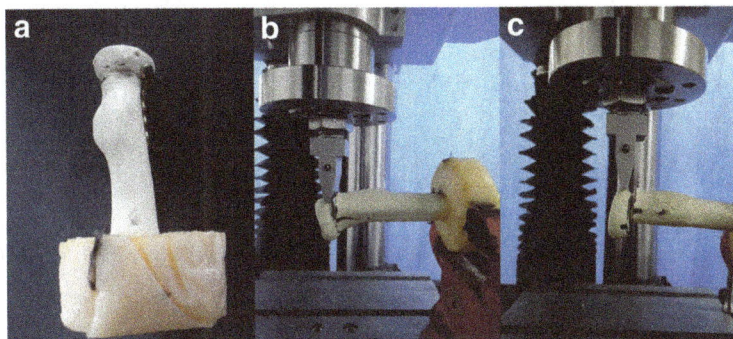

Fig. 6 Different failure mode of the plate (a), crossed screw (b), and parallel screw (c)

Although the parallel screw has not been used in clinical practice yet, the biomechanical results for this fixation method are considerable. In clinical practice, the wound exposure of the screw treatment of the radial head and neck fracture is less than for the plate fixation method. While the crossed screws need to be taken from both sides of the radial head and although the wound exposure is small, the two entry points cannot simultaneously be exposed without rotating the forearm of the fixed operation. Moreover, this may lead to complications when the two screws collide with each other, or when the two screws are not in the center of the radius occurred (i.e., occurrence of an offset). Also, the parallel-screw method only requires a small wound exposure, the two screws being inserted in parallel at a 45° angle with the radial axis in order to fix the fracture site. The biomechanical results obtained in the parallel-screw group are just slightly less than those obtained for the crossed-screw group. Therefore, we can consider using two parallel screws to fix a simple radial neck fracture.

Although our study provides interesting results regarding the biomechanical properties of three different fixation methods, it also has some limitations. First, since the biomechanical properties of the standard bone were investigated without any muscle and other corresponding soft tissue attachment, it cannot simulate the real human elbow joint force transmission and role. Second, our sample size was relatively small. Bending load and torsion direction of the body cannot completely simulate the real daily activities of the human body or the mechanical injury mechanism. In addition, it should be noted that there is a subtle difference in screw orientation in the coronal plane. We attempted to control for this by predrilling the screw trajectory with a custom-made jig, but our funds were limited, and we could not proceed this way. Also, the biomechanical analysis provided in this study only reports bending, torsional, and failure loads. The observed index only includes bending and torsional stiffness as a trade-off. Other biomechanical performance indicators are lacking. Finally, the use of synthetic bone models as opposed to cadaveric specimens could also be seen as a limitation of this study.

Conclusion

Results of this biomechanical study suggest that the crossed-screw fixation is optimal for Mason II radial neck fractures among the three internal fixation strategies analyzed in this study (crossed screws, parallel screws, and plate). Alternatively, the parallel-screw method also constitutes a good internal fixation strategy. The stiffness of the plate was the weakest among the three investigated techniques and was also the one that required the largest wound exposure. However, our conclusion needs to be supported by additional large sample size studies investigating its biomechanical and clinical application.

Abbreviations
ORIF: Open reduction with internal fixation; PMMA: Polymethylmethacrylate

Acknowledgements
The authors are grateful for the assistance from Yiwu high-level personnel for scientific research projects and for technical support and equipment from the Tianjin Institute of Orthopedics.

Funding
This research was supported by the Yiwu high-level personnel for scientific research projects (No. 201603). The funders had no role in the study design, data collection or analysis, decision to publish, or preparation of the manuscript.

Authors' contributions
XCS, JP, and DYW designed the study. HWC, DYW, and XCS obtained the funding. PJ, RZ, and HWC collected the data. XCS, JP, and TLP analyzed the data. TLP, XCS, and DYW interpreted the data. TLP, DYW, and RZ composed the article. All authors read and approved the final manuscript.

Competing interests
The authors declare that they have no competing interests.

Author details

[1]Department of Orthopaedics Surgery, Yiwu People's Hospital, NO.699, Jiangdong Road, Yiwu, Zhejiang Province 322007, China. [2]Department of Orthopaedics Surgery, The Second Affiliated Hospital and Yuying Children's Hospital of Wenzhou Medical University, NO.109, Xue Yuan West Road, Wenzhou, Zhejiang Province 325027, China.

References

1. Duckworth AD, Clement ND, Jenkins PJ, Aitken SA, Court-Brown CM, MM MQ. The epidemiology of radial head and neck fractures. J Hand Surg Am. 2012 Jan;37(1):112–9.
2. Rhyou IH, Kim KC, Kim KW, Lee JH, Kim SY. Collateral ligament injury in the displaced radial head and neck fracture: correlation with fracture morphology and management strategy to the torn ulnar collateral ligament. J Shoulder Elb Surg. 2013;22(2):261–7.
3. Rosenblatt Y, Athwal GS, Faber KJ. Current recommendations for the treatment of radial head fractures. Orthop Clin North Am. 2008;39(2):173–85. vi
4. Shepard MF, Markolf KL, Dunbar AM. Effects of radial head excision and distal radial shortening on load-sharing in cadaver forearms. J Bone Joint Surg Am. 2001;83-A(1):92–100.
5. Esser RD, Davis S, Taavao T. Fractures of the radial head treated by internal fixation: late results in 26 cases. J Orthop Trauma. 1995;9(4):318–23.
6. Geel CW, Palmer AK, Ruedi T, Leutenegger AF. Internal fixation of proximal radial head fractures. J Orthop Trauma. 1990;4(3):270–4.
7. Sanders RA, French HG. Open reduction and internal fixation of comminuted radial head fractures. Am J Sports Med. 1986;14(2):130–5.
8. Zwingmann J, Welzel M, Dovi-Akue D, Schmal H, Sudkamp NP, Strohm PC. Clinical results after different operative treatment methods of radial head and neck fractures: a systematic review and meta-analysis of clinical outcome. Injury. 2013;44(11):1540–50.
9. Mason ML. Some observations on fractures of the head of the radius with a review of one hundred cases. Br J Surg. 1954;42(172):123–32.
10. Broberg MA, Morrey BF. Results of treatment of fracture-dislocations of the elbow. Clin Orthop Relat Res. 1987;216:109–19.
11. Johnston GW. A follow-up of one hundred cases of fracture of the head of the radius with a review of the literature. Ulster Med J. 1962;31:51–6.
12. Burkhart KJ, Mueller LP, Krezdorn D, Appelmann P, Prommersberger KJ, Sternstein W, Rommens PM. Stability of radial head and neck fractures: a biomechanical study of six fixation constructs with consideration of three locking plates. J Hand Surg Am. 2007;32(10):1569–75.
13. Capo JT, Svach D, Ahsgar J, Orillaza NS, Sabatino CT. Biomechanical stability of different fixation constructs for ORIF of radial neck fractures. Orthopedics. 2008 Oct;31(10)
14. Giffin JR, King GJ, Patterson SD, Johnson JA. Internal fixation of radial neck fractures: an in vitro biomechanical analysis. Clin Biomech (Bristol, Avon). 2004 May;19(4):358–61.
15. Patterson JD, Jones CK, Glisson RR, Caputo AE, Goetz TJ, Goldner RD. Stiffness of simulated radial neck fractures fixed with 4 different devices. J Shoulder Elb Surg. 2001;10(1):57–61.
16. Smith AM, Morrey BF, Steinmann SP. Low profile fixation of radial head and neck fractures: surgical technique and clinical experience. J Orthop Trauma. 2007;21(10):718–24.
17. Smith GR, Hotchkiss RN. Radial head and neck fractures: anatomic guidelines for proper placement of internal fixation. J Shoulder Elb Surg. 1996;5(2 Pt 1):113–7.
18. Gutowski CJ, Darvish K, Ilyas AM, Jones CM. Comparison of crossed screw versus plate fixation for radial neck fractures. Clin Biomech (Bristol, Avon). 2015 Nov;30(9):966–70.
19. Berschback JC, Lynch TS, Kalainov DM, Wysocki RW, Merk BR, Cohen MS. Clinical and radiographic comparisons of two different radial head implant designs. J Shoulder Elb Surg. 2013;22(8):1108–20.
20. Duckworth AD, McQueen MM, Ring D. Fractures of the radial head. Bone Joint J. 2013;95-B(2):151–9.
21. Hall JA, McKee MD. Posterolateral rotatory instability of the elbow following radial head resection. J Bone Joint Surg Am. 2005;87(7):1571–9.
22. Ikeda M, Oka Y. Function after early radial head resection for fracture: a retrospective evaluation of 15 patients followed for 3–18 years. Acta Orthop Scand. 2000;71(2):191–4.
23. Karlsson MK, Herbertsson P, Nordqvist A, Besjakov J, Josefsson PO, Hasserius R. Comminuted fractures of the radial head. Acta Orthop. 2010;81(2):224–7.
24. Ring D. Open reduction and internal fixation of fractures of the radial head. Hand Clin. 2004;20(4):415–27. vi
25. Ikeda M, Sugiyama K, Kang C, Takagaki T, Oka Y. Comminuted fractures of the radial head. Comparison of resection and internal fixation. J Bone Joint Surg Am. 2005;87(1):76–84.
26. Li SL, Lu Y, Wang MY. Is cross-screw fixation superior to plate for radial neck fractures? Bone Joint J. 2015;97-B(6):830–5.

23

Femoral nonunion with segmental bone defect treated by distraction osteogenesis with monolateral external fixation

Qun Zhang*, Wei Zhang*, Zhuo Zhang, Licheng Zhang, Hua Chen, Ming Hao, Junhao Deng and Peifu Tang

Abstract

Background: Currently, the common treatment for femoral nonunion with large segmental bone defect is difficult and complex. The effective surgical methods are rare, include vascularized bone grafting, Masquelet technique and Ilizarov distraction osteogenesis. The objective of this study is to investigate the outcomes of segmental femoral defects treated with monolateral external fixation using the distraction osteogenesis.

Methods: We retrospectively analyzed patients with femoral nonunion with segmental bone defects (> 6 cm) between January 2010 and January 2014 in our single trauma center. All patients were treated by distraction osteogenesis with monolateral external fixation. All surgeries were performed by the same surgeon. Bone union, duration of distraction osteogenesis in days, time to consolidation in months, external fixation index (EFI), complications, and additional surgical interventions were recorded postoperatively. The modified Application of Methods of Illizarov (ASAMI) criteria were used to evaluate the operative effectiveness.

Results: Forty-one patients were enrolled in this study for analysis. The length of the bone defect ranged from 6 to 17 cm. All patients eventually achieved healing, and no patient experienced recurrence of infection or newly developed infection. The average time needed for healing was 13 months. In terms of the incidence of complications, 3 cases axial deviations, 5 cases docking site nonunion, 23 cases pin-tract infection, 14 cases knee joint stiffness or their joint mobility declined, 2 cases osteogenesis insufficient in the distraction area,1 case refracture, and 2 cases loose external fixation pins. In terms of the evaluations of fracture healing and function, 30 patients excellent, 6 patients good, 5 patients fair, and 0 patient poor. In terms of postoperative function evaluations, 21 patients excellent, 9 patients good, 7 patients fair, and 4 patients poor.

Conclusion: For patients with femoral nonunion with large segmental bone defects, the monolateral external fixation can provide effective stability, improve compliance, and reduce complications.

Keywords: Monolateral external fixation, Distraction osteogenesis, Bone defects, Femoral nonunion

Background

The common causes of posttraumatic femoral nonunion with large segmental bone defect (> 6 cm) include acute bone loss, bone ischemia atrophy in nonunion sites, and surgical removal of dead bone and sclerotic bone after infection [1, 2].Current treatment for the disease, in addition to the need of addressing the issue of bone nonunion with bone defect, soft tissue defect, nearby

joint stiffness, deformities (rotation, angulation, and shortening), infection and many other issues should also be treated simultaneously [3–5]. At present, the common treatments include vascularized bone grafts (such as ribs, ilium, and fibula), intramembranous osteogenesis technique (Masquelet technique), and Ilizarov distraction osteogenesis [6–10]. Among them, Ilizarov distraction osteogenesis can simultaneously address the issues of infection, bone and soft tissue defects, and correction of deformities and eventually achieves the fracture healing. It is one of the most effective therapeutic strategies for posttraumatic complex nonunion [5, 9, 10].Clinically,

* Correspondence: zhang_qun2017@163.com; zwtyrran@163.com
Qun Zhang and Wei Zhang are co-first authors.
Qun Zhang and Wei Zhang contributed equally.
Department of Orthopaedics, Chinese PLA General Hospital, No. 28 Fuxin Road, Beijing 100853, People's Republic of China

the Ilizarov circular frame, the Taylor spatial frame (TSF), the semicircular Ilizarov pin fixator, and the conventional external fixation are applied to distraction osteogenesis [11–15]. However, complications associated with external fixation systems are high. Moreover, the compliance of patients is relatively poor. Although the monolateral external fixation can provide good stability and compliance is high, there are relatively few reports that describe the outcomes of femoral nonunion treated with this external fixation system [16–18].

Therefore, we retrospectively analyzed patients with femoral nonunion with segmental bone defects who were treated with the monolateral external fixator between January 2010 and January 2014 to evaluate the effectiveness, stability, and complications of the monolateral external fixator.

Methods

The inclusion criteria were as follows: (1) posttraumatic femoral nonunion, (2) segmental bone defect > 6 cm preoperatively and/or intraoperatively, and (3) Ilizarov technique with the monolateral external fixator. Patients who met the above criteria were included in this study. The exclusion criteria were as follows: (1) nonunion caused by primary or secondary tumor, congenital bone disease, metabolic bone disease, or severe vascular origin disease; (2) nonunion for which physiotherapy or drug therapy was used during the treatment to promote fracture healing; (3) nonunion that was combined with severe systemic organ failure; and (4) nonunion that was combined with a mental disorder.

Surgical procedure

After successful anesthesia, for patients who originally had fixation objects, the internal and external fixation objects were firstly removed to expose the nonunion site (Fig. 1a-g2). Then, dead bone, sclerotic bone, fibrous scar tissue, and infected tissue were completely debrided, and a pendulum saw was used to clean up the nonunion site until fresh bleeding healthy bone tissue was reached. By now, the length of bone defect was measured. On the basis of radical debridement, the placement of external fixation pins was initiated. The hydroxyapatite-coated external fixation pins and the extendable monolateral external fixation frame were from Orthofix, Italy. Under the image intensifier, 8–9 parallel pins were inserted at the lateral side of the femur, perpendicular to its long axis. Three pins were fixed at the proximal and distal ends of the femur, respectively, and 2–3 pins were inserted on the transported bone segment. Make sure all pins are on the same coronal plane. The external extendable monolateral fixation frame was then installed. After the osteotomy plane was determined, small-incision low-energy subperiosteal osteotomy was

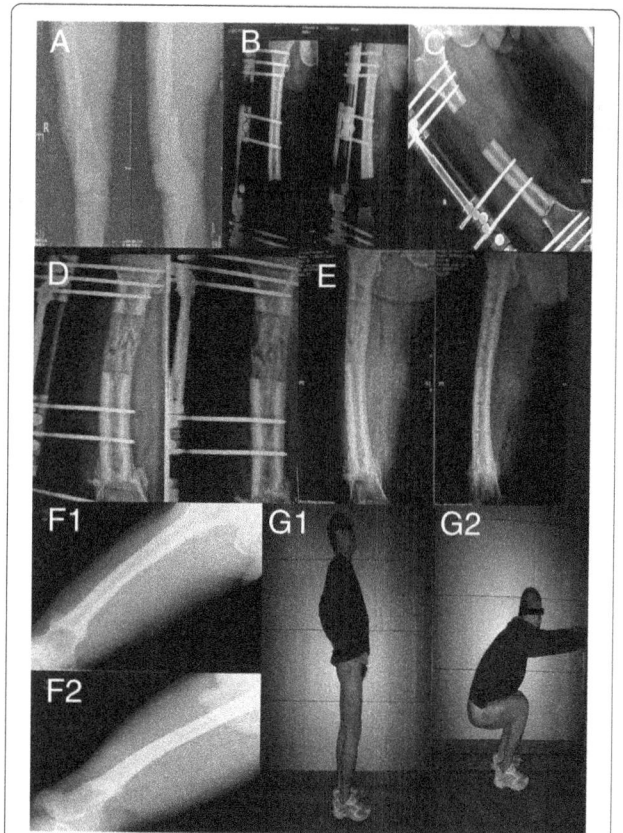

Fig. 1 Sixty-year-old male, suffered a 2-year-long postoperative infection after fracture of left femoral shaft. a The X-ray showed refractures occurred 2 years later; b the patient was given the debridement of lesions, single-arm external fixator, and bone transport. The postoperative presentation of the X-ray demonstrated a 10-cm-long bone defect of femur. c The 5-month-later presentation of the X-ray demonstrated the femur length became normal. d The 1-year-later presentation of the X-ray demonstrated the bone grew well in the region of distraction osteogenesis and the docking site healed well. e The 18-month-later presentation of the X-ray with external fixator removed. f The 4-year-later X-ray presentation showed no infection recurred. g The patient showed a good function of flexion and extension of knee joint

performed, and compression was applied at the osteotomy site. Finally, the incision was closed. If the soft tissue could not be closed during the primary phase or infection was severe, a vacuum-assisted closure device was used to cover the wound, and the wound would be closed during the second phase. The suspected tissue was taken from multiple sites during the procedure and was sent for bacteriological culture to guide postoperative antibiotic use. The surgeries were completed by the same experienced senior surgeon.

Postoperative management

For aseptic nonunion, patients were treated with broad-spectrum antibiotics for 3 days. For septic nonunion, anti-infection treatment was administered for 14 days

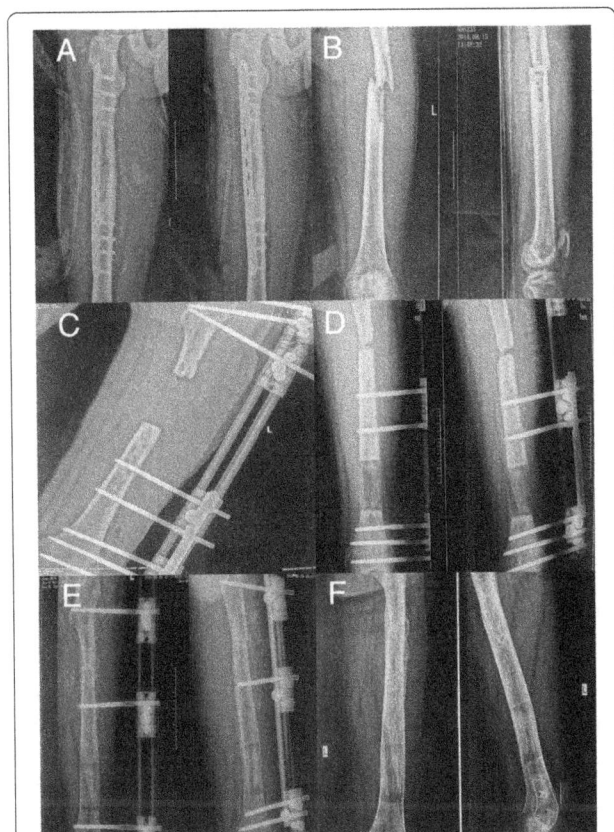

Fig. 2 Twenty six-year-old male, suffered a 14-month-long infection after the operation using bone plates of fracture of left femoral shaft. **a** The X-ray presentation after the open debridement combined with irrigation outside the hospital. **b** After removing the internal fixator due to the runaway infection, the postoperative presentation of the X-ray demonstrated the nonunion of fracture and evident displacement, and some sequestra with bone defects could be seen locally. **c** The 1-week-later X-ray presentation after bone transport: single-arm external fixator served well, and there existed a 6-cm-long bone defect after thorough removal of sequestra and infectious tissues. **d** The 2-month-later X-ray presentation after bone transport: bone growth could be seen in the region of distraction osteogenesis, but both sides of docking site were significantly hardened. **e** The 14-month-later X-ray presentation after bone transport: the docking site healed well after debridement, autogenous bone graft, and compression. The bone grew well in the region of distraction osteogenesis and external fixation pins were partly removed. **f** The 20-month-later X-ray presentation after bone transport: no infection recurred

according to the drug sensitivity results (Fig. 2a-f). Disinfection care for the pin tract was conducted every day to prevent infection. Seven to 10 days postoperatively, bone transport was initiated, with the extension based on 0.25 mm four times per day. Three days postoperatively, the patients began partial weight-bearing activities with crutches. X-rays were taken and reviewed every 2 weeks to observe the growth condition of the distraction area and whether there was axial deviation of the transported bone segment. X-ray monitoring was stopped when the limb length was achieved or when the

docking site made contact. Before removing the external fixator, the compression or distraction force was gradually eliminated to ensure that the frame connection was neutral so that there was no tension in any direction. The removal of the external fixation was based on the following findings: osteogenesis is sufficient in the distraction area, fracture healing was reliable, and no deformations were found at the nonunion site and distraction area when the patient walked on full weight-bearing activities.

All relevant complications were recorded, and the corresponding treatments were clarified. Postoperative pin-tract infection was classified according to Marsh's description [19]. The assessment of clinical efficacy was conducted by the modified Application of Methods of Illizarov (ASAMI) criteria [20].

Results

According to the inclusion and exclusion criteria, our study enrolled 43 patients (Additional file 1). Two patients were lost to follow-up, and 41 patients were eventually included for analysis. The patients ranged in age from 26 to 76 years old, with an average age of 44 years old. There were 31 males and 10 females. Twenty-eight patients had previous open fractures, and 13 patients had previous closed fractures. The duration from the time of injury to the present ranged from 10 to 60 months, with an average of 23.4 months. The patients had received 1–9 previous surgeries: 7 patients had initial internal fixations, 21 patients had intramedullary (IM) nailing, and 13 patients had external fixation. The length of the bone defect ranged from 6 to 17 cm, with an average length of 10.1 cm. There were 33 cases of septic nonunion (21 draining and 12 quiescent nonunion) and 8 cases of aseptic nonunion. Fifteen injured limbs had combinations of rotation deformities, and 11 cases had angulation deformities. Eight patients had knee joint dysfunction. The demographic characteristics of the patients studied can be seen in Table 1.

The postoperative follow-up time ranged from 20 to 60 months (average 35 months). All fractures eventually achieved healing, and no patient experienced recurrence of infection or newly developed infection. The duration of distraction osteogenesis (DOG) was 60–191 days (average 110 days). The time needed for healing was 6–20 months (average 13 months). The external fixation index (EFI) was 1.15–1.52 months/cm (average 1.30 months/cm). In terms of complications, 3 patients had axial deviations, which were corrected by surgical adjustment and enhanced fixation; 5 patients had docking site nonunion, of whom 3 patients were given autologous cancellous bone grafting combined with continuous compression at the docking site to achieve healing, and 2 patients underwent the "accordion technique" to achieve healing. There were 23 cases of pin-

Table 1 Demographic characteristics of the patients studied

Variable	Number
Total number	41
Age (years)	26–76
Gender	
Male	31
Female	10
Time since injury (months)	10–60
Number of surgeries	1–9
Patterns of initial fractures	
Open	28
Closed	13
Patterns of initial surgeries	
Plating	7
IM nail	21
External fixation	13
Patterns of bone nonunion	
Infection	33
Aseptic	8
Length of bone loss (cm)	6–17
Other types of deformities	
Rotation	15
Angular	11

Table 2 Details of the outcomes and complications

Variable	
Follow-up in months	35(20–60)
Duration of DOG in days	110(60–191)
Time to consolidation in months	13(6–20)
EFI (months/cm)	1.30(1.15–1.52)
The number of union	41
The number of complications	
Pin-track infection	23
Wire/pin loosening	2
Reinfection in fraction site	0
Vascular/nerve injury	0
Axial deviation	3
Docking site nonunion	5
Refraction	1
Osteogenesis insufficient in distraction area	2
Knee joint rigidity	14
The number of additional surgical interventions	
Bone grafting	4
Knee arthrolysis	10
Accordion technique	3
External fixator adjustment	3
Remove/change external fixation pin	2
Fixation in refraction	1

DOG distraction osteogenesis, EFI external fixation index

tract infection, of which 15 cases were type A, 7 cases were type B, and 1 case was type C; 10 of those cases mainly occurred at the greater trochanter site, while the pins of 3 patients were removed and replaced, after which control was gained over the infection. Fourteen patients had knee joint stiffness and a range of knee motion declined; according to the differences in the patients' living requirement, joint arthrolysis was performed later for 10 patients. Two patients had osteogenesis insufficient in the distraction area; 1 patient was treated with autologous cancellous bone grafting, while the other patient was treated with the "accordion technique." One patient experienced refracture when he accidentally fell down 1 year after the external fixation frame was removed; the refracture occurred at the docking site. Since this patient previously had an infectious bone nonunion, an external fixation frame was used for fixation again, and refracture healing was achieved with the "accordion technique." Two patients had loose external fixation pins, which were replaced with new fixation pins (see Table 2). In terms of the evaluations of fracture healing and function, 30 patients excellent, 6 patients good, and 5 patients fair. In terms of postoperative function evaluations, 21 patients excellent, 9 patients good, 7 patients fair, and 4 patients poor (see Table 3).

Discussion

The incidence of femoral nonunion is increasing, with a recent report published in JAMA indicating that it is as high as 13.9% [21]. This increase may be related to the increasing number of patients with severe fractures (higher degrees of open and comminuted fracture) caused by high-energy injuries (traffic, high-level fall, and crush injuries). When this condition is combined with large bone segment defects (> 6 cm) and infection, it becomes even more difficult to solve [1]. Traditional treatment requires multiple operations at different

Table 3 Evaluation of the bone and functional results

Grades	Bone results[a]	Functional results[b]
Excellent	30	21
Good	6	9
Fair	5	7
Poor	0	4

[a]Excellent result was defined as union, no infection, deformity of 7° and limb length discrepancy (LLD) of 2.5 cm; good was defined as union, with any two of the other three criteria; fair result was defined as union, with one of the other three criteria; and poor result was defined as nonunion
[b]Excellent result was defined as active, without the other four criteria; good was defined as active, with 1–2 of the other four criteria; fair was defined as active, with 3–4 of the other four criteria; and poor was defined as inactive

stages. Only under the premise that a thorough debridement is conducted to control the infection or there is clearly no infection can the next step in the treatment strategy for bone defect repair be determined. Traditional surgical methods often cannot effectively and simultaneously solve a series of problems including bone and soft tissue defects, lower limb deformity (rotation, angulation, and shortening), fracture nonunion, and infection.

In terms of femoral nonunion with segmental bone defects, the frequently used treatment methods include vascular pedicle autologous bone grafting (such as ribs, ilium, and fibula), intramembranous osteogenesis technique (Masquelet technique), and Ilizarov distraction osteogenesis. All of these methods have their advantages and limitations. Autologous bone grafting with a vascular pedicle requires high level of microsurgical techniques; the bone supply is limited, and it will cause a secondary damage to the donor site; failure of revascularization of the transplanted bone segment will lead to the failure of fracture healing, and insufficient femoralization of the transplanted bone segment will result in poor bone strength, which then becomes prone to refracture [6, 7, 22].

Compared with the above traditional surgical method, the Masquelet and Ilizarov techniques are the main surgical methods for the treatment of large segmental bone defects of the femur [9]. With the internal fixation, the Masquelet technique allows the patients to avoid carrying a bulky circular external fixator and its associated complications, thereby increasing patient's compliance. However, this technique has a higher requirement for the integrity of muscle soft tissue; it requires multiple operations (at least 2) and a large amount of autologous bone; it has a higher risk of re-infection and failure of revascularization and ossification of the transplanted bone region; and it is poor at correcting severe deformities [8, 9, 23]. Therefore, its surgical indications should be selected cautiously and strictly. The Ilizarov technology has unique advantages in the treatment of femoral nonunion, especially with large-segment bone defect, as it can simultaneously address infection, bone and soft tissue defects, and corrections of deformities at the primary stage. It is suitable for various types of nonunion with a lower requirement for soft tissue covering and a higher fracture healing rate [9–12, 16–18]. Our study achieved a 100% fracture healing rate, and the functional rates of good/excellent were achieved by 73.2% of patients.

The common external fixation systems with the Ilizarov technique include the Ilizarov circular frame, the TSF, the semicircular Ilizarov pin fixator, and the conventional external fixator. However, they are often full-circular or hybrid external fixation frames, which are

bulky for patients to carry and affect the exercise of adjacent joints; they also have high demands in terms of the surgeon's technique. Therefore, Harshwal used monolateral external fixation frames to treat 7 cases of femoral nonunion, and 5 cases achieved fracture healing with good function [16]. R. Rohilla compared monolateral external fixation with circular external fixation for the treatment of tibial nonunion and found that although the circular external frame could provide better stability with less screw path infection, there were no significant statistical differences in terms of fracture healing rate and functions in the two groups [24].

On the basis of our own study, we found that the monolateral external fixator has the following advantages: (1) the surgical procedure is simpler, and it is easy to promote to lower-level medical trauma centers; (2) patients have a better tolerance, and the functional exercises are more convenient, which can facilitate improved knee joint function so that the patient can return to family and society earlier; (3) it is more suitable for patients with senile or disuse osteoporosis, and the hydroxyapatite-coated external fixation pins have stronger holding power so that the risks of loosening and failure of cutting are probably lower; and (4) since the external fixation pins are fixed from the lateral side of the femur, the risk of neurovascular damage may be lower than that associated with the circular external frame. The drawback is that, compared with the circular external frame, when the soft tissue coverage of the healthy active bone tissue at the proximal and distal femur is insufficient or when the affected limb has deformities in all three-dimensional planes, the monolateral external fixation frame cannot be used. All of the 41 patients in our study group used the monolateral external fixation frame and could perform out-of-bed functional exercises early to achieve fracture healing; furthermore, the incidence of complications was lower.

It has been reported that when distraction osteogenesis was used for the treatment of femoral nonunion, the incidence of surgical complications was very high [12, 18, 25, 26], with the mean complications per patient ranging from 1.33 (20/15) to 3.55 (71/20) [18]. Our study result was 1.22 (50/41), and the average length (10.1 cm) of bone defects of the included patients was much larger than the lengths in previously reported studies (6–8.3 cm). Under a much longer treatment cycle and with more complex conditions, the incidence of complications of this study was even lower. The most common complication was still pin-tract infection, though the incidence (56.1%) of pin-tract infection in our study was also lower than those described in other reports (63–100%) [25]. This difference may be associated with better patient education, more stable fixation by external fixation pins, and less interference with soft tissue (the use of the monolateral external fixation avoids contralateral soft tissue piercing). The second common complication was knee joint stiffness. In our study, 8 patients had preoperative joint stiffness, and only 6 patients had newly developed postoperative joint stiffness or functional decline. This low incidence was probably because there was no obstruction by the external frame behind the knee joint with the monolateral external fixation, which allows the patients to be able to perform early postoperative full-range joint exercise. However, for patients with preoperative joint stiffness, circular or hybrid external fixation also have unique advantages. The surgeon can simultaneously place a trans-articular external fixation to perform traction treatment on the stiff joint, which is a defect of the monolateral external fixation. The surgeon can choose a circular external fixation to perform simultaneous correction of joint stiffness at the primary stage according to the condition of the patient's joint function and the surgical requirement, or the surgeon can perform joint release or joint traction at the second stage after fracture healing.

In addition, the incidence of other complications is relatively lower. However, we should pay more attention to docking site nonunion and insufficient osteogenesis in the distraction area, especially in longer bone defect and poorer soft tissue condition and elderly patients with poorer osteogenic capacity. The "accordion technique" is an effective method. By giving repeated compression-distraction stimulation at the docking site or distraction area, it can induce intramembranous and endochondral osteogenesis, thereby promoting fracture healing [27]. When necessary, autologous iliac bone graft can also be a surgical option, but this procedure is often associated with damage to the donor area and insufficient bone supply. When the lengthening bone segment experiences axial deviation, an external fixation should be adjusted immediately. By increasing the contact area of the docking site and correcting poor alignment of the affected limb, the incidence of docking site nonunion can be reduced. If necessary, a small incision can be made to clean up any fibrous scar tissue at the docking site, and a limited decortication can be performed to improve the rate of fracture healing [5, 28].

This study also has some limitations. First, this study is a retrospective small-sample single-center study with a low level of evidence. Secondly, since there is no control group, we can only evaluate the advantages and shortcomings of the monolateral external fixation, which cannot prove that it is superior to circular external fixation. All of these observations require further confirmation in large-sample multi-center prospective randomized controlled trials.

Conclusion

Compared with the traditional circular or hybrid external fixation, even for patients with large segmental femoral defects, the monolateral external fixation can provide effective mechanical stability, make better compliance for patients, and reduce operation-associated complications. Despite the associated surgical complications being still high, correct understanding and reasonable treatment strategies can minimize the pain experienced by patients and improve the surgical success rate.

Abbreviations
ASAMI: Association for the Study and Application of the Method of Ilizarov; DOG: Distraction osteogenesis; EFI: External fixation index; IM: Intra-medullary; JAMA: The Journal of the American Medical Association; LLD: Limb length discrepancy; TSF: Taylor spatial frame

Acknowledgements
This work is supported by the Chinese PLA general hospital, and we really appreciate the help given by related departments and participators.

Funding
No external funding was received.

Authors' contributions
ZQ was involved in overall study design and funding. ZQ and ZW contributed equally to this work and should be considered co-first authors. ZW, ZZ, ZLC, DJH, and HM designed and wrote the analysis plan for the current paper. ZW undertook the statistical analyses. All authors were involved in the interpretation of data. ZQ and ZW wrote the first draft of the manuscript. All authors critically read the manuscript to improve intellectual content. All authors have approved the final manuscript in its present form.

Competing interests
The authors declare that they have no competing interests.

References
1. Nikolaos KK, Theodoros HT, Peter VG. Surgical management of infected non-unions: an update. Injury. 2016;46:25–32.
2. Kyu-Hyun Y, Yougun W, Sang BK, et al. Plate augmentation and autologous bone grafting after intramedullary nailing for challenging femoral bone defect: a technical note. Arch Orthop Trauma Surg. 2016;136:1381–5.
3. Anastasios DK, Panayaotis NS. Management of nonunion with distraction osteogenesis. Injury. 2006;37:51–5.
4. Ioannis DG, Angelos NP, Christina MA, et al. Diagnostic and treatment modalities in nonunions of the femoral shaft. a review. Injury. 2012;43:980–8.
5. Robert R S, Jacob SP, Austin TF, et al. Repair of tibial nonunions and bone defect with the Taylor spatial frame. J Orthop Trauma. 2008;22:88–95.
6. Wei FC, TA El-G, Lin CH, Ueng WN. Free fibula osteoseptocutaneous graft for reconstruction of segmental femoral defects. J Trauma. 1997;43:784–92.
7. Yajima H, Tamai S, Mizumoto S, One H. Vascularised fibular grafts for reconstruction of the femur. J Bone Joint Surg (Br). 1993;75:123–8.
8. Masquelet AC, Begue T. The concept of induced membrane for reconstruction of long bone defects. Orthop Clin N Am. 2010;41:27–37.
9. Giannoudis, PV. Treatment of bone defects: bone transport or the induced membrane technique? Injury. 2016;47:291–2.
10. Papakostidis C, Bhandari M, Giannoudis PV. Distraction osteogenesis in the treatment of long bone defects of the lower limbs: effectiveness, complications and clinical results; a systematic review and meta analysis. Bone Joint J. 2013;95:1673–80.

11. Wael A, Mohamed ES. Ilizarov distraction osteogenesis over the preexisting nail for treatment of nonunited femurs with significant shortening. Eur J Orthop Surg Traumatol. 2016;26:319–28.

12. Saridis A, Panagiotopoulos E, Tyllianakis M, et al. The use of the Ilizarov method as a salvage procedure in infected nonunion of the distal femur with bone loss. J Bone Joint Surg (Br). 2006;88:232–7.

13. Kucukkaya M, Karakoyun O, Armagan R, Kuzqun U. Correction of complex lower extremities deformities with use of the Ilizarov–Taylor spatial frame. Acta Orthop Traumatol Turc. 2009;43:1–6.

14. Khanfour AA, Mohamed ME. Efficacy of a compliant semicircular Ilizarov pin fixator module for treating infected nonunion of the femoral diaphysis. Strat Traum Limb Recon. 2014;9:101–9.

15. Chanchit S. Distraction osteogenesis for the treatment of post traumatic complications using a conventional external fixator: a novel technique. Injury. 2005;36:185–93.

16. Raj KH, Sohan SS, Divesh J. Management of nonunion of lower-extremity long bones using mono-lateral external fixator—report of 37 cases. Injury. 2014;45:560–7.

17. Sailhan F. Bone lengthening (distraction osteogenesis): a literature review. Osteoporos Int. 2011;22:2011–5.

18. Peng Y, Lihai Z, Tongtong L, et al. Infected nonunion of tibia and femur treated by bone transport. J Orthop Surg Res. 2015;10:49–59.

19. Marsh JL, Nepola JV, Mefffert R. Dynamic external fixation for stabilization of non union. Clin Orthop. 1992;278:200–6.

20. Paley D, Catagni MA, Argnani F. Ilizarov treatment of tibial nonunions with bone loss. Clin Orthop. 1989;241:146–65.

21. Robert Z, Ze X, Thomas E, et al. Epidemiology of fracture nonunion in 18 human bones. JAMA Surgery. 2016;9:1–12.

22. Hou SM, Liu TK. Reconstruction of skeletal defects in the femur with "two-strut" free vascularized fibular grafts. J Trauma. 1992;33:840–5.

23. Olesen UK, Eckardt H, Bosemark P, et al. The Masquelet technique of induced membrane for healing of bone defects: a review of 8 cases. Injury. 2015;46:44–7.

24. Rohilla R, Wadhwani J, Devag A, et al. Prospective randomized comparison of ring versus rail fixator in infected gap nonunion of tibia treated with distraction osteogenesis. Bone Joint J. 2016;10:1399–405.

25. Blum AL, BongioVanni JC, Morgan SJ, et al. Complications associated with distraction osteogenesis for infected nonunion of the femoral shaft in the presence of a bone defect: a retrospective series. J Bone Joint Surg. 2010;92:565–70.

26. Nikolaos G, Badri N, Selvadurai N. Distraction osteogenesis and nonunion of the docking site: is there an ideal treatment option? Injury. 2007;38:100–7.

27. Asim MM, Adrian SC, Juan SR, et al. The accordion maneuver: a noninvasive strategy for absent or delayed callus formation in cases of limb lengthening. Adv Orthop. 2015;3:1–8.

28. Paley D, Maar DC. Ilizarov bone transport treatment for tibial defects. J Orthop Trauma. 2000;14:76–85.

24

Predictability of the effects of facet joint infiltration in the degenerate lumbar spine when assessing MRI scans

Ulf Krister Hofmann[1]*, Ramona Luise Keller[2], Christian Walter[1] and Falk Mittag[1]

Abstract

Background: Imaging results are frequently considered as hallmarks of disease by spine surgeons to plan their future treatment strategy. Numerous classification systems have been proposed to quantify or grade lumbar magnetic resonance imaging (MRI) scans and thus objectify imaging findings. The clinical impact of the measured parameters remains, however, unclear. To evaluate the pathological significance of imaging findings in patients with multisegmental degenerative findings, clinicians can perform image-guided local infiltrations to target defined areas such as the facet joints.
The aim of the present retrospective study was to evaluate the correlation of MRI facet joint degeneration and spinal stenosis measurements with improvement obtained by image-guided intraarticular facet joint infiltration.

Methods: Fifty MRI scans of patients with chronic lumbar back pain were graded radiologically using a wide range of classification and measurement systems. The reported effect of facet joint injections at the site was recorded, and a comparative analysis performed.

Results: When we allocated patients according to their reported pain relief, 27 showed no improvement (0–30%), 16 reported good improvement (31–75%) and 7 reported excellent improvement (> 75%). MRI features assessed in this study did, however, not show any relevant correlation with reported pain after facet joint infiltration: Values for Kendall's tau ranged from $\tau = -0.190$ for neuroforaminal stenosis grading as suggested by Lee, to $\tau = 0.133$ for posterior disc height as proposed by Hasegawa.

Conclusion: Despite the trend in evidence-based medicine to provide medical algorithms, our findings underline the continuing need for individualised spine care that, along with imaging techniques or targeted infiltrations, includes diagnostic dimensions such as good patient history and clinical examination to formulate a diagnosis.

Trial registration: ClinicalTrials.gov, NCT03308149, retrospectively registered October 2017

Keywords: Lumbar spinal stenosis, Lumbar degenerative disease, MRI, Facet joint degeneration, Facet joint injection

Background

Chronic lumbar back pain and sciatica are common symptoms of degenerative conditions of the spine that lead to enormous costs to the health care systems of industrialised countries [1–4]. The diagnosis and resulting conservative or operative treatment is based on the patient's medical history and concerns, physical examination and radiographic imaging, especially X-rays and magnetic resonance imaging (MRI) scans. On the basis of improvements in diagnostic imaging and surgical techniques, therapeutic strategies have become increasingly focused on surgical treatment [5, 6]. Despite all improvements, however, especially in patients with chronic multisegmental lumbar disease and spinal stenosis observed on MRI, clinicians still cannot reliably predict the success of spinal decompression and/or fusion surgery. Since it has been established that neither clinical findings [7, 8] nor radiologic facet joint pathology [9–11] can be used to reliably diagnose a painful facet joint, local targeted infiltrations can be additionally used to temporarily simulate the effect of surgery through local

* Correspondence: ulf.hofmann@med.uni-tuebingen.de
[1]Department of Orthopaedic Surgery, University Hospital of Tübingen, Hoppe-Seyler-Strasse 3, 72076 Tübingen, Germany
Full list of author information is available at the end of the article

administration of local analgesic and anti-inflammatory agents to the facet joints [12–16].

So far, no consensus has been established about whether radiologic imaging can predict the response to diagnostic or therapeutic facet joint blocks (reviewed by Cohen and Raja (2007)) [17]. In their 2010 study, Stojanonic et al. described a possible association between MRI spinal stenosis and successful extra-articular medial branch block infiltrations. Even though these study results failed to reach statistical significance, this finding might offer an additional perspective on how to consider the effects observed by facet joint infiltrations [18].

In the present study, we aimed to systematically evaluate the quality of different measurement and classification systems for spinal stenosis and facet joint degeneration on MRI for their ability to predict reported pain relief after facet joint infiltration in patients with chronic lumbar back pain. We hypothesised that, as pathological grading increased in MRI scans, pain alleviation would also increase after bilateral facet joint infiltration.

Methods
Study design
All patients who had received inpatient gradual diagnostics [12, 13] from 2005 to 2016 for chronic lumbar back pain were screened for inclusion in the study. Inclusion criteria included undergoing a monosegmental facet joint infiltration on the first day of inpatient gradual diagnostics and clearly stated pain relief in percentage (%) for that specific infiltration in the medical documentation. Moreover, the pain level prior to infiltration needed to be clearly documented and a high-quality MRI available before infiltration. Patients were excluded if they had a positive history of lumbar surgery or the presence of artificial implants in the area of interest.

Various measurement and grading techniques were used to evaluate facet joint degeneration, neuroforaminal stenosis or spinal canal stenosis on the MR images. All measurements were performed blinded by the same observer, who was familiar with and had practiced all tested measurement techniques.

Full departmental, institutional and local ethical committee approvals were obtained before commencement of the study (project number 503/2016BO2).

Infiltration technique and reported pain relief
An analgesic (0.5 ml bupivacaine 0.25%) and a corticosteroid (0.5 ml triamcinolone 10 mg/ml) were injected intraarticularly into the facet joint under fluoroscopic guidance. Patients were then asked on the following day to report the pain relief obtained by the infiltration in terms of percentage (%) of the total pain present before infiltration.

Measurement technique
Degeneration of the facet joints was classified by using the method of Weishaupt et al. [19, 20], which uses T2 images to evaluate the presence of osteophytes, subchondral cysts, bone erosions and possible joint space narrowing to allocate degeneration grades ranging from 0 to 3. Because infiltrations were performed bilaterally, the higher degeneration grade was used for further statistical analyses.

To stratify stenosis of the spinal canal and the neuroforamen, we performed both qualitative and quantitative techniques. Again, the higher pathological value from both sides was used for further analyses.

Quantitative neuroforaminal stenosis measurements:

I. In sagittal T2 images, posterior disc height [21] was measured after the central position of the spinal canal in the axial plane was identified (Fig. 1a).

II. The minimum antero-posterior diameter of the neuroforamen was measured in axial T2 images in two ways: First, it was measured in the axial plane where the root can be seen to traverse it [22] (Fig. 1b). The second measurement was performed at the level where the location of the intervertebral disc was confirmed in sagittal T2 images. If several images were available that met these criteria, the more cranial one was analysed (Fig. 1c).

III. The minimum cross-sectional area of the foraminal zone was measured on sagittal T1 images. As suggested by Sipola et al. [23], the key area of interest was the zone below the pedicle because of the cranial transition of the nerve root in the foramen. Therefore, no space below a line parallel to the lower end plate was included (Fig. 1d).

Using sagittal T1 images, we qualitatively graded neuroforaminal stenosis, as proposed by Lee et al. [24, 25], whereby stages 0–3 are allocated according to the degree of nerve root compression at the narrowest point at the medial margin of the pedicle in the subpedicular zone.

Quantitative spinal canal stenosis measurements:

I. Axial T2 images at the level of the intervertebral disc were used to measure the ligamentous interfacet distance [26]. This distance covers a line connecting the ventral joint space of the facet joints between the inner surface of the flaval ligaments. If two adjacent images were available at the disc level, the narrower distance was measured (Fig. 1e).

II. Antero-posterior constriction was measured as the mid-sagittal diameter of the dural sac at its narrowest level in axial T2 images (Fig. 1f).

III. The smallest cross-sectional area of the dural sac at the infiltrated level was measured in T2 axial images [27–29]. The lateral margins in the neuroforaminal

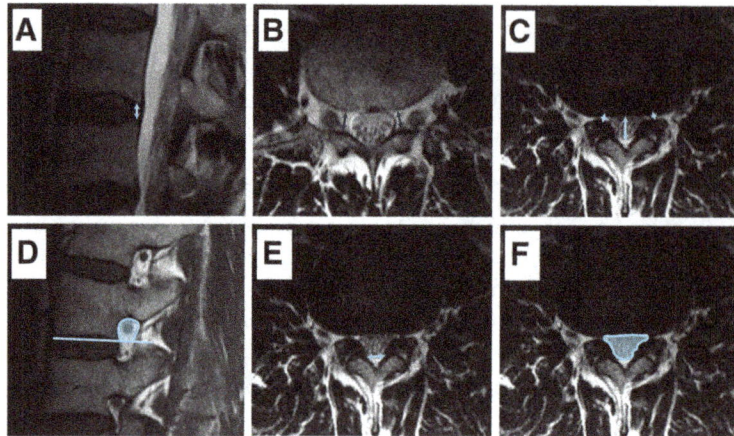

Fig. 1 Quantitative measurements: **a** Sagittal T2, **b**, **c**, **e**, **f** axial T2 and **d** sagittal T1 images. **a** Posterior disc height [21]. **b** Neuroforaminal antero-posterior distance at the level where the root can be seen to traverse it [22] and **c** at the level of the intervertebral disc. The blue median arrow shows the sagittal diameter of the dural sac at that level. **d** Cross-sectional area of the neuroforamen [23], **e** ligamentous interfacet distance [26] as a line connecting the ventral joint space of the facet joints between the inner surface of the flaval ligaments and **f** cross-sectional area of the dural sac [27–29] at the level of the intervertebral disc. The lateral margins of the dura in the neuroforaminal area were extrapolated from the images above and below

area were extrapolated from the images above and below (Fig. 1f).

We qualitatively graded spinal canal stenosis, as suggested by Schizas et al.,[30] in axial T2 images, whereby categories A1-4 were subsumed as A.

Imaging

All three Tesla or 1.5 Tesla MRIs were available in digital form and analysed on an Eizo RadiForce RS110 48-cm Class Colour LCD screen (Eizo Nanao Corporation, Hakusan, Ishikawa, Japan) with a centricity PACS Radiology RA1000 workstation (GE Healthcare, Barrington, IL, USA).

Statistical analysis

Distributions of variables for all parameters were assessed as histograms. Categorical variables are described as absolute frequencies. Depending on normality, data are reported as mean (standard deviation) or median (minimum-maximum). Differences between two groups were calculated by t test for independent samples and Mann-Whitney U test. To evaluate the association of reported pain relief and imaging findings, we calculated Kendall's tau correlation coefficient. For further analyses, pain relief was additionally categorised into three groups: no (below 30%), good (30–74%) and excellent (75–100%) pain relief.

All reported p values have a two-tailed significance level of alpha = 0.05. No adjustment for multiple testing was performed. Graphic illustration of the results was performed by using bar diagrams, boxplots and scatterplots. Statistical analysis was conducted with IBM SPSS version 22.

Results

In total, 50 patients met all inclusion criteria (30 women and 20 men). The median age was 57 (28–95) years (Fig. 2a). From the time of MRI to infiltration, the median elapsed time was 54 (0–295) days. The preinfiltration pain

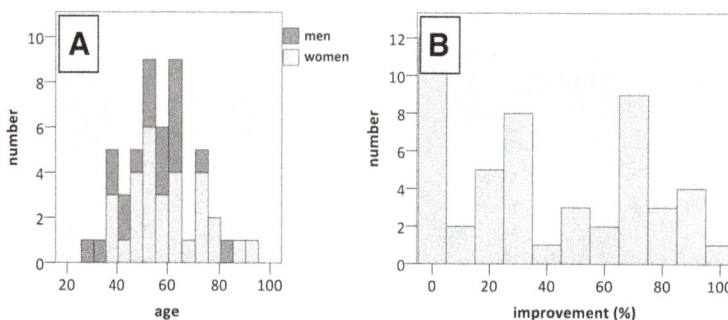

Fig. 2 a Histogram displaying patient age with a peak around 55 years. **b** Heterogeneous improvement after facet joint infiltration ranging from 0 to 100%, with a median improvement of 30%

level on a numeric rating scale was 4 (3–9), with a median improvement after facet joint infiltration of 30% (0–100%) (Fig. 2b). When we allocated patients according to their reported pain relief, 27 showed no improvement (0–30%), 16 reported good improvement (31–75%) and 7 reported excellent improvement (>75%). Twenty-four patients received infiltrations on facet joints L4/5, 22 on L5/S1 and 2 on L2/3 and L3/4.

No relevant connection could be observed between reported improvement after infiltration and MRI findings for any of the analysed parameters (Table 1, Figs. 3 and 4).

Even when we performed a subgroup analysis between those patients with maximum improvement (100%, $n = 7$) and those with no improvement at all (0%, $n = 12$), no significant difference was notable (Table 2). The original study data are available as Additional file 1.

Discussion

When we analysed the relationship between reported pain relief after fluoroscopy-guided facet joint infiltrations and qualitative or quantitative radiomorphometric parameters, no relevant connection could be found. In 2007, Gorbach et al. described a lack of correlation between success of facet joint infiltration and imaging grading of facet joint degeneration when using the system suggested by Weishaupt [31]. In 2010, Stojanovic et al. also described only a weak correlation of MRI facet joint hypertrophy and a positive response to diagnostic medial branch blocks [18].

With further improvements in imaging techniques that allow detailed visualisation of spinal structures, radiographic findings are increasingly considered to be solid evidence, similar to laboratory test results or histopathological findings. This anticipated confidence might dispose surgeons to largely base their recommendations for treatment strategies on such imaging. The correlation between radiological and clinical findings to distinguish

between symptomatic and asymptomatic patients is, however, limited and unreliable for all common modalities such as X-ray, computed tomography, MRI scan or single-photon emission computed tomography (SPECT) scan [32–35]. This applies to both facet joint degeneration [36, 37] and spinal stenosis, independent of whether quantitative [38, 39] or qualitative stenosis classifications [40] are used. Clear correlations are usually described only for different parameters of the same technique: the occurrence of intraarticular fluid of the facet joints, for example, is known to increase with degenerative spondylolisthesis [41, 42] and appears to be associated with lumbar instability [42, 43]. Of note, this observation does not describe a clinical symptom. In addition, when examining the literature on that topic critically, one must not ignore that reported positive correlations between two phenomena such as clinical and radiologic findings bear an intrinsic publication bias, so that it is only after the initial euphoria in the scientific community that clear clinical relevance can be established.

Efforts nevertheless continue in order to improve diagnostic predictability of imaging techniques: although the supine MRI technique still predominates, upright imaging might improve the results because of the weight-bearing condition. Still, it does not provide dynamic, but only static information. Another difficulty with the correct interpretation of imaging results occurs in circumstances in which adaptational processes are difficult or even impossible to visualise. This can especially be noted when the clinical presentation of acute minor nuclear prolapses is compared with those of elderly patients with a long history of what is, in many cases, asymptomatic severe spinal stenosis. One explanation for such differences might be the triggered inflammatory processes that lead to swelling or intraarticular synovial fluid collection, which in peripheral joints is easily recognisable clinically, whereas the zygapophyseal joints do not offer

Table 1 Correlation analysis of radiomorphometric measurements or qualitative classifications and pain relief after facet joint injection

Variable	Kendall's tau	p value
Qualitative measurements		
Facet joint degeneration (Weishaupt) [20]	− 0.020	0.866
Neuroforaminal stenosis (Lee) [58]	− 0.190	0.103
Spinal canal stenosis (Schizas) [30]	0.036	0.767
Quantitative measurements		
Posterior disc height [21]	0.133	0.195
Neuroforaminal antero-posterior distance [22]	− 0.007	0.946
Neuroforaminal cross-sectional area [23]	0.085	0.402
Ligamentous interfacet distance [26]	− 0.026	0.799
Minimum sagittal antero-posterior diameter of the spinal canal	0.030	0.767
Minimum cross-sectional area of the spinal canal [27–29]	− 0.022	0.826

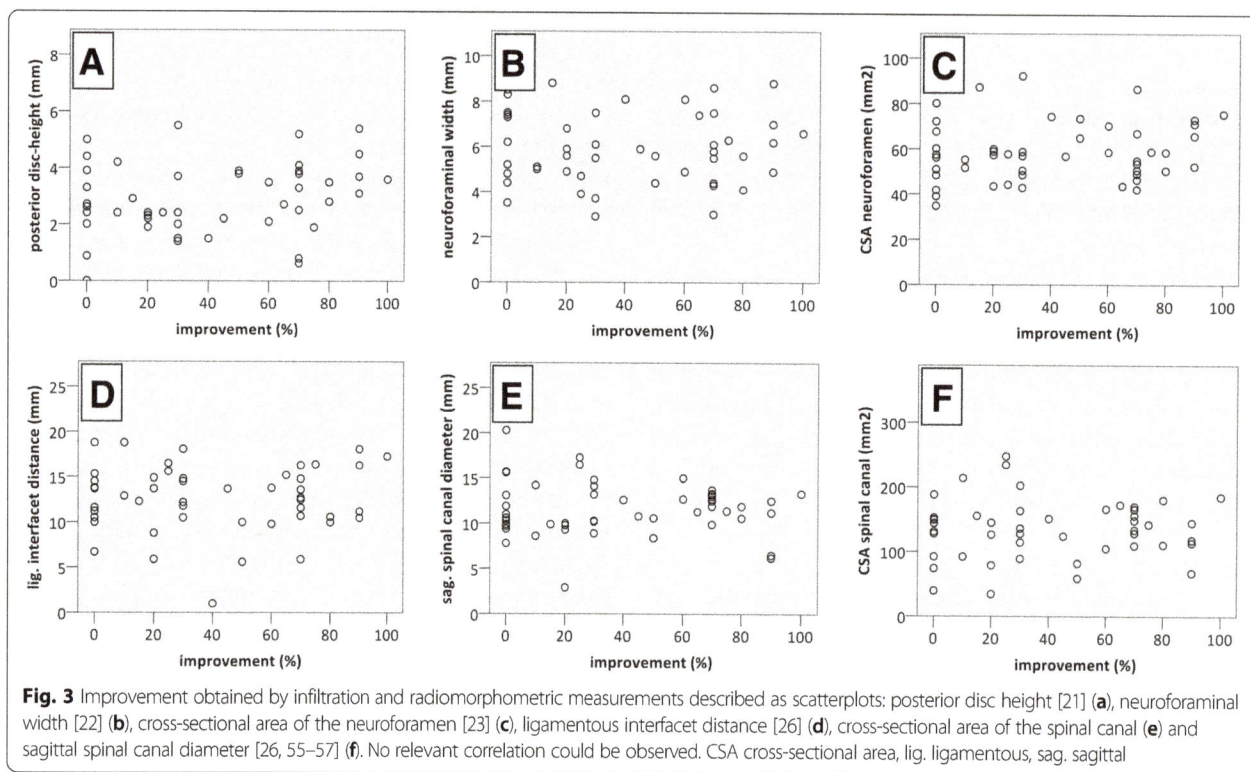

Fig. 3 Improvement obtained by infiltration and radiomorphometric measurements described as scatterplots: posterior disc height [21] (**a**), neuroforaminal width [22] (**b**), cross-sectional area of the neuroforamen [23] (**c**), ligamentous interfacet distance [26] (**d**), cross-sectional area of the spinal canal (**e**) and sagittal spinal canal diameter [26, 55–57] (**f**). No relevant correlation could be observed. CSA cross-sectional area, lig. ligamentous, sag. sagittal

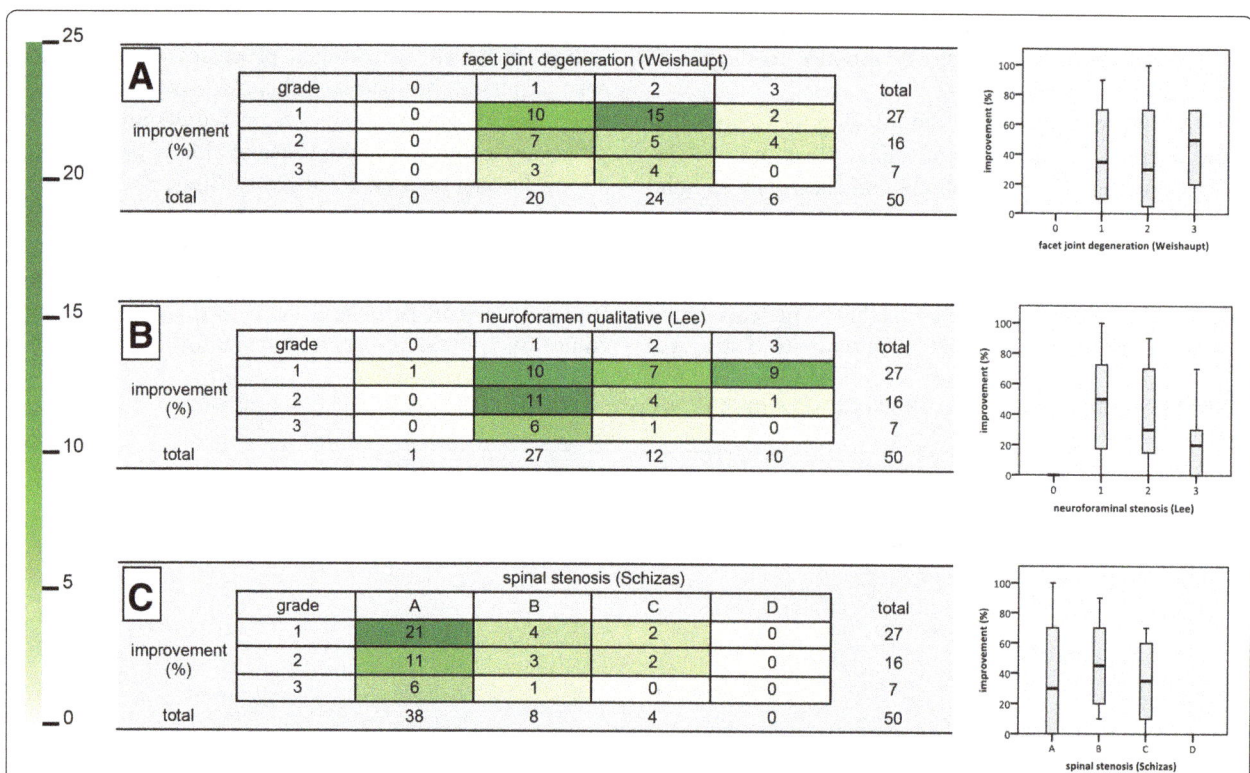

Fig. 4 Correlation of observed improvement by infiltrations with qualitative facet joint degeneration and spinal stenosis classifications in the form of heat maps (left column) and boxplots (right column). **a** Facet joint degeneration (Weishaupt [20]), **b** neuroforaminal stenosis (Lee [25]) and **c** spinal stenosis (Schizas [30]). Pain relief obtained by the infiltrations is grouped into three categories: 1, no improvement (below 30%); 2, good (30–74%); and 3, excellent (75–100%) improvement. Colour intensity in the heat maps is shown according to absolute frequencies

Table 2 Analysis of patients with maximum pain relief and no response

Variable	0% pain relief (n = 18)	100% pain relief (n = 11)	p value
Infiltrated motion segments			0.711[a]
Qualitative measurements			
Facet joint degeneration (Weishaupt) [20]			0.837[a]
Neuroforaminal stenosis (Lee) [58]			0.432[a]
Spinal canal stenosis (Schizas) [30]			0.902[a]
Quantitative measurements			
Posterior disc height [21]	2.8 (2.1)	3.8 (0.9)	0.266[b]
Neuroforaminal antero-posterior distance [22]	6.3 (1.6)	6.2 (1.5)	0.860[b]
Neuroforaminal cross-sectional area [23]	58.3 (16.9)	63.9 (10.1)	0.439[b]
Ligamentous interfacet distance [26]	13.5 (4.1)	13.4 (3.6)	0.973[b]
Minimum sagittal antero-posterior diameter of the spinal canal	12.1 (3.5)	10.3 (2.8)	0.260[b]
Minimum cross-sectional area of the spinal canal [27–29]	155.3 (81.3)	131.4 (41.7)	0.482[b]

No difference in motion segments between those two groups was observed. Values are reported as means (standard deviation)

[a] Mann-Whitney U test

[b] t test for independent samples

such a clinical feature. In addition, fluid production in the facet joints seen on MRI is presently interpreted as a sign of instability [41–43] rather than a sign of inflammation. Perhaps the activation of the degenerative stage could be visualised by imaging of metabolic processes, using, for example, SPECT-CT or positron emission tomography-CT [44]. It is still a matter of discussion whether the response to infiltration and the prognostic value of facet joint degeneration in these imaging modalities is increased compared with those for MRI. Furthermore, the power of imaging often lies in its ability to rule out other differential diagnoses, such as fracture, infection or neoplasm, rather than to prove a symptomatic condition.

In compensation for this diagnostic imaging gap, image-guided diagnostic facet joint infiltrations have been established, for which evidence is considered strong (level II) to isolate the facet joint as a pain generator [45]. To the best of our knowledge, a study evaluating the prognostic value of diagnostic facet joint infiltrations for the outcome of spinal fusion surgery is still lacking and thus, preoperative diagnostic infiltrations remain an eminence-based procedure. First data are, however, available on the prognostic value of facet joint infiltrations before lumbar facet radiofrequency denervation that show that a correct prognosis was made in about 60–70% of analysed patients [46]. The role of such infiltrations has nonetheless been recently questioned. Schütz et al. [47] performed a triple cross-over study to investigate the effects obtained by diagnostic facet joint infiltrations compared with those by placebo and sham infiltrations. They found no relevant difference between the three modalities and thus questioned the diagnostic value of medial branch blocks. Indeed, a high

false positive rate for facet joint infiltrations is described in the literature [48]. When the data are examined closely, however, one general problem with most studies on the topic must be recognised: patients with chronic lumbar back pain usually do not present with monosegmental problems but rather with multisegmental changes, which in a chronic form must be considered a complex syndrome compared with monosegmental facet joint pathology. This consideration also includes the locus of nociception: whereas nociception in facet joint syndrome has been suggested to originate in the synovial membrane, hyaline cartilage, bone or fibrous capsule of the facet joint [17], in chronic conditions, structures other than the facet joints themselves, such as myofascial trigger points or even reactive overexcitability of nociceptive neurons in the central nervous system [49], can provide the nociceptors. Moreover, dual innervation of the facet joint with overlapping zones of referred pain [50–52] makes medial branch blocks inadequate for diagnosis of a single motion segment's facet joints. In contrast to intraarticular injections (as in the present study), medial branch blocks also seem to anaesthetise not just the joint but also the muscles, ligaments and periosteum that they innervate [53]. Although this does not argue against performing medial branch blocks per se, this information needs to be considered when interpreting data from the literature.

Given the uncertainty surrounding both the interpretability of MRI findings and the diagnostic value of facet joint infiltrations, it is clear that future studies should first concentrate on patients with monosegmental problems. Only when a clear determination of sensitivity, specificity, validity and reliability has been obtained can multisegmental problems be addressed. In view of the given uncertainty of both modalities, the results obtained in the present study could be interpreted in two ways. First, it is possible that either of these techniques or both are completely useless. Second, the results could imply that the information that both modalities provide is complementary. There is no completely reliable gold standard with which to compare a diagnostic test (or injection) when the absence of pain is the end point [54]. It is therefore clear that, for the time being, not only the sum of findings from one modality such as imaging, but also a thorough clinical examination, medical history and—in select cases—infiltration results will allow the development of a solid therapeutic recommendation.

Study limitations

All infiltrations were guided by fluoroscopy. Nevertheless, it is possible that some of the infiltrations were not applied intraarticularly, but periarticularly. The clear difference between the effects obtained by intraarticular and periarticular infiltrations is yet to be demonstrated. A general critical feature of most studies addressing patients with chronic lumbar back pain is the mostly multisegmental underlying pathology that makes it difficult to analyse monosegmental effects. A crucial consideration for the correct interpretation of our findings is that the results described apply only to chronic conditions.

Conclusion

Although imaging results are frequently considered as hallmarks of disease by specialists to plan their future treatment strategy, a clear correlation of symptoms and imaging results is not yet possible with current techniques. The prognostic value of facet joint infiltrations for surgical outcome has also recently been questioned. Our results show an absolute lack of correlation between imaging results with MRI and effects obtained by targeted facet joint infiltration. In view of the trend in evidence-based medicine to provide medical algorithms, our findings underline the continuing need for individualised spine medicine that, along with imaging techniques or targeted infiltrations, includes diagnostic dimensions such as good patient history and clinical examination.

Abbreviations
MRI: Magnetic resonance imaging; SPECT: Single-photon emission computed tomography

Acknowledgements
We thank Barbara Every, ELS, of BioMedical Editor, for English language editing.

Funding
No funding was received for the study.

Authors' contributions
UKH designed the study, performed the statistical analyses and wrote the manuscript; RLK performed the measurements and helped with the statistical analyses; CW helped to write the manuscript; and FM supervised the study and helped to write the manuscript. All authors read and approved the final manuscript.

Authors' information
Not applicable.

Competing interests
The authors declare that they have no competing interests.

Author details
[1]Department of Orthopaedic Surgery, University Hospital of Tübingen, Hoppe-Seyler-Strasse 3, 72076 Tübingen, Germany. [2]Faculty of Medicine, Julius-Maximilians University of Würzburg, Josef-Schneider-Str.2, 97080 Würzburg, Germany.

References
1. Deyo RA, Mirza SK. Trends and variations in the use of spine surgery. Clin Orthop Relat Res. 2006;443:139–46.
2. Patel AT, Ogle AA. Diagnosis and management of acute low back pain. Am Fam Physician. 2000;61(6):1779–86. 1789-1790
3. Rubin DI. Epidemiology and risk factors for spine pain. Neurol Clin. 2007;25(2):353–71.
4. Schmidt CO, Raspe H, Pfingsten M, Hasenbring M, Basler HD, Eich W, Kohlmann T. Back pain in the German adult population: prevalence, severity, and sociodemographic correlates in a multiregional survey. Spine (Phila Pa 1976). 2007;32(18):2005–11.
5. Deyo RA, Gray DT, Kreuter W, Mirza S, Martin BI. United States trends in lumbar fusion surgery for degenerative conditions. Spine (Phila Pa 1976). 2005;30(12):1441–5. discussion 1446-1447
6. Deyo RA, Mirza SK, Turner JA, Martin BI. Overtreating chronic back pain: time to back off? J Am Board Fam Med. 2009;22(1):62–8.
7. Manchikanti L, Pampati V, Fellows B, Bakhit CE. Prevalence of lumbar facet joint pain in chronic low back pain. Pain Physician. 1999;2(3):59–64.
8. Schwarzer AC, Wang SC, Bogduk N, McNaught PJ, Laurent R. Prevalence and clinical features of lumbar zygapophysial joint pain: a study in an Australian population with chronic low back pain. Ann Rheum Dis. 1995;54(2):100–6.
9. Cohen SP, Hurley RW, Christo PJ, Winkley J, Mohiuddin MM, Stojanovic MP. Clinical predictors of success and failure for lumbar facet radiofrequency denervation. Clin J Pain. 2007;23(1):45–52.
10. Jackson RP, Jacobs RR, Montesano PX. 1988 Volvo award in clinical sciences. Facet joint injection in low-back pain. A prospective statistical study. Spine (Phila Pa 1976). 13(9):966–71.
11. Schwarzer AC, Wang SC, O'Driscoll D, Harrington T, Bogduk N, Laurent R. The ability of computed tomography to identify a painful zygapophysial joint in patients with chronic low back pain. Spine (Phila Pa 1976). 1995;20(8):907–12.
12. Hofmann UK, Gesicki M, Mittag F. Inpatient gradual diagnostics and its relevance for determining treatment strategies in lumbar back pain. BMC Musculoskelet Disord. 2016;17:275.
13. Kayser R, Mahlfeld K, Heyde CE. Concepts of in-patient gradual diagnostics for patients with lumbar back-pain. Orthopade. 2008;37(4):285–99.
14. Jerosch J, Tappiser R, Assheuer J. MRI-controlled facet block—technique and initial results. Biomed Tech (Berl). 1998;43(9):249–52.
15. Peh W. Image-guided facet joint injection. Biomed Imaging Interv J. 2011;7(1):e4.
16. Makki D, Khazim R, Zaidan AA, Ravi K, Toma T. Single photon emission computerized tomography (SPECT) scan-positive facet joints and other spinal structures in a hospital-wide population with spinal pain. Spine J. 2010;10(1):58–62.
17. Cohen SP, Raja SN. Pathogenesis, diagnosis, and treatment of lumbar zygapophysial (facet) joint pain. Anesthesiology. 2007;106(3):591–614.

18. Stojanovic MP, Sethee J, Mohiuddin M, Cheng J, Barker A, Wang J, Palmer W, Huang A, Cohen SP. MRI analysis of the lumbar spine: can it predict response to diagnostic and therapeutic facet procedures? Clin J Pain. 2010;26(2):110–5.

19. Pathria M, Sartoris DJ, Resnick D. Osteoarthritis of the facet joints: accuracy of oblique radiographic assessment. Radiology. 1987;164(1):227–30.

20. Weishaupt D, Zanetti M, Boos N, Hodler J. MR imaging and CT in osteoarthritis of the lumbar facet joints. Skelet Radiol. 1999;28(4):215–9.

21. Hasegawa T, An HS, Haughton VM, Nowicki BH. Lumbar foraminal stenosis: critical heights of the intervertebral discs and foramina. A cryomicrotome study in cadavera. J Bone Joint Surg Am. 1995;77(1):32–8.

22. Beers GJ, Carter AP, Leiter BE, Tilak SP, Shah RR. Interobserver discrepancies in distance measurements from lumbar spine CT scans. AJR Am J Roentgenol. 1985;144(2):395–8.

23. Sipola P, Leinonen V, Niemelainen R, Aalto T, Vanninen R, Manninen H, Airaksinen O, Battie MC. Visual and quantitative assessment of lateral lumbar spinal canal stenosis with magnetic resonance imaging. Acta Radiol. 2011;52(9):1024–31.

24. Kunogi J, Hasue M. Diagnosis and operative treatment of intraforaminal and extraforaminal nerve root compression. Spine (Phila Pa 1976). 1991;16(11):1312–20.

25. Lee S, Lee JW, Yeom JS, Kim KJ, Kim HJ, Chung SK, Kang HS. A practical MRI grading system for lumbar foraminal stenosis. AJR Am J Roentgenol. 2010;194(4):1095–8.

26. Herzog RJ, Kaiser JA, Saal JA, Saal JS. The importance of posterior epidural fat pad in lumbar central canal stenosis. Spine (Phila Pa 1976). 1991;16(6 Suppl):S227–33.

27. Hamanishi C, Matukura N, Fujita M, Tomihara M, Tanaka S. Cross-sectional area of the stenotic lumbar dural tube measured from the transverse views of magnetic resonance imaging. J Spinal Disord. 1994;7(5):388–93.

28. Laurencin CT, Lipson SJ, Senatus P, Botchwey E, Jones TR, Koris M, Hunter J. The stenosis ratio: a new tool for the diagnosis of degenerative spinal stenosis. Int J Surg Investig. 1999;1(2):127–31.

29. Schonstrom N, Lindahl S, Willen J, Hansson T. Dynamic changes in the dimensions of the lumbar spinal canal: an experimental study in vitro. J Orthop Res. 1989;7(1):115–21.

30. Schizas C, Theumann N, Burn A, Tansey R, Wardlaw D, Smith FW, Kulik G. Qualitative grading of severity of lumbar spinal stenosis based on the morphology of the dural sac on magnetic resonance images. Spine (Phila Pa 1976). 2010;35(21):1919–24.

31. Gorbach C, Schmid MR, Elfering A, Hodler J, Boos N. Therapeutic efficacy of facet joint blocks. AJR Am J Roentgenol. 2006;186(5):1228–33.

32. Boden SD, Wiesel SW. Lumbar spine imaging: role in clinical decision making. J Am Acad Orthop Surg. 1996;4(5):238–48.

33. Dreyfuss PH, Dreyer SJ, Herring SA. Lumbar zygapophysial (facet) joint injections. Spine (Phila Pa 1976). 1995;20(18):2040–7.

34. Jensen MC, Brant-Zawadzki MN, Obuchowski N, Modic MT, Malkasian D, Ross JS. Magnetic resonance imaging of the lumbar spine in people without back pain. N Engl J Med. 1994;331(2):69–73.

35. Weiner BK, Patel R. The accuracy of MRI in the detection of lumbar disc containment. J Orthop Surg Res. 2008;3:46.

36. Kalichman L, Li L, Kim DH, Guermazi A, Berkin V, O'Donnell CJ, Hoffmann U, Cole R, Hunter DJ. Facet joint osteoarthritis and low back pain in the community-based population. Spine (Phila Pa 1976). 2008;33(23):2560–5.

37. Schwarzer AC, Aprill CN, Derby R, Fortin J, Kine G, Bogduk N. Clinical features of patients with pain stemming from the lumbar zygapophysial joints. Is the lumbar facet syndrome a clinical entity? Spine (Phila Pa 1976). 1994;19(10):1132–7.

38. Goni VG, Hampannavar A, Gopinathan NR, Singh P, Sudesh P, Logithasan RK, Sharma A, Bk S, Sament R. Comparison of the oswestry disability index and magnetic resonance imaging findings in lumbar canal stenosis: an observational study. Asian Spine J. 2014;8(1):44–50.

39. Kim YU, Kong YG, Lee J, Cheong Y, Kim S, Kim HK, Park JY, Suh JH. Clinical symptoms of lumbar spinal stenosis associated with morphological parameters on magnetic resonance images. Eur Spine J. 2015;24(10):2236–43.

40. Yuan S, Zou Y, Li Y, Chen M, Yue Y. A clinically relevant MRI grading system for lumbar central canal stenosis. Clin Imaging. 2016;40(6):1140–5.

41. Chaput C, Padon D, Rush J, Lenehan E, Rahm M. The significance of increased fluid signal on magnetic resonance imaging in lumbar facets in relationship to degenerative spondylolisthesis. Spine (Phila Pa 1976). 2007;32(17):1883–7.

42. Lattig F, Fekete TF, Grob D, Kleinstuck FS, Jeszenszky D, Mannion AF. Lumbar facet joint effusion in MRI: a sign of instability in degenerative spondylolisthesis? Eur Spine J. 2012;21(2):276–81.

43. Rihn JA, Lee JY, Khan M, Ulibarri JA, Tannoury C, Donaldson WF 3rd, Kang JD. Does lumbar facet fluid detected on magnetic resonance imaging correlate with radiographic instability in patients with degenerative lumbar disease? Spine (Phila Pa 1976). 2007;32(14):1555–60.

44. Shur N, Corrigan A, Agrawal K, Desai A, Gnanasegaran G. Radiological and radionuclide imaging of degenerative disease of the facet joints. Indian J Nucl Med. 2015;30(3):191–8.

45. Sehgal N, Dunbar EE, Shah RV, Colson J. Systematic review of diagnostic utility of facet (zygapophysial) joint injections in chronic spinal pain: an update. Pain Physician. 2007;10(1):213–28.

46. Cohen SP, Moon JY, Brummett CM, White RL, Larkin TM. Medial branch blocks or intra-articular injections as a prognostic tool before lumbar facet radiofrequency denervation: a multicenter, case-control study. Reg Anesth Pain Med. 2015;40(4):376–83.

47. Schutz U, Cakir B, Dreinhofer K, Richter M, Koepp H. Diagnostic value of lumbar facet joint injection: a prospective triple cross-over study. PLoS One. 2011;6(11):e27991.

48. Manchukonda R, Manchikanti KN, Cash KA, Pampati V, Manchikanti L. Facet joint pain in chronic spinal pain: an evaluation of prevalence and false-positive rate of diagnostic blocks. J Spinal Disord Tech. 2007;20(7):539–45.

49. Mense S. Muscle pain: mechanisms and clinical significance. Dtsch Arztebl Int. 2008;105(12):214–9.

50. Fukui S, Ohseto K, Shiotani M, Ohno K, Karasawa H, Naganuma Y. Distribution of referred pain from the lumbar zygapophyseal joints and dorsal rami. Clin J Pain. 1997;13(4):303–7.

51. Maldjian C, Mesgarzadeh M, Tehranzadeh J. Diagnostic and therapeutic features of facet and sacroiliac joint injection. Anatomy, pathophysiology, and technique. Radiol Clin N Am. 1998;36(3):497–508.

52. Marks RC, Houston T, Thulbourne T. Facet joint injection and facet nerve block: a randomised comparison in 86 patients with chronic low back pain. Pain. 1992;49(3):325–8.

53. Murtagh R. The art and science of nerve root and facet blocks. Neuroimaging Clin N Am. 2000;10(3):465–77.

54. Saal JS. General principles of diagnostic testing as related to painful lumbar spine disorders: a critical appraisal of current diagnostic techniques. Spine (Phila Pa 1976). 2002;27(22):2538–45. discussion 2546

55. Kalichman L, Cole R, Kim DH, Li L, Suri P, Guermazi A, Hunter DJ. Spinal stenosis prevalence and association with symptoms: the Framingham study. Spine J. 2009;9(7):545–50.

56. Ullrich CG, Binet EF, Sanecki MG, Kieffer SA. Quantitative assessment of the lumbar spinal canal by computed tomography. Radiology. 1980;134(1):137–43.

57. Verbiest H. The significance and principles of computerized axial tomography in idiopathic developmental stenosis of the bony lumbar vertebral canal. Spine (Phila Pa 1976). 1979;4(4):369–78.

58. Lee GY, Lee JW, Choi HS, KJ O, Kang HS. A new grading system of lumbar central canal stenosis on MRI: an easy and reliable method. Skelet Radiol. 2011;40(8):1033–9.

25

In vivo evaluation of microglia activation by intracranial iron overload in central pain after spinal cord injury

Fan Xing Meng[1,2†], Jing Ming Hou[2,3†] and Tian Sheng Sun[1,2*]

Abstract

Background: Central pain (CP) is a common clinical problem in patients with spinal cord injury (SCI). Recent studies found the pathogenesis of CP was related to the remodeling of the brain. We investigate the roles of iron overload and subsequent microglia activate in the remodeling of the brain after SCI.

Methods: An SCI-induced CP model was established in Sprague-Dawley rats that were randomly assigned to SCI, sham operation, deferoxamine (DFX), minocycline, and nitric oxide synthase inhibitor treatment groups. At 12 weeks, pain behavior and thermal pain threshold were evaluated in each group, and *iron transferrin receptor* (*TfR*)*1* and *ferritin* (*Fn*) mRNA, as well as iron-regulatory protein (IRP)1, FN, lactoferrin, and nuclear factor (NF)-κB protein levels in the rat brains were measured. Microglia proliferation and differentiation and IRP1 expression were evaluated by immunohistochemistry.

Results: Autophagy was observed in rats after SCI, accompanied by reduced latency of thermal pain, increased iron content and IRP1 and NF-κB levels in the hindlimb sensory area, hippocampus, and thalamus, and decreased Fn levels in the hindlimb sensory area. *TfR1* mRNA expression was upregulated in activated microglia. Treatment with an iron-chelating agent, or inhibitors of nitric oxide synthase or microglia suppressed microglia proliferation.

Conclusions: SCI may induce intracranial iron overload, which activates microglia via NF-κB signaling. Microglia secrete inflammatory factors that induce neuronal damage and lead to CP. Treatment with an iron-chelating agent or NF-κB or microglia inhibitors can relieve CP resulting from SCI.

Keywords: Central pain, Spinal cord injury, Iron, Microglia, NF-κB

Background

Around 60–90% of patients with spinal cord injury (SCI) develop central pain (CP) [1, 2], which is defined as pain hypersensitivity resulting from central nervous system injury. Pain in the lower limbs is often persistent and difficult to endure [3, 4], making CP a major problem for patients and physicians. It is thought that structural and functional remodeling of the brain after SCI can cause CP; however, the mechanisms underlying the development of CP are poorly understood [5–9].

In our previous work, we used magnetic susceptibility weighted imaging to investigate the functional remodeling of the brain in SCI patients. We found that iron-overloaded regions—including the sensory regions of the cortex, thalamus, and cingutate (unpublished data)—were remodeled, implying that intracranial iron overload is involved in the pathogenesis of CP.

Intracranial iron overload plays an important role in the occurrence and development of Alzheimer's and Parkinson's disease and cerebral hemorrhage [10–12]. The toxicity of iron may be linked to oxidative stress injury induced by the Fenton reaction. Iron overload can activate brain microglia, which initiate and amplify neuronal damage [13]. Activated microglia also regulate the levels of cytokines such as interleukin-1β, tumor necrosis factor (TNF)-α, and nitrous oxide; the ensuing formation of reactive oxygen species and amplification of

* Correspondence: suntiansheng-@163.com
†Equal contributors
[1]Third Military Medical University, No. 30 Gaotanyan Street, Chongqing 400038, China
[2]Department of Orthopedics, Chinese PLA Army General Hospital, Dongcheng District, Nanmencang No. 5, Beijing 100700, China
Full list of author information is available at the end of the article

the proinflammatory cytokine cascade can lead to neuronal damage or loss [14, 15]. In addition, activated microglia may induce nuclear factor (NF)-κB signaling in neurons [16, 17].

The present study investigated the causes of intracranial iron overload and its relationship with CP pathogenesis. Our findings provide a basis for the treatment of CP following SCI through the use of iron-chelating agents and NF-κB and microglia inhibitors.

Methods

Experimental design

In this experiment, we selected L-arginine as the nitric oxide synthase (NOS) inhibitors, deferoxamine (DFX) as the iron chelator, and minocycline as the microglia activation inhibitors.

Female Sprague-Dawley rats ($n = 75$; 230.0 ± 15.4 g) were randomly divided into five groups ($n = 15$ each): sham operation (laminectomy only without SCI or drug treatment); control (CP rats after SCI without drug treatment); L-arginine treatment (1.5 mg/kg by intraperitoneal (i.p.) injection on the day after surgery, followed by once-weekly injections until the end of the experiment); DFX treatment (100 mg/kg by i.p. injection 1 day after surgery, followed by once-weekly injections until the end of the experiment); and minocycline treatment (45 mg/kg by i.p. injection immediately after surgery repeated over 12 h, followed by 22.5 mg/kg by i.p. injection twice daily for two consecutive days).

Rat model of CP after SCI

Rats were anesthetized with 10% chloral hydrate (3 ml/kg) and subjected to T10 laminectomy under sterile surgical conditions by making a 3-cm incision around the T10 vertebra. The skin and muscle were cut, and the T9–T11 spine and lamina and spinal cord dorsal epidura were exposed over an area of about 2–3 mm. Using the Allen hitting method and guided by a plastic catheter, the blunt end of a 30-g stainless steel rod was dropped vertically from a height of 15 cm onto the gasket in order to induce SCI, which was confirmed by observing the twitching of the rat's hindlimbs and tail. The incision was then sutured shut. Sham-operated animals were subjected to the same procedure but without the weight drop. After the operation, rats were placed in individual cages and administered 0.6 g lincomycin by intramuscular injection for 3 days to prevent incision infection and assisted with urination if necessary.

Assessment of pain behavior

Following surgery, rats were observed for spontaneous pain behaviors, including trimming, scratching, licking of the hindlimbs and tail, and vocalizations.

Determination of thermal pain hypersensitivity

The latency of thermal pain hypersensitivity was measured for each group at 2, 4, 8, 12, 16, and 24 h and then once daily after surgery. Each rat's foot was placed on a hot plate (55 °C), and the time until the rat lifted its foot was recorded. Both feet were tested with a 3-min interval between each measurement. The procedure was repeated three times, and the average value was determined.

Determination of cerebral cortex iron content

The iron content of the whole rat brain and various brain regions was determined by atomic absorption spectrophotometry. The whole brains or hindlimb sensory areas, thalamus, and hippocampus were collected and weighed, immersed in 20 mmol/1 HEPES buffer (1:20, w/v), and homogenized. A 30-μl volume of homogenate was mixed with an equal volume of ultrapure nitric acid and digested in a 50 °C water bath for 48 h, then diluted with 3.12 mmol/l nitrate at a 1:10 ratio. A standard curve was prepared using iron solution (50 mg/l) diluted with 5% nitric acid. The blank and actual samples were read three times at 248.3 nm.

Determination of transferrin receptor (TfR)1 mRNA levels by real-time (RT-)PCR

TfR1 mRNA expression in various brain regions, including the hindlimb sensory cortex, hippocampus, and thalamus ($n = 3$ rats/group) was determined by RT-PCR. RNA was extracted from tissue with TRIzol reagent (Invitrogen, Carlsbad, CA, USA) according to the manufacturer's instructions, and 20 μg were treated with 10 U DNaseI (Takara Bio, Otsu, Japan) for 30 min at 37 °C. cDNA was synthesized using oligo dT primer, and 1 μl was added to the reaction containing 27.5 μl Real-Time PCR Master Mix(TOYOBO), 15 pmol of primers, and 7.5 pmol TaqMan probe, for a total volume of 30 μl. Primers and probes for *TfR1* and *ferritin* (*Fn*) were designed with Primer Premier 5.0 software and synthesized by Shenggong Biotechnology (Shanghai, China). The sequences were as follows: Tfrc-F, CGT GGA GAC TAC TTC CGT GC, and Tfrc-R, GCC AGA GCC CCA GAA GAT GTG; GAPDH-F, CGGCAAGTTCAACGGCACAG, and GAPDH-R CCATGGTGGTGAAGACGCCA.

Determination of TfR1 and Fn levels in the brain by enzyme-linked immunosorbent assay (ELISA)

Tissue from the hindlimb sensory cortex, hippocampus, and thalamus of five rats was homogenized in radioimmunoprecipitation assay buffer containing protease and phosphatase inhibitors and phenylmethylsulfonyl fluoride at 4 °C. The homogenate was centrifuged at 10,000 rpm for 30 min, and the supernatant was collected and stored at −70 °C. The protein content of each sample was determined with the bicinchoninic acid assay. TfR1 and Fn levels were determined by ELISA(ab-cam). Each sample was prepared in triplicate, and optical density values were calculated as mean ± standard deviation.

Determination of iron-regulatory protein (IRP)1, Fn, lactoferrin (Lf), and NF-κB levels by western blotting

IRP1, Fn, Lf, and NF-κB protein levels in the hind-limb sensory cortex of rats in each group were determined by western blotting. Briefly, 50 μg protein from brain tissue lysates were resolved by 10% non-denaturing sodium dodecyl sulfate polyacrylamide gel electrophoresis and transferred to a nitrocellulose membrane, which was confirmed by Ponceau S staining. The membrane was blocked with skim milk powder at room temperature for 2 h, followed by overnight incubation at 4 °C with rat anti-human IRP1 (Santa Cruz Biotechnology,USA) (1:100), rabbit anti-human Fn (1:100, PLLABS), rabbit anti-rat NF-κB (1:400, abcam), rabbit anti-rat LF (Santa Cruz Biotechnology,USA) (1:200), and anti-β-actin (1:100) antibodies. After three washes with tris-buffered saline containing 0.05% Tween 20, the membrane was incubated with horseradish peroxidase-conjugated secondary antibody (1:500) at room temperature. The enhanced chemiluminescence detection kit (Pierce, Rockford, IL, USA) was used to detect protein bands, which were analyzed using ImageJ software (National Institutes of Health, Bethesda, MD, USA).

Effect of abnormal iron deposition on microglia activation

At predetermined time points, rats underwent transcardial perfusion with 4% paraformaldehyde. The brain was dissected and fixed in paraformaldehyde at 4 °C for 4–6 h, followed by immersion in 20 and 30% sucrose solutions. After the brains were saturated, they were embedded in optimal cutting temperature medium and sectioned at a thickness of 7 μm. Sections were incubated overnight with the following primary antibodies: rabbit anti-rat Anti Iba1 (WAKO,Japan) (1:200) and rat anti-

human IRP1 (Santa Cruz Biotechnology,USA) (1:100). After three washes with phosphate-buffered saline, sections were incubated with biotin-conjugated secondary antibody for 90 min, washed three times, and incubated for 90 min with horseradish peroxidase-conjugated secondary antibody. After rinsing, sections were treated with diaminobenzidine (Stable DAB, Research Genetics, USA), washed with water, dehydrated, mounted, and visualized by microscopy.

Statistical analysis

Data were analyzed with SPSS v.17.0 software. Data are presented as mean ± standard deviation. Univariate analyses were used to compare group means. $P < 0.05$ was considered as statistically significant.

Results

Detection of CP in a rat model

Spontaneous pain in animal models is characterized by scratching and biting below the level of injury. After SCI, rats were observed to scratch, bite, and excessively groom body parts below the level of injury, i.e., hindlimbs and tail, which was not exhibited by rats in the sham operation group.

Average thermal pain latency values were as follows: 1.55 ± 0.14 s for SCI, 2.19 ± 0.09 s for sham operation, and 1.9 ± 0.11, 1.89 ± 0.10, and 1.66 ± 0.09 s for arginine, DFX, and minocycline treatment groups, respectively, (Fig. 1a). Thermal pain threshold was higher for sham-operated animals than that for the other groups ($P <$ 0.05), while that of the SCI group was decreased relative to the other groups ($P < 0.05$). The sham operation group had the highest latency values, while the SCI group had the lowest values, at the time points examined (Fig. 1b).

Determination of intracranial iron content

Whole brain iron content was 11.5 ± 2.1 μg/g for SCI, 12.3 ± 2.6 μg/g for sham operation, and 11.4 ± 1.8, 11.8 ± 3.1, and 12.4 ± 2.4 μg/g for arginine, DFX, and

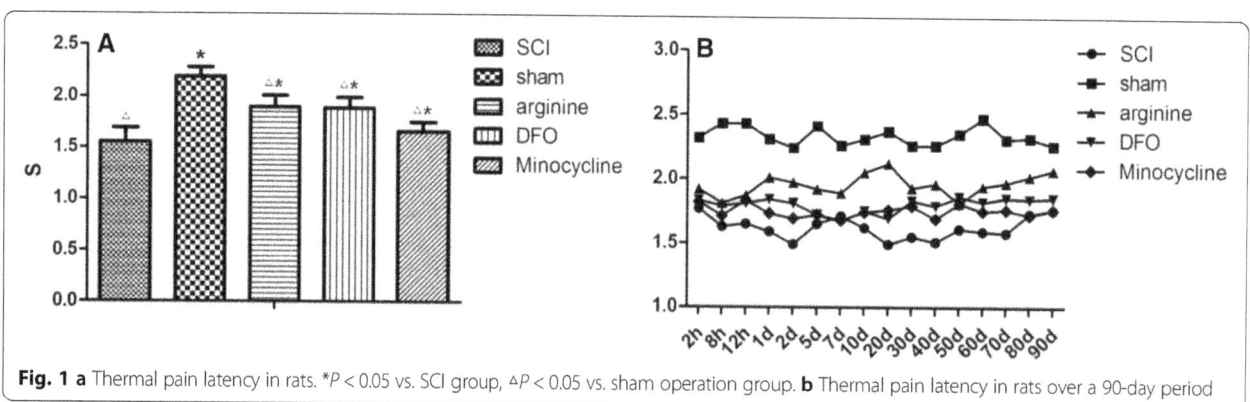

Fig. 1 a Thermal pain latency in rats. *$P < 0.05$ vs. SCI group, △$P < 0.05$ vs. sham operation group. **b** Thermal pain latency in rats over a 90-day period

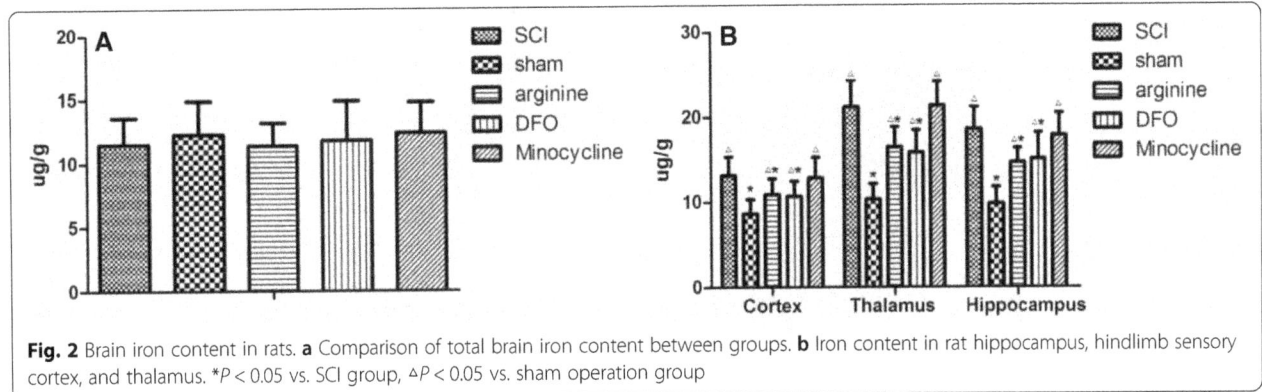

Fig. 2 Brain iron content in rats. **a** Comparison of total brain iron content between groups. **b** Iron content in rat hippocampus, hindlimb sensory cortex, and thalamus. *$P < 0.05$ vs. SCI group, △$P < 0.05$ vs. sham operation group

minocycline treatment groups, respectively, (Fig. 2a). There were no differences in the whole-brain iron content among groups. However, the iron contents of the hindlimb sensory area, hippocampus, and thalamus were lower in the sham operation as compared to the other groups ($P < 0.05$), while the brain iron contents of the SCI and minocycline treatment groups were higher than those of the other groups ($P < 0.05$) (Fig. 2b and Table 1).

Expression of IRP1 and NF-κB in the brain

IRP1 and NF-κB levels were lower, while Fn levels were higher, in the hindlimb sensory cortex of sham-operated rats as compared to those of other groups ($P < 0.05$) (Fig. 3). IRP1 levels were lower, while those of NF-κB and Fn were higher, in the SCI than in the sham operation, or arginine or DFX treatment groups ($P < 0.05$). These results suggest that arginine treatment decreases IRP1 and NF-κB and increases Fn levels after SCI, whereas DFX treatment decreases NF-κB and increases Fn levels but does not affect IRP1 expression. Minocycline treatment had no effect on the expression of any of these proteins, and there were no differences in LF level among groups.

TfR1 and Fn levels in the hindlimb sensory cortex, thalamus, and hippocampus

TfR1 levels were lower, whereas Fn levels were higher, in sham-operated animals than in the other groups ($P < 0.05$) (Fig. 4). In the SCI group, TfR1 expression was higher, whereas Fn expression was lower, than in the sham operation and arginine and DFX treatment groups ($P < 0.05$). Arginine treatment lowered TfR1 expression ($P < 0.05$)

and increased Fn levels ($P < 0.05$) after SCI. DFX treatment increased Fn levels ($P < 0.05$) but had no effect on TfR1 expression, while minocycline had no effect on TfR1 or Fn levels ($P > 0.05$).

TfR1 gene expression in the hindlimb sensory cortex, thalamus, and hippocampus

TfR1 gene expression in the rat hindlimb sensory area, thalamus, and hippocampus was determined by RT-PCR (Fig. 5). *TfR1* levels in the various brain regions were lower in sham-operated rats as compared to those in the other groups ($P < 0.05$), but were higher in the SCI than in the sham and arginine treatment groups ($P < 0.05$). These results indicate that arginine and DFX treatment decrease *TfR1* gene expression after SCI, with the former showing a greater effect.

Microglia distribution and IRP1 expression in the brain following SCI

The number (Fig. 6a, b) and activation (Fig. 6c, d) of microglia in the hindlimb sensory cortex was markedly increased after SCI. Treatment with arginine, DFX, and minocycline decreased microglia number and activation (Fig. 6e–g). Accordingly, the number of IRP1-positive cells was increased after SCI (Fig. 7a, b), an effect that was abrogated in the presence of arginine (Fig. 7c).

Discussion

CP is also known as central dysesthesia syndrome [18] and is a common complication after SCI, hindering patients' rehabilitation and diminishing their quality of life [19]. One study reported that 40% of SCI patients were willing to sacrifice sexual, gut, and bladder functions for a reduction in

Table 1 Iron content in the sensory cortex, hippocampus, and thalamus of different groups ($\bar{x} \pm s$)

Group	SCI	sham	arginine	DFO	Minocycline
Hindlimb cortex	13.2 ± 2.2	8.6 ± 1.7	10.9 ± 1.9	10.7 ± 1.8	12.9 ± 2.4
Thalamus	21.2 ± 3.1	10.3 ± 1.9	16.5 ± 2.4	15.9 ± 2.6	21.4 ± 2.8
Hippocampus	18.6 ± 2.6	9.8 ± 2.1	14.7 ± 1.7	15.1 ± 3.1	17.9 ± 2.6

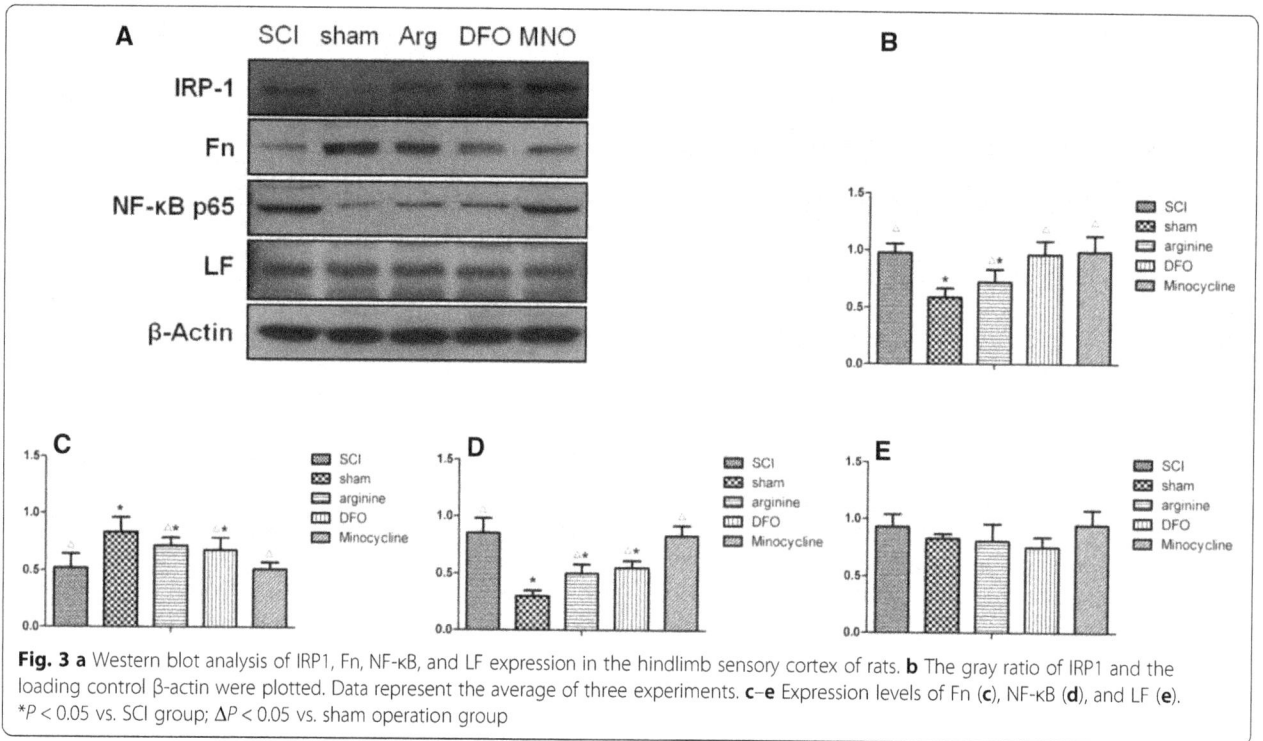

Fig. 3 a Western blot analysis of IRP1, Fn, NF-κB, and LF expression in the hindlimb sensory cortex of rats. **b** The gray ratio of IRP1 and the loading control β-actin were plotted. Data represent the average of three experiments. **c–e** Expression levels of Fn (**c**), NF-κB (**d**), and LF (**e**). *$P < 0.05$ vs. SCI group; Δ$P < 0.05$ vs. sham operation group

pain [20]. Since the etiology of CP after SCI is not well understood, there are no means of effectively diagnosing or treating this condition. Currently available treatments include physical therapy, drugs (non-steroidal anti-inflammatory analgesics, anticonvulsants, antidepressants, or opioids), and surgery [21]. These methods are only effective in 20–30% of cases [22]. Moreover, drugs are frequently associated with side effects and can lead to addiction. Blocking nerve fibers at the posterior root of the spinal nerve by nerve root cutting or anhydrous alcohol injection may have analgesic effects; however, this method is imprecise and is associated with a high rate of postoperative pain recurrence as well as organ dysfunction.

It has been suggested that CP following SCI arises from imbalances in the sensory pathway [23] or inhibitory and excitatory receptors [24, 25]; in addition, pattern theory [26] and the central nervous system immune response have also been proposed as explanations [27]. Some brain regions including the somatic sensory center, thalamus, and limbic system undergo structural and functional remodeling after SCI to compensate for the loss of sensory function; this may be an underlying cause of CP [5–9]. Patients with partial spinal cord transection may also experience pain in the distal part of the injured spine; although, pain severity is not directly related to whether or not there is total injury [28, 29], suggesting that the source of pain is likely proximal to the injury site. In this study we used Allen's weight-drop method [30] to establish an SCI model. Rats with CP were treated with DFX, arginine, or minocycline, which

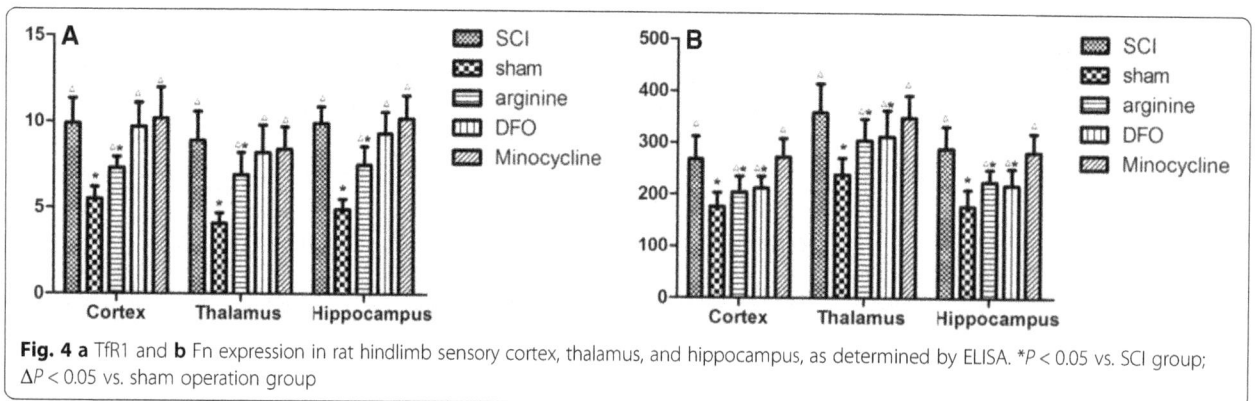

Fig. 4 a TfR1 and **b** Fn expression in rat hindlimb sensory cortex, thalamus, and hippocampus, as determined by ELISA. *$P < 0.05$ vs. SCI group; Δ$P < 0.05$ vs. sham operation group

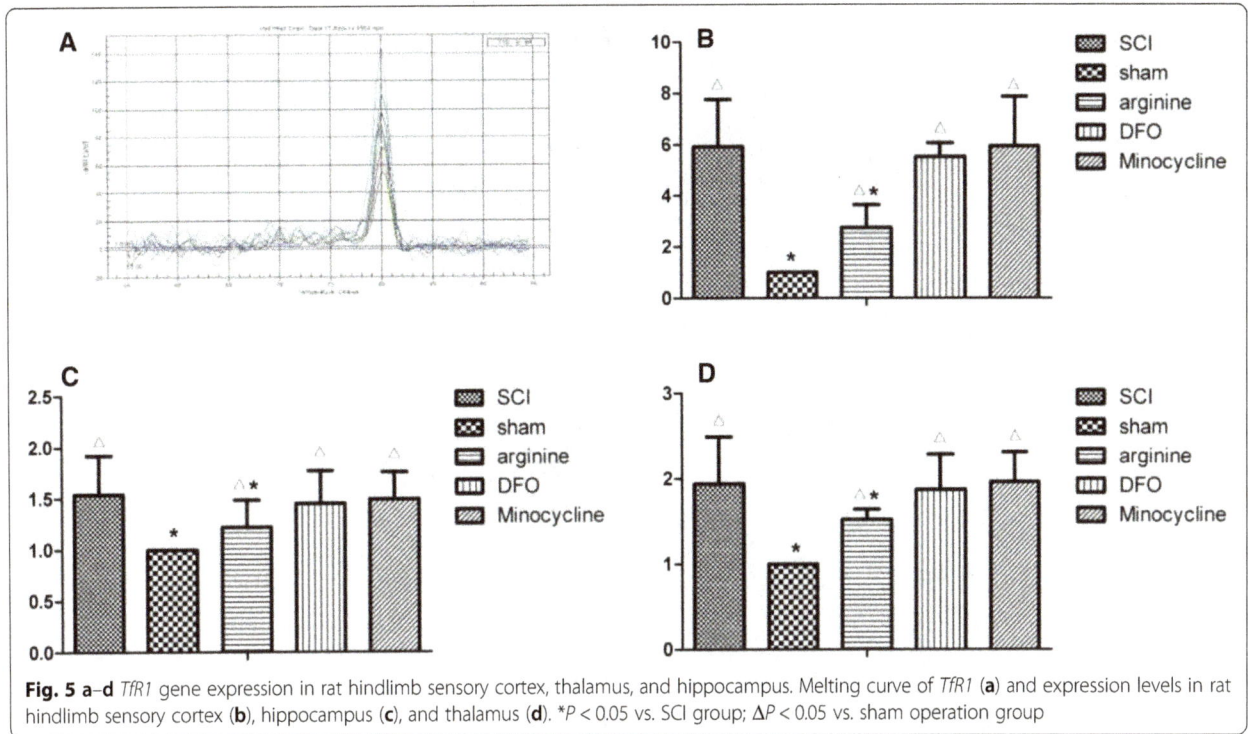

Fig. 5 a–d *TfR1* gene expression in rat hindlimb sensory cortex, thalamus, and hippocampus. Melting curve of *TfR1* (**a**) and expression levels in rat hindlimb sensory cortex (**b**), hippocampus (**c**), and thalamus (**d**). *$P < 0.05$ vs. SCI group; $\Delta P < 0.05$ vs. sham operation group

reduced the excessive grooming behavior indicative of CP in SCI rats while increasing the thermal pain threshold.

Intracranial iron is involved in RNA and protein synthesis in the brain as well as myelination and dopamine production. However, excessive iron in the brain has been linked to neurodegenerative disorders [31, 32] due to its role in the generation of hydroxyl free radicals via the Fenton reaction [33] ($Fe^{2+} + H_2O_2 \rightarrow Fe^{3+} \cdot OH + OH^-$), which causes oxidative stress-induced damage to cells and

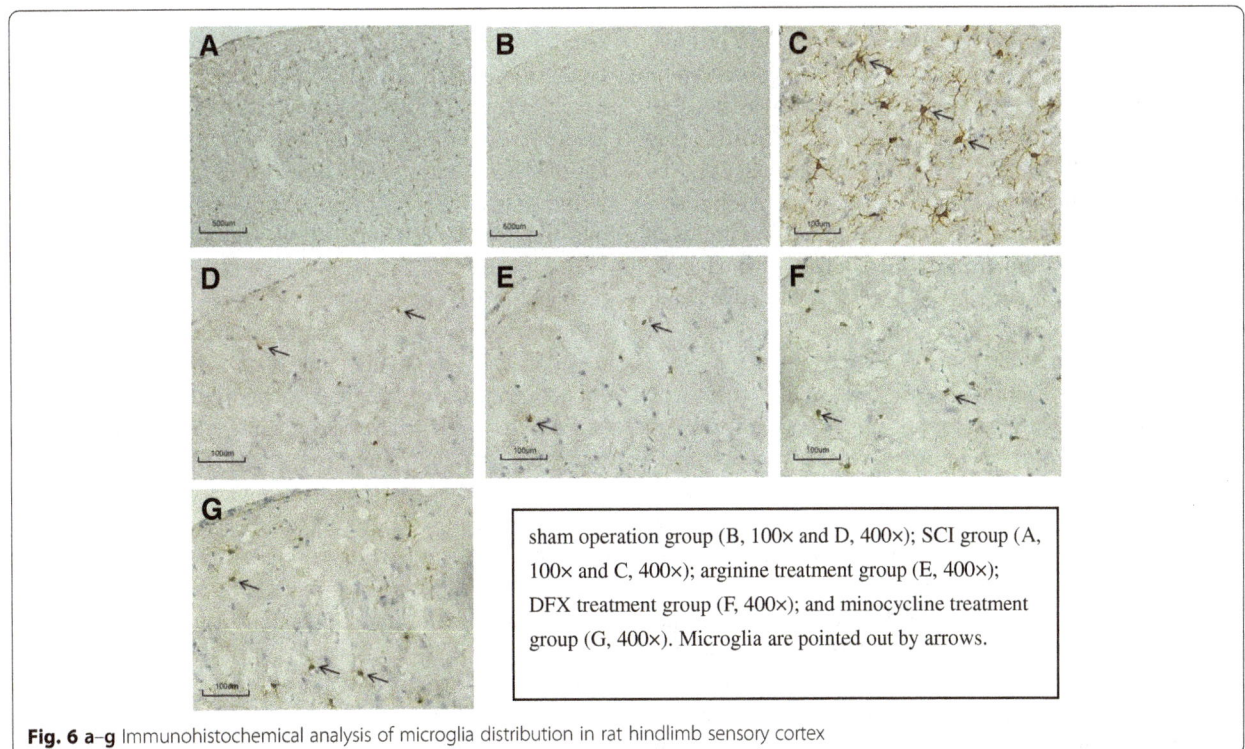

sham operation group (B, 100× and D, 400×); SCI group (A, 100× and C, 400×); arginine treatment group (E, 400×); DFX treatment group (F, 400×); and minocycline treatment group (G, 400×). Microglia are pointed out by arrows.

Fig. 6 a–g Immunohistochemical analysis of microglia distribution in rat hindlimb sensory cortex

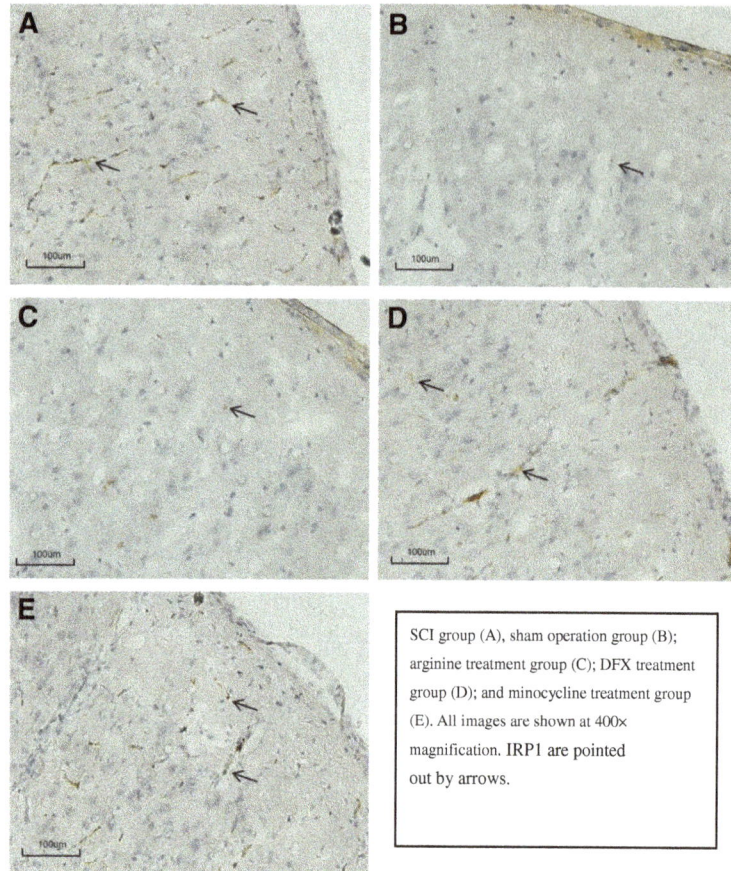

Fig. 7 a–e Immunohistochemical analysis of IRP1 expression in rat hindlimb sensory cortex

SCI group (A), sham operation group (B); arginine treatment group (C); DFX treatment group (D); and minocycline treatment group (E). All images are shown at 400× magnification. IRP1 are pointed out by arrows.

tissue. The redistribution of intracranial iron and iron deposition in specific brain regions has been observed in some neurodegenerative diseases such as Alzheimer's, Parkinson's, and Huntington's disease and Hallervorde-Spatz syndrome [34–36]. Brain iron levels are also elevated by physical stress, including heat and exercise stress and seasickness [37, 38]. Recent studies have found mutations in genes associated with brain iron metabolism, strongly suggesting that increased brain iron levels is a causative factor in some neurodegenerative diseases [39].

We used atomic absorption spectrophotometry to determine brain iron content and found that iron levels in the thalamus, hippocampus, and hindlimb sensory area were elevated for up to 12 weeks in all SCI groups relative to sham-operated animals, similar to what is observed in some neurodegenerative disorders. These results suggest an association between retention of iron in specific brain structures and CP.

Iron metabolism in the brain depends on the expression of various iron metabolism proteins. The passage of iron through the blood-brain barrier and its uptake by neurons is mainly mediated by the Tf/TfR interaction [40–44]. We found that *TfR1* expression in the hindlimb

sensory cortex, hippocampus, and thalamus was increased in all SCI rats, indicating that an increase in iron uptake via the Tf/TfR pathway may underlie iron overloading. Fn is a natural iron chelator that is widely expressed in neurons and glia in humans and rodents. It is the major form of brain iron storage, accounting for one-third to three-fourth of all iron stored in the brain [45]. Fn can be of the H or L type [46, 47]; the former is involved in the rapid uptake and reuse of iron, while the latter is associated with long-term iron storage [48]. Although iron levels are increased in Parkinson's and Alzheimer's disease, there is no corresponding increase in Fn levels [49], which is known to limit iron-induced brain damage [42]. Here, we found that Fn expression was decreased in the thalamus, hippocampus, and hindlimb sensory area of rats in the SCI as compared to the control group, indicating that iron storage capacity in these brain regions was impaired in the CP model, which may have resulted in an increase in free iron content. Fn and TfR expression is mainly regulated by the iron response element/IRP system. We found that IRP1 levels in the thalamus, hippocampus, and hindlimb sensory area of rats were elevated by SCI, corresponding to increased TfR and decreased Fn 1 expression. However, LF levels in these brain regions were unaffected by SCI, suggesting that LF-mediated iron uptake is not involved in intracranial iron overloading and CP following SCI.

DFX is an iron chelator that can pass through the blood-brain barrier and accumulate in the brain parenchyma, preventing the release of iron from Fn and thereby reducing oxidative damage caused by iron overload [26]. In this study, DFX treatment abrogated the increase in iron levels in the hippocampus, hindlimb sensory area, and thalamus of rats resulting from SCI.

NF-κB has been shown to be activated by Fe^{2+} in macrophages [50, 51], and in turn activates microglia [50]; application of an NF-κB inhibitor can abolish this effect and limit the damage to neurons caused by SCI [52, 53]. We found that NF-κB levels were elevated in the hindlimb sensory area of rats after SCI; however, this effect was mitigated by treatment with DFX or NF-κB inhibitor.

The presence of activated microglia is a hallmark of central nervous system diseases characterized by the loss of neurons, such as Parkinson's and Alzheimer's disease [54]. Long-term use of anti-inflammatory drugs that target the cytokines released by microglia can reduce the rate of AD and PD by about 50% [55, 56]. In animal models of neuropathic pain, it was found that peripheral nerve injury activates microglia; conversely, inhibiting microglia activation reduced the occurrence of hyperalgesia and evoked pain. Microglia can capture free iron in the brain and store these ions in Fn molecules. Injection of $FeCl_2$ into the hippocampus of rats delayed injury to neurons, but also induced the activation of microglia [57]. In the present study, minocycline treatment suppressed the activation of microglia in the hindlimb sensory area of rats after SCI.

Analysis of behavioristics and the intracranial iron content, however, revealed that the NOS inhibitors treatment was slightly better compared with iron chelator and the microglia activation inhibitors, although this difference was not statistically significant. One could make a feasible explanation that remodeling of the brain after SCI contains multiple mechanisms and factors, and several pathways could be inhibited at upstream by blocking NOS pathway.

Conclusions

The results presented here indicate that after SCI, activation of IRP can lead to intracranial iron overload, which activates microglia via the NF-κB signaling pathway. The proinflammatory cytokines secreted by these microglia causes neuronal damage and loss, leading to CP. This effect can be abrogated by treatment with an iron-chelating agent, NF-κB inhibitor, or microglia inhibitor, suggesting that these agents can effectively relieve CP in SCI patients. There are mechanisms of CP out of scope of this article; therefore, further research is required.

Abbreviations
CP: Central pain; DFX: Deferoxamine; Fn: Ferritin; IRP1: Iron-regulatory protein1; Lf: Lactoferrin; NOS: Nitric oxide synthase; SCI: Spinal cord injury; TfR1: Transferrin receptor 1

Acknowledgements
The present study was supported by the National Natural Science Foundation of China (grants no. 81301679 and 81671211).

Funding
Funded by NSFC (Natural Science Foundation of China). The funding body did nothing in the design of the study; collection, analysis, and interpretation of the data; and in writing the manuscript.

Authors' contributions
FXM contributed to the conduct of the study and manuscript preparation and helped design the study. JMH contributed to the study design and helped prepare the manuscript. STS helped design the study. All authors read and approved the final manuscript.

Competing interests
The authors declare that they have no competing interests.

Author details
[1]Third Military Medical University, No. 30 Gaotanyan Street, Chongqing 400038, China. [2]Department of Orthopedics, Chinese PLA Army General Hospital, Dongcheng District, Nanmencang No. 5, Beijing 100700, China. [3]Department of Rehabilitation, Southwest Hospital, Third Military Medical University, No. 30 Gaotanyan Street, Chongqing 400038, China.

References
1. Bonica JJ. History of pain concepts and pain therapy. Mt Sinai J Med. 1991;58(3):191–202.
2. Donnelly C, Eng JJ. Pain following spinal cord injury: the impact on community reintegration. Spinal Cord. 2005;43(5):278–82.
3. Yezierski RP. Pain following spinal cord injury: the clinical problem and experimental studies. Pain. 1996;68(2–3):185–94. Review.
4. Klega A, Eberle T, Buchholz HG, et al. Central opioidergic neurotransmission in complex regional pain syndrome. Neurology. 2010;75(2):129–36.
5. Buckalew N, Haut MW, Morrow L, et al. Chronic pain is associated with brain volume loss in older adults: preliminary evidence. Pain Med. 2008;9(2):240–8.
6. Gustin SM, Wrigley PJ, Siddall PJ, et al. Brain anatomy changes associated with persistent neuropathic pain following spinal cord injury. Cereb Cortex. 2010;20(6):1409–19.
7. Likavcanova K, Urdzikova L, Hajek M, et al. Metabolic changes in the thalamus after spinal cord injury followed by proton MR spectroscopy. Magn Reson Med. 2008;59(3):499–506.
8. Peyron R, Schneider F, Faillenot I, et al. An fMRI study of cortical representation of mechanical allodynia in patients with neuropathic pain. Neurology. 2004;63(10):1838–46.
9. Wrigley PJ, Press SR, Gustin SM, et al. Neuropathic pain and primary somatosensory cortex reorganization following spinal cord injury. Pain. 2009;141(1–2):52–9.
10. Jin L, Wang J, Zhao L, et al. Decreased serum ceruloplasmin levels characteristically aggravate nigral iron deposition in Parkinson's disease. Brain. 2011;134(Pt 1):50–8.
11. Chen Z, Gao C, Hua Y, et al. Role of iron in brain injury after intraventricular hemorrhage. Stroke. 2011;42(2):465–70.

12. Duce JA, Tsatsanis A, Cater MA, et al. Iron-export ferroxidase activity of beta-amyloid precursor protein is inhibited by zinc in Alzheimer's disease. Cell. 2010;142(6):857–67.

13. Mairuae N, Connor JR, Cheepsunthorn P. Increased cellular iron levels affect matrix metalloproteinase expression and phagocytosis in activated microglia. Neurosci Lett. 2011;500(1):36–40.

14. Chen CW, Chen QB, Ouyang Q, et al. Transient early neurotrophin release and delayed inflammatory cytokine release by microglia in response to PAR-2 stimulation. J Neuroinflammation. 2012;9:142.

15. Smith JA, Das A, Ray SK, et al. Role of pro-inflammatory cytokines released from microglia in neurodegenerative diseases. Brain Res Bull. 2012;87(1):10–20.

16. Kim BW, Koppula S, Hong SS, et al. Regulation of microglia activity by glaucocalyxin-A: attenuation of lipopolysaccharide-stimulated neuroinflammation through NF-κ B and p38 MAPK signaling pathways. PLoS One. 2013;8(2):e55792.

17. Dalal NV, Pranski EL, Tansey MG, et al. RNF11 modulates microglia activation through NF-κ B signalling cascade. Neurosci Lett. 2012;528(2):174–9.

18. Beric A. Central dysesthesia syndrome in spinal cord injury patients. Pain. 1988;34:109–16.

19. Masri R. Keller chronic pain following spinal cord injury. Adv Exp Med Biol. 2012;760:74–88.

20. Nepomuceno C, Fine PR, Richards JS, et al. Pain in patients with spinal cord injury. Arch Phys Med Rehabil. 1979;60(12):605–9.

21. Attal NL, Mazaltarine G, Perrouin-Verbe B, et al. Chronic neuropathic pain management in spinal cord injury patients. What is the efficacy of pharmacological treatments with a general mode of administration? (oral, transdermal, intravenous). Ann Phys Rehabil Med. 2009;52(2):124–41.

22. Baastrup C, Finnerup NB. Pharmacological management of neuropathic pain following spinal cord injury. CNS Drugs. 2008;22(6):455–75.

23. Miki K, Iwata K, Tsuboi Y, et al. Dorsal column-thalamic pathway is involved in thalamic hyperexcitability following peripheral nerve injury: a lesion study in rats with experimental mononeuropathy. Pain. 2000;85(1–2):263–71.

24. Sokal DM, Chapman V. Effects of spinal administration of muscimol on C- and A-fibre evoked neuronal responses of spinal dorsal horn neurones in control and nerve injured rats. Brain Res. 2003;962(1–2):213–20.

25. Dougherty PM, Palecek J, Paleckova V, et al. The role of NMDA and non-NMDA excitatory amino acid receptors in the excitation of primate spinothalamic tract neurons by mechanical, chemical, thermal, and electrical stimuli. Neurosci. 1992;12(8):3025–41.

26. Melzack R, Loeser JD. Phantom body pain in paraplegics: evidence for a central "pattern generating mechanism" for pain. Pain. 1978;4(3):195–210.

27. Evseev VA, Davydova TV, Vetrile LA. Common neuroimmunological features of drug addiction, alcoholism, epilepsy, and neurogenic pain syndromes. Vestn Ross Akad Med Nauk. 2006;(7):38–43.

28. Richards JS, Meredith RL, Nepomuceno C, et al. Psycho-social aspects of chronic pain in spinal cord injury. Pain. 1980;8(3):355–66.

29. Summers JD, Rapoff MA, Varghese G, Porter K, Palmer RE. Psychosocial factors in chronic spinal cord injury pain. Pain. 1991;4:7183–9.

30. Thompson FJ, Reier PJ, Lucas CC, Parmer R, et al. Altered patterns of reflex excitability subsequent to contusion injury of the rat spinal cord. J Neurophysiol. 1992;68(5):1473–86.

31. Atwood CS, Obrenovich ME, Liu T, Chan H, Perry G, Smith MA, Martins RN. Amyloid-beta: a chameleon walking in two worlds: a review of the trophic and toxic properties of amyloid-beta. Brain Res Brain Res Rev. 2003;43(1):1–16.

32. Bush AI. The metallobiology of Alzheimer's disease. Trends Neurosci. 2003;26(4):207–14.

33. Maulik N. Redox signaling of angiogenesis. Antioxid Redox Signal. 2002;4(5):805–15.

34. Aisen P, et al. Iron metabolism. Curr OPin Chem Biol. 1999;3:200–6.

35. Jellinger KA. The role of iron in neuro degeneration. Drugs Aging. 1999;14:115–14.

36. Qian ZM, Wang Q. Expression of iron transport prote in sand excessiveiron accumulation of iron in the brain in neuro degenerative disorders. Brain Res Rev. 1998;27:257–67.

37. Wang L, Wang W, Zhao M, Ma L, Li M. Psychological stress induces dysregulation of iron metabolism in rat brain. Neuroscience. 2008;155(1):24–30.

38. Berg D, Youdim MB. Role of iron in neurodegenerative disorders. Top Magn Reson Imaging. 2006;17(1):5–17.

39. Qian ZM, Shen X. Brain iron transport and neurodegeneration. Trends Mol Med. 2001;7(3):103–8.

40. Curtis AR, Fey C, Morris CM. Mutation in the gene encoding ferritin light polypeptide causes dominant adult-onset basal ganglia disease. Nat Genet. 2001;28(4):350–4.

41. Bradbury MW. Transport of iron in the blood-brain-cerebrospinal fluid system. Neurochem. 1997;69(2):443–54.

42. Moos T, Morgan EH. Evidence for low molecular weight, non-transferrin-bound iron in rat brain and cerebrospinal fluid. J Neurosci Res. 1998;54(4):486–94.

43. Attieh ZK, Mukhopadhyay CK, Seshadri V. Ceruloplasmin ferroxidase activity stimulates cellular iron uptake by a trivalent cation-specific transport mechanism. J Biol Chem. 1999;274(2):1116–23.

44. Hulet SW, Powers S, Connor JR. Distribution of transferrin and ferritin binding in normal and multiple sclerosis human brains. J Neurol Sci. 1999;165(1):48–55.

45. Hallgren B. The effect of age on the nonhaemin iron in the human brain. J Neurochem. 1958;3:41–51.

46. Connor JR, Snyder BS, Arosio P. A quantitative analysis of isoferritins in select regions of aged, parkinsonian, and Alzheimer's diseased brains. J Neurochem. 1995;65(2):717–24.

47. Harrison PM, Arosio P. The ferritins: molecular properties, iron storage function and cellular regulation. Biochim Biophys Acta. 1996;1275(3):161–203.

48. Levi S, Yewdall SJ, Harrison PM, et al. Evidence that H- and L- chains have cooperative roles in the iron-uptake mechanism of human ferritin. Bioehem J. 1992;288:591–6.

49. Fleming J, Joshi JG. Ferritin: isolation of aluminum-ferritin complex from brain. Proc Natl Acad Sci U S A. 1987;84(22):7866–70.

50. Filipov NM, Seegal RF, Lawrence DA. Manganese potentiates in vitro production of proinflammatory cytokines and nitric oxide by microglia through a nuclear factor kappa B-dependent mechanism. Toxicol Sci. 2005;84(1):139–48.

51. Xiong S, She H, Takeuchi H, et al. Signaling role of intracellular iron in NF-kappaB activation. J Biol Chem. 2003;278(20):17646–54.

52. Kauppinen TM, Swanson RA. Poly(ADP-ribose) polymerase-1 promotes microglial activation, proliferation, and matrix metalloproteinase-9-mediated neuron death. J Immunol. 2005;174(4):2288–96.

53. Klegeris A, McGeer PL. Interaction of various intracellular signaling mechanisms involved in mononuclear phagocyte toxicity toward neuronal cells. J Leukoc Biol. 2000;67(1):127–33.

54. Jellinger K, Paulus W, Grundke-Iqbal I, Riederer P, Youdim MB. J Neural Transm Park Dis Dement Sect. 1990;2(4):327–40.

55. Vlad SC, Miller DR, Kowall NW, Felson DT. Neurology. 2008;70(19):1672–7.

56. Chen H, Jacobs E, Schwarzschild MA. Nonsteroidal antiinflammatory drug use and the risk for Parkinson's disease. Ann Neurol. 2005;58(6):963–7.

57. Wang J, Tsirka SE. Tuftsin fragment 1–3 is beneficial when delivered after the induction of intracerebral hemorrhage. Stroke. 2005;36(3):613–8. Epub 2005 Feb 3.

26

Early developed ASD (adjacent segmental disease) in patients after surgical treatment of the spine due to cancer metastases

Grzegorz Guzik

Abstract

Background: The causes of ASD are still relatively unknown. Correlation between clinical status of patients and radiological MRI findings is of primary importance. The radiological classifications proposed by Pfirmann and Oner are most commonly used to assess intradiscal degenerative changes.
The aim of the study was to assess the influence of the extension of spine fixation on the risk of developing ASD in a short time after surgery.

Methods: A total of 332 patients with spinal tumors were treated in our hospital between 2010 and 2013. Of these patients, 287 underwent surgeries. A follow-up MRI examination was performed 12 months after surgical treatment. The study population comprised of 194 patients. Among metastases, breast cancer was predominant (29%); neurological deficits were detected in 76 patients. Metastases were seen in the thoracic (45%) and lumbar (30%) spine; in 25% of cases, they were of multisegmental character. Pathological fractures concerned 88% of the patients. Statistical calculations were made using the $\chi 2$ test. Statistical analysis was done using the Statistica v. 10 software. A p value <0.05 was accepted as statistically significant. The study population was divided on seven groups according to applied treatment.

Results: Clinical signs of ASD were noted in only seven patients. Two patients had symptoms of nerve root irritation in the lumbar spine. Twenty-two patients (11%) were diagnosed with ASD according to the MRI classifications by Oner, Rijt, and Ramos, while the more sensitive Pfirmann classification allowed to detect the disease in 46 patients (24%). Healthy or almost healthy discs of Oner type I correlated with the criteria of Pfirmann types II and III. The percentage of the incidence of ASD diagnosed 1 year after the surgery using the Pfirmann classifications was significantly higher than diagnosed according to the clinical examination.

Conclusions: The incidence of ASD in patients after spine surgeries due to cancer metastases does not differ between the study groups. ASD detectability based on clinical signs is significantly lower than ASD detectability based on MR images according to the system by Pfirrmann et.al. ASD risk increase among patients with multilevel fixation.

Keywords: Metastases, Spinal tumors, Surgical treatment of the spine, Spinal tumor resections, Spine stabilizations

Correspondence: grzegorz.guzik@vp.pl
Orthopedic Oncology Department, Specialist Hospital in
Brzozów-Podkarpacki Oncology Center, ul Bielawskiego 18, 36-200 Brzozów,
Poland

Background

Adjacent segmental disease following surgery of the spine represents a serious diagnostic and therapeutic problem. There are many factors causing intervertebral disc degeneration or its accelerated development. The ones that are mentioned as most important are age, location, natural aging processes, increased mobility of the segments bordering with the fusion site, changes in the forces imposed on the endplates and in their springiness, changes in intradiscal pressure, and others. It is of essential importance whether symptoms of disc and endplate degeneration occurred before the surgical treatment. What is also relevant is the level and extent of spine stabilization, treatment method and how much time elapsed since surgery. One of the most significant causes of disc degeneration is sagittal imbalances [1–4].

Diagnostics of adjacent segmental disease is particularly difficult. It should be stressed that only 25% of radiologically diagnosed abnormalities are associated with clinical signs of the disease [5–9]. The systems of classification proposed by Oner, Rijt, and Ramos and Pfirmann are of the most frequently used [8, 9]. The classification result should be compared with the clinical condition of a patient. The understanding of risk factors associated with adjacent segmental disease, and its accelerated development is of key importance for optimizing methods of the surgical treatment of spinal diseases and improving its outcomes [10–13].

The aim of the study was to assess influence of extension and type of spine stabilizations on the risk of adjacent segmental disease (ASD) in a short time after surgery. We also try to determine the correlation between the clinical and radiological symptoms of ASD and the incidence of different types of ASD in two classifications based on MRI. The analysis includes MRI and clinical findings in surgically treated patients with metastatic tumors.

Methods

A total of 332 patients with spinal tumors were treated in our hospital between 2010 and 2013. Of these patients, 287 underwent surgeries. A retrospective examination of the patients operated on the lumbar and/or the thoracic section of the spine was carried out. The patients that underwent surgeries of the cervical spine and the patients in whom only vertebral biopsy was performed were excluded from the study. The study population comprised of a total of 247 operated patients.

The majority of the treated patients were women, representing 64% of the study population. The mean age was 63 for women and 68 for men.

Among the metastases, breast cancer dominated (29%), followed by prostate cancer (7%), multiple myeloma (12%), lung cancer (9%), kidney cancer (6%), lymphoma (3%), thyroid cancer (3%), cancer of unknown primary site (14%), and others (17%).

Neurological deficits were detected in 76 patients. Complete paralysis of the limbs, classified as Frankel A, was found in nine patients. Acute pareses diagnosed in 15 patients were classified as Frankel B, while in 26 patients as Frankel C. Minor pareses (Frankel grade D) occurred in 26 patients. There were no quadriplegic patients in our series.

In 45% of the patients, the metastases were located in the thoracic spine, while in 30% of the patients the lumbar region was involved. The patients with involvement of more than one segment of the spine accounted for 25% of cases.

The posterior elements of the spine were mainly affected, being involved in 63% of the patients. Both posterior and anterior elements were involved in 32% of the patients, and the posterior elements alone were affected in 5% of the patients.

Pathological fractures were diagnosed in 80% of the patients; while in 20% of them, the metastases did not result in fractures. Spinal instability, assessed based on the Kostiuk and Taneichi scale, was diagnosed in 64% of the patients.

Each patient had classical radiograms, CT, and MRI scans of the spine, and the following characteristics were evaluated: type, location and extent of the pathological lesions, spinal axis disorder, shape and type of fractures, and dislocation and stability of spinal segments.

The patients were divided into the following groups depending on the type of surgery: group A—patients after posterior stabilization of the spine, group B—posterior stabilization combined with laminectomy, group C—spinal laminectomy, group D—resection of the vertebral bodies through posterior approach combined with implantation of a vertebral body prosthesis and posterior stabilization, group E—resection of the vertebral body through anterior approach combined with implantation of a vertebral body prosthesis, group F—implantation of

Table 1 Number of operated patients in different groups and their participation in a follow-up MRI performed 12 months after the surgery

Group	Group A	Group B	Group C	Group D	Group E	Group F	Group G
Number of operated patients (247)	36	118	7	16	9	38	23
Number of patients who had a follow-up MRI (194)	31	87	6	12	9	31	18

Table 2 Different types of radiologically detected (MRI) adjacent segment degenerative changes classified according to the systems by Oner, Rijt, and Ramos in relation to surgical options in the treatment of 194 follow-up patients

Group	Group A	Group B	Group C	Group D	Group E	Group F	Group G
Number of patients N(%)	31(16)	87(45)	6(3)	12(6)	9(5)	31(16)	18(9)
Type 1	28	76	6	9	8	28	17
Type 2	1	3	–	1	–	1	1
Type 3	1	3	–	1	–	–	–
Type 4	–	1	–	–	–	–	–
Type 5	–	–	–	1	–	1	–
Type 6	1	4	–	–	1	1	–

a vertebral body prosthesis with posterior stabilization, group G—anterior approach with vertebral body prosthesis and posterior stabilization. Only titanium implants were used, which allowed for the performance of subsequent CT and MRI examinations.

Due to limited survival of the patients, follow-up was 12 months after the surgery. Final analysis involved 194 patients. The rest of the patients were treated outside our center or did not respond to physician's examination call (Table 1).

Four-level spine stabilization was the shortest one and concerned 12 patients. Five-level stabilization was done in 21 patients, sixe-level in 52 patients, seven-level in 62 patients, eight-level in 24 patients, and nine-level in 23 patients.

MRI and clinical examinations were performed to detect signs of damage to the discs in the segments adjacent to the surgically treated section of the spine. Attention was paid to increased pain intensity, its location, pain on palpation, and the range of spinal mobility. The shape of the spine, spinal axis disorders with special attention given to the sagital axis, and distortions of the natural curvatures of the spine were evaluated. What was also considered was the shape and morphology of the endplates adjacent to the stabilization site as well as disc degeneration classified using the systems by Oner, Rijt, and Ramos and Pfirmann.

The categorical variables were expressed as percentages. The inter-group differences were tested using the $\chi2$ test. All statistical analyses were performed by using Statistica 10. A value of $P < 0.05$ was considered statistically significant.

The research has been performed in accordance with the declaration of Helsinki. As this retrospective analysis consists of anonymised clinical routine data, the Research Ethics Committee deems the application for and issue of an ethics approval not necessary. All the patients gave a written consent to the use of data for research, name of ethics committee: Ethics Committee in Cracov, ul Krupnicza.

Results

A total of 194 patients had a follow-up MRI of the spine. Only seven patients in our material presented clinical signs of ASD. The patients reported chronic spinal pain. Clinical examination revealed pain on palpation of the spinous processes adjacent to the stabilized segment of the spine. Signs of nerve root irritation in the lumbar section occurred in two patients.

ASD was diagnosed in 22 (11%) patients based on the classification systems by Oner, Rijt, and Ramos. The table below demonstrates the incidence of different types of the characteristic of ASD degenerative changes classified according to the beforementioned systems (Table 2).

Table 3 Different types of radiologically detected (MRI) adjacent segment degenerative changes classified according to the Pfirmann and Metzdorf scale in relation to surgical options in the treatment of 194 follow-up patients

Group	Group A	Group B	Group C	Group D	Group E	Group F	Group G
Number of patients N(%)	31(16)	87(45)	6(3)	12(6)	9(5)	31(16)	18(9)
Grade 1	25	67	5	6	7	24	14
Grade 2	2	6	–	1	1	3	2
Grade 3	1	4	1	2	–	1	1
Grade 4	1	3	–	1	–	1	1
Grade 5	1	4	–	–	1	1	–
Others	1	3	–	2	–	1	–

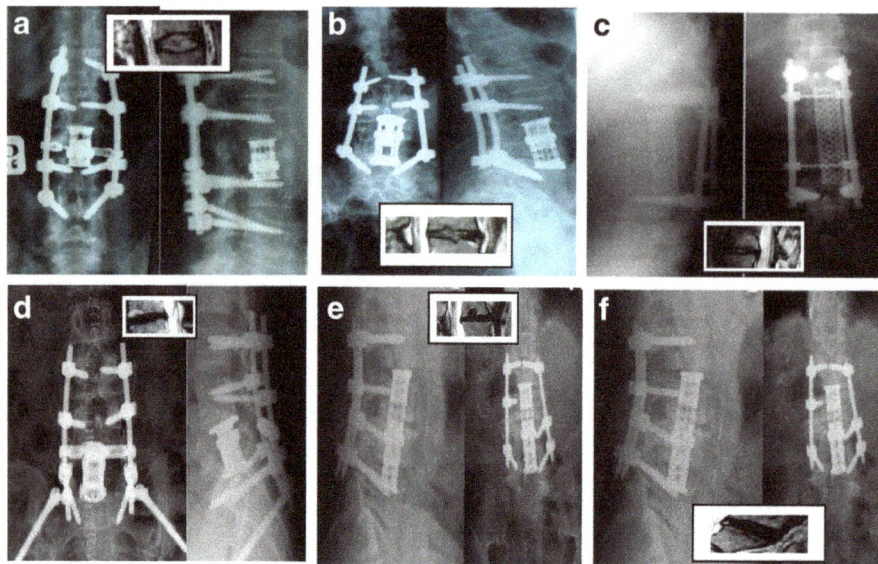

Fig. 1 a–f Examples of six postoperative radiograms and MRI scans focused on different types of ASD

The incidence of various types of disc degeneration according to the Pfirmann and Metzdorf classification is presented in Table 3. It must be pointed out that following this system may entail difficulties in precise classification of some of the pathologic changes. Oner III and IV types were excluded from the Pfirmann classification and defined differently. Oner type I included healthy or almost healthy discs, of which some were classified as type II and III by Pfirmann. This resulted in an increased detectability of ASD up to a level of 46 cases (24%).

Figure 1(a–f) shows radiograms performed 1 year after surgery and MRI scans of adjacent segment in patients with metastatic tumor.

The study population was divided into different surgical treatment groups. No statistically significant differences in the incidence of ASD were found between these groups of patients (according to both the Pfirrmann and the Oner classifications) (Table 4).

Our study found significant statistical difference between the incidence of ASD cases diagnosed by the clinical examination and the incidence of ASD cases diagnosed by MRI according to the Pfirrmann et al. classification (Table 5).

Tables 6, 7, 8, and 9 present the incidence of various types of ASD related to the extent of spine stabilizations.

We did not find any correlation between the incidence of an early developed ASD and the type of the primary tumor.

New foci of metastatic lesions in the spine were detected in 11 out of 46 patients with radiological signs of ASD. No features of spinal destabilization and local recurrence of the tumor were noted, nor were pathological fractures within the adjacent vertebrae. Ten patients were diagnosed with distortion of the sagital axis of the spine which presented as lumbar lordosis flattening or worsened thoracic kyphosis.

Discussion

The available literature lacks data on the incidence of ASD in patients surgically treated due to metastases to

Table 4 Statistical analysis of the incidence of ASD diagnosed by MRI in different groups of patients

Group	A	B	C	D	E	F	G
Number of ASD diagnosed by MRI according to the Oner, Rijt, and Ramos classifications							
N (%)	31 (16)	87 (45)	6 (3)	12 (6)	9 (5)	31 (16)	18 (9)
ASD N (%)	3 (10)	11 (13)	0 (0)	3 (25)	1 (11)	3 (10)	1 (6)
Number of ASD diagnosed by MRI according to the Pfirrmann and Metzdorf classifications							
N (%)	31 (16)	87 (45)	6 (3)	12 (6)	9 (5)	31 (16)	18 (9)
ASD N (%)	6 (19)	20 (23)	1 (17)	6 (50)	2 (22)	7 (23)	4 (22)

Results are presented as a number and percent
ASD adjacent segment disease
$p < 0.05$ for inter-group difference χ^2

Table 5 Statistical analysis of the incidence of ASD based on MRI and clinical examination

Detected ASD in clinical examination and MRI according to different types of radiological scale

Scale	Oner, Rijt, and Ramos	Pfirmann and Metzdorf	Clinical signs
ASD N (%)	22 (11)	46 (24)*	7 (4)

Results are presented as a number and percent
ASD adjacent segmental disease
*$p < 0.05$ for inter-group difference χ^2

Table 7 Statistical analysis of the incidence of ASD according to stabilization extension

Oner, Rijt, and Ramos	Levels 4–6	Levels 7–9	P value
Types 1, 2, and 3	82	101	ns
Types 4, 5, and 6	3	9	<0.05

ns not significant

the spine. Further research concerning this subject may provide valuable information on the etiological factors of the disease and improve treatment outcomes. Surgical treatment for spinal tumors is characterized by numerous differences compared with surgeries due to injuries or pathological changes. It is generally accepted to avoid bone grafting. The objective is to achieve a primary efficient stabilization, effective to the end of patient's life. The principle is to stabilize long sections of the spine. Bone losses are filled with implants—vertebral prostheses or bone cement [14–21].

Studies on the etiology, diagnostics, and treatment of adjacent segmental disease are of vital importance because of a steady growth in spinal surgeries volumes. They are of particular relevance to young people surgically treated for disc disease, spine defects, or injuries. Studies involving patients operated on for oncological reasons in whom long sections of the spine are stabilized afford the opportunity to broaden the knowledge of the disease with additional aspects being evaluated [1–5, 7].

Harrop estimates the current state of knowledge of the factors responsible for the etiology of the disease at 35%. Among these factors, he mentions the following: reduced mobility of segments, changes in load, changes in compressibility, and pressure within a disc [5].

Lopez and Espina perceive increasing stress on the discs and endplates adjacent to the operated spinal segment as the main cause of the disease, which is confirmed by Eck [7].

Sears and Sergides et al. indicated decreased risk of ASD after spinal surgery without instrumentation.

Prevalence of ASD after one-level fixation was 1.7% and 5% after three-level fixation. Laminectomy caused a 2.4 fold increase in ASD [22].

Lee et al. indicated that patients over 60 years old had a 2.5 fold increase in ASD [23].

Seevedra-Pozo et al. presented correlation between ADS and number of stabilized levels [24].

Radcliff i Kepler et al. based on MRI scans reported that the risk of ASD is 2–3% per year [25].

The early development of ASD (before 1 year) after surgery was reported by Dynesys et al and Etebar et al. They compare ASD frequency after posterior stabilization with elastic and stiff rod. In their study, MRI scans revealed ASD 9 months after surgery. Similarly Masevnin et al. (after evaluation of 120 patients) found ASD in 10 cases after two-level stabilization and 19 cases after 360 degree stabilization [26].

According to Park et al. study, the incidence of ASD increased with time from surgery. After posterior stabilization due to spondylolisthesis ASD was diagnosed in 5.2% after 36 months and among 100% after 369 months [27].

The MRI image of load-induced changes is typical. The types of degenerative changes have been demonstrated by Pfirmann and Metzdoff. They have singled out five types of the visible on MRI changes resulting from a natural progression of disc degeneration [28].

Oner, Rijt, and Ramos have differentiated between the six types of degenerative changes visible in the sagital MRI projection: type 1—normal, type 2—black disc in T2 signal, Type 3—Schmorl-type, type 4 - anterior collapse, type 5—central herniation, and type 6—degenerated disc [8].

Table 6 Frequency of ASD according to Oner, Rijt, and Ramos classification in patient with multilevel spine fixation

	4-level	5-level	6-level	7-level	8-level	9-level
Oner, Rijt, and Ramos						
Type 1	10	19	50	56	18	19
Type 2	1		1	3	1	1
Type 3			1	1	2	1
Type 4					1	
Type 5					1	1
Type 6	1	2		2	1	1

Table 8 Frequency of ASD according to Pfirmann and Metzdorf scale in patients with multilevel spine fixation

	4-level	5-level	6-level	7-level	8-level	9-level
Pfirmann and Metzdorf						
Grade 1	9	17	37	51	16	18
Grade 2	2	1	7	3	1	1
Grade 3		1	2	4	2	1
Grade 4		1	3	1	1	1
Grade 5		1	1	1	3	1
Others	1		2	2	1	1

Table 9 Statistical analysis of the incidence of ASD according to stabilization extension

Pfirmann and Metzdorf	Levels 4–6	Levels 7–9	P value
Grades 1 and 2	74	97	<0.05
Grades 3, 4, and 5	11	19	<0.05

Boden points out that 57% of patients with symptoms of ASD present no clinical signs of the disease [5].

Levin and Hale's studies have revealed the seen on MRI radiological signs of adjacent segmental disease of the lumbar spine in 70% of cases, while clinical signs in only 36% of patients after spinal stabilization [7].

Our study has demonstrated a high incidence of ASD 1 year after spine surgeries due to cancer metastases. The most prevalent types of changes were Oner types II, III, and IV and Pfirmann types II and III. It should be noted that the criteria proposed by the authors do not overlap, and some degeneration types of Oner do not equal the types of Pfirmann. No statistically significant differences in the incidence of ASD cases were found between the study groups. The incidence of ASD cases diagnosed according to the criteria by Pfirrmann et al. (46–24%) was noticeably higher (statistically significant) than the incidence of ASD cases diagnosed according to the clinical criteria (7–3.6%). The number of clinically diagnosed ASD cases, accounting for merely 3.6% of the total study population (7/194), was significantly lower and constituted 31% of the cases diagnosed according to the Onner system and 15 of the cases diagnosed according to the Pfirrmann system. The incidence of early ASD after seven to nine levels spine stabilizations was significantly higher than after four to six levels. Our study showed higher rate of ASD 1 year after multilevel spine stabilizations than other studies.

Conclusions

1. The prevalence of early ASD after multilevel spine stabilizations in patients with metastatic tumors is significantly higher than after surgical treatment with different underlying condition.
2. Oner types II, III, and IV and Pfirmann types II and III were most prevalent.
3. The number of ASD cases diagnosed by MRI according to the Pfirrmann classification differs from the number of ASD cases diagnosed by the clinical examination.
4. No statistically significant differences in the incidence of ASD cases between the surgical treatment groups were found.

Abbreviation
ASD: Adjacent segmental disease

Acknowledgements
None.

Authors' contributions
I am the only author of this work.

Competing interests
The author declares that he/she has no competing interests.

References
1. Hilibrand AS, Robbins M. Adjacent segment degeneration and adjacent segment disease: the consequences of spinal fusion? Spine J. 2004;4:190–4.
2. Asdourian PL. Metastatic disease of the spine. In: Bridwell WH, De Wald RL, editors. The Textbook of Spinal Surgery. II wyd. Philadelphia: Lippincott – Raven Publishers; 1997. p. 2007–50.
3. Askar Z, Wardlaw D, Muthukumar T, et al. Correlation between intervertebral disc morphology and the results in patients undergoing graf ligament stabilisation. Eur Spine J. 2004;13:714–8.
4. Boriani S, Weinstein JN, Biagini R. Spine update: primary bone tumors of the spine: terminology and surgical staging. Spine. 1997;22:1036–44.
5. Cheh G, Bridwell KH, Lenke LG, et al. Adjacent segment disease followinglumbar/ thoracolumbar fusion with pedicle screw instrumentation: a minimum 5-year follow-up. Spine. 2007;32:2253–7.
6. Dickman CA, Fehlings MG, Gokaslan ZL. Spinal Cord and Spinal Column Tumors Principles and Practise. Thieme New York; 2004. p. 303–333.
7. Ecker RT, et al. Diagnosis and treatment of vertebral column metastases. Mayo Clinic Proc. 2005;80(9):1177–86.
8. Eleraky M, Papanastassiou I, Tran ND, et al. Comparison of polymethylmethacrylate versus expandable cage in anterior vertebral column reconstruction after posterior extracavitary corpectomy in lumbar and thoracolumbar metastatic spine tumors. Eur Spine J. 2011; 20(8):1363–70.
9. Fisher CG, DiPaola CP, Ryken TC, et al. A novel classification system for spinal instability in neoplastic disease: an evidence-based approach and expert consensus from the Spine Oncology Study Group. Spine. 2010;35(22): 1221–9.
10. Frankel BM, Jones T, Wang C. Segmental polymethylmethacrylate augmented pedicle screw fixation in patients with bone softening caused by osteoporosis and metastatic tumor involvement: a clinical evaluation. Neurosurgery. 2007;61(3):531–8.
11. Galasko CSB, Norris HE, Crank S. Spinal instability secondary to metastatic cancer. J Bone Joint Surg. 2000;82A:570–6.
12. Ghiselli G, Wang JC, Bhatia NN, et al. Adjacent segment degeneration in the lumbar spine. J Bone Joint Surg Am. 2004;86-A:1497–503.
13. Guzik G. Przerzuty do kręgosłupa – diagnostyka i leczenie. Bielsko Biała: Alfa Medica Press; 2015.
14. Helgeson MD, Bevevino AJ, Hilibrand AS. Update on the evidence for adjacent degeneration and disease. Spine J. 2013;13:342–51.
15. Kaloostian PE, Yurter A, Zadnik PL, et al. Current paradigms for metastatic spinal disease: an evidence-based review. Ann Surg Oncol. 2014;21(1):248–62.
16. Kelley SP, Ashford RU, Rao AS, Dickson RA. Primary bone tumours of the spine: a 42-year survey from the Leeds Regional Bone Tumour Registry. Eur Spine J. 2007;16:405–9.
17. Kim DH, Chang UK, Kim SH, Bilsky MH. Tumors of the Spine. Philadelphia: Saunders Elsevier; 2008.
18. Kumar A, Beastall J, Hughes J, Karadimas EJ, Nicol M, Smith F, Wardlaw D. Changes in the disc space after fractures of the thoracolumbar spine. Spine. 2008;33(26):2909–14.
19. Levin DA, Hale JJ, Bendo JA. Adjacent segment degeneration following spinal fusion for degenerative disc disease. Biuletin NYU Hosp Joint Dis. 2007;65(1):29–36.

20.   Metcalfe S, Gbejuade H, Patel NR. The posterior transpedicular approach for circumferential decompression and instrumented stabilization with titanium cage vertebrectomy reconstruction for spinal tumors: consecutive case series of 50 patients. Spine. 2012;37(16):1375–83.

21.   Niosi CA, Zhu QA, Wilson DC, et al. Biomechanical characterization of the three-dimensional kinematic behaviour of the dynesys dynamic stabilization system: an in vitro study. Eur Spine J. 2006;15:913–22.

22.   Sears WR, Sergides IG, Kazemi N, et al. Incidence and prevalence of surgery at segments adjacent to a previous posterior lumbar artrodesis. Spine J. 2011;11(1):11–20.

23.   Lee JC, Kim Y, Soh JW, et al. Risc factors of adjacent segment disease requiring surgery after lumbar spinal fusion: comparison of posterior lumbar interbody fusion and posterolateral fusion. Spine. 2014;39(5):339–45.

24.   Saavedra-Pozo FM, Deusdara RA, Benzel EC. Adjacent segment disease perspective and review of the literature. Ochsner J. 2014;14:78–83.

25.   Radcliff KE, Kepler CK, Jakoi A, Sidhu GS, Rihn J, Vaccaro AR. Adjacent segment disease in the lumbar spine following different treatment interventions. Spine J. 2013;13:1339–49.

26.   Masevnin S, Ptashnikov D, Michaylov D, Meng H, Smekalenkov O, Zaborovskii N. Risk factors for adjacent segment disease development after lumbar fusion. Asian Spine J. 2015;9:239–44.

27.   Park P, Garton HJ, Gala VC, Hoff JT, McGillicuddy JE. Adjacent segment disease after lumbar or lumbosacral fusion: review of the literature. Spine (Phila Pa 1976). 2004;29:1938–44.

28.   Fourney DR, Frangou EM, Ryken TC, et al. Spinal instability neoplastic score: an analysis of reliability and validity from the spine oncology study group. J Clin Oncol. 2011;29(22):3072–7.

27

Prospective clinical and radiographic evaluation of an allogeneic bone matrix containing stem cells (Trinity Evolution® Viable Cellular Bone Matrix) in patients undergoing two-level anterior cervical discectomy and fusion

Timothy A. Peppers[1], Dennis E. Bullard[2], Jed S. Vanichkachorn[3], Scott K. Stanley[4], Paul M. Arnold[5], Erik I. Waldorff[6], Rebekah Hahn[6], Brent L. Atkinson[7], James T. Ryaby[6] and Raymond J. Linovitz[8*]

Abstract

Background: Trinity Evolution® (TE), a viable cellular bone allograft, previously demonstrated high fusion rates and no safety-related concerns after single-level anterior cervical discectomy and fusion (ACDF) procedures. This prospective multicenter clinical study was performed to assess the radiographic and clinical outcomes of TE in subjects undergoing two-level ACDF procedures.

Methods: In a prospective, multicenter study, 40 subjects that presented with symptomatic cervical degeneration at two adjacent vertebral levels underwent instrumented ACDF using TE autograft substitute in a polyetheretherketone (PEEK) cage. At 12 months, radiographic fusion status was evaluated by dynamic motion plain radiographs and thin cut CT with multiplanar reconstruction by a panel that was blinded to clinical outcome. Fusion success was defined by angular motion ($\leq 4°$) and the presence of bridging bone across the adjacent vertebral endplates. Clinical pain and function assessments included the Neck Disability Index (NDI), neck and arm pain as evaluated by visual analog scales (VAS), and SF-36 at both 6 and 12 months.

Results: At both 6 and 12 months, all clinical outcome scores (SF-36, NDI, and VAS pain) improved significantly ($p < 0.05$) compared to baseline values. There were no adverse events or infections that were attributed to the graft material, no subjects that required revisions, and no significant decreases to mean neurological evaluations at any time as compared to baseline. At 12 months, the per subject and per level fusion rate was 89.4 and 93.4%, respectively. Subgroup analysis of subjects with risk factors for pseudoarthrosis (current or former smokers, diabetic, or obese/extremely obese) compared to those without risk factors demonstrated no significant differences in fusion rates.

Conclusions: Patients undergoing two-level ACDF with TE in combination with a PEEK interbody spacer and supplemental anterior fixation had a high rate of fusion success without any serious adverse events related to the graft material.

Trial registration: Trinity Evolution in Anterior Cervical Discectomy and Fusion (ACDF) NCT00951938

Keywords: ACDF, PEEK cage, Allograft, Multilevel, Arthrodesis, Cervical spine, Spine fusion

* Correspondence: raylinovitz@gmail.com
[8]PO Box 1671, Rancho Santa Fe, CA 92067, USA
Full list of author information is available at the end of the article

Background

Symptomatic cervical disc degeneration includes a multitude of pathologic processes including decreased disc height, disc herniation, and spondylosis resulting in radiculopathy and/or myelopathy. Anterior cervical discectomy and fusion (ACDF) is an established surgical treatment that achieves good to excellent clinical results in patients with symptomatic cervical degenerative disc disease [1]. Although multilevel ACDF is a safe and reliable procedure, multilevel procedures are associated with an increased rate of reoperation, higher non-union rates and longer time to fusion as compared to single-level procedures [2–6]. Additionally, patients who use tobacco [7] and particularly smokers who had a 2-level ACDF [8] have been associated with increased rates of pseudoarthrosis.

To minimize this risk of pseudoarthrosis, surgeons may select from a variety of bone graft materials with various qualities. Few bone graft substitutes contain all three essential bone-forming elements of autograft (osteogenicity, osteoconductivity, and osteoinductivity) [9] in a single, off-the-shelf product. Trinity Evolution® (TE) is a cellular bone allograft that consists of viable cellular cancellous bone matrix and demineralized cortical bone. TE possesses all three essential elements that are required for successful bone grafting, physiologic numbers of osteogenic cells (including mesenchymal stem cells and osteoprogenitor cells), osteoinductive proteins, and an osteoconductive matrix to which the cells are attached [10]. In a prospective study that evaluated the safety and effectiveness of TE in single-level ACDF, the fusion rate was 93.5% at 12 months, no serious allograft-related events occurred and comparisons to the literature revealed that TE may help negate any comorbid physiological barriers to fusion associated with risk factors such as smoking and diabetes [11].

The primary aim of this multicenter clinical study was to prospectively assess the safety and effectiveness of the TE viable cellular bone allograft in combination with a polyetherethereketone (PEEK) interbody spacer in two-level ACDF using patient reported and radiological outcome measures. To better assess effectiveness, the fusion rates were compared with the international literature that described a comparable surgical approach using other graft materials. A secondary aim of the study was to compare fusion rates between patients with and without risk factors for pseudoarthrosis.

Methods

Study design

From October 2009 to June 2012, a prospective, multicenter study was conducted at five investigational sites to evaluate the safety and effectiveness of a cellular bone allograft (Trinity Evolution® (TE)) in combination with a PEEK interbody spacer for ACDF surgery. All patients 18 years of age or older with symptomatic cervical degeneration at two adjacent vertebral levels between C3 and T1 were eligible for the study and those enrolled underwent ACDF with supplemental fixation and a PEEK interbody spacer (Orthofix, Inc., Lewisville, TX). TE was packed within and around the spacer. Exclusion criteria included the use of any other bone graft or bone graft substitute in addition to or in place of TE in and around the interbody spacer or arthrodesis at a single level only or at more than two levels. IRB approval was obtained for each site prior to the initiation of enrollment.

Surgical procedures

All operations were performed by five surgeons using comparable surgical techniques. A standard Smith-Robinson approach to the cervical spine was carried out through a transverse incision. After removal of disc material and endplate cartilage, subchondral bone was perforated and the neural structures were decompressed. During distraction, a PEEK cage (Orthofix Inc. Lewisville, TX) packed with TE was inserted into the intervertebral space. Additionally, TE was packed around the cage if space permitted. Rigid anterior plate-screw fixation was performed in all patients.

Postoperative management and data collection

Subjects were discharged from the hospital on the day of surgery or the day after surgery and were treated with comparable postoperative protocols. All subjects were allowed to ambulate on the first day after surgery. Postoperative immobilization in a cervical collar or brace was prescribed at the surgeon's discretion.

Information regarding subject age, gender, body mass index (BMI), smoking status and the presence or absence of diabetes was collected. Subjects were evaluated clinically and radiographically at 6 (+/−1) weeks, 6 months (+/−1) and 12 (+/−1) months. At all timepoints, plain radiographs (flexion/extension, AP and lateral) and neurological evaluations (motor, sensory, or reflex) were collected. Neurologic evaluations included motor assessments of elbow flexors, wrist extensors, elbow extensors and finger extensions using a 0–5 scoring system. For sensory function, each cervical segment was assessed for absence, impaired, or normal function. For reflex assessment, biceps, brachioradialis, and triceps were evaluated using a four-point scale. Thin cut (≤1 mm) computed tomography with multiplanar reformatting (CT) was also performed for every subject at 12 months according to the study protocol.

Clinical endpoints included three health measurement instruments: the Neck Disability Index (NDI), visual analogue scale (VAS) (neck and arm), and the SF-36v2, which evaluated pain, function and quality of life (QOL).

The NDI ranged from 0–50 points with higher scores representing greater functional improvement. The VAS scale ranged from 0 to 100 mm with 0 representing no pain and 100 representing severe pain on activity. The SF-36, an eight-scale profile of functional health and well-being scores, was summarized to obtain the physical composite score (PCS) and the mental composite score (MCS). In contrast to NDI and VAS, higher scores for SF-36 represent less disability.

Radiographic evaluation

At 12 months, the criteria for fusion required the presence of bridging bone across the adjacent endplates on thin cut CT scans with multiplanar reformatting and $\leq 4°$ angular motion on flexion/extension plain radiographs. Both levels were required to be fused in order for the subject to be judged as fused. Radiographic fusion status was determined via an independent review by three qualified reviewers who possessed substantial orthopedic experience and either an MD or a PhD. All three reviewers had to independently agree that bridging bone was present in order for the site to be judged as fused. All radiographic evaluations were performed by reviewers blinded to the patient's clinical outcomes. At 6 months, fusion was assessed by bony bridging based on plain radiographs.

The quantitative assessments of intervertebral motion were produced by trained analysts using specialized motion analysis software, QMA™ (Quantitative Motion Analysis; Medical Metrics, Inc., Houston, TX). QMA™ has been validated to produce measurements of intervertebral rotation and translation and is accurate to within 1 degree and 1 mm [12, 13]. The reproducibility of the measurements has also been validated [12, 13].

International literature search

The literature search was conducted using PubMed with search terms for ACDF, PEEK, and two- or multilevel. Publications that were included must have reported a two-level ACDF procedure using a PEEK cage with supplemental fixation, the specific graft material, the follow-up times that fusion was assessed and the fusion incidence. Publications that were excluded were reports that described one-, three-, and four- level ACDF procedures or two-level ACDF reports that utilized autograft or allograft interbody spacers, a PEEK cage without graft material or a PEEK cage without rigid supplemental fixation (e.g., "stand-alone").

Statistical methods

The data in the figures and the results are presented as the mean and standard error (SE) and mean and standard deviation (SD), respectively. A multiple paired t test with a subsequent Bonferroni correction was done for subject reported outcome measures. The Fisher's exact test was used to compare fusion rates among subjects with risk factors for pseudoarthrosis. Significance was set at $p \leq 0.05$. The statistical analyses were performed using SAS (version 9.3, Cary, NC).

Results

Forty subjects were enrolled in the study and arthrodesis was performed on 80 levels. Thirty-five and 38 subjects completed their 6 and 12 month study visits, respectively.

Baseline characteristics

The mean age and standard deviation was 48.5 +/–9 years and the age range was 26–65 years of age. Demographics are described in Table 1. Twenty-six (65.0%), thirteen (32.5%), and one (2.5%) subject received arthrodesis at C5-C7, C4-C6, and C3-C5, respectively.

Fusion

The per subject fusion rate increased over time and was determined to be 65.7% of subjects fused at 6 months and 89.4% at 12 months (Table 2; Fig. 1). The per level fusion rate mirrored the increase over time that was observed in the per subject fusion rate and was 54.3 and 93.4% at 6 and 12 months, respectively (Table 2; Fig. 1). The fusion rates at 12 months for subjects that were current or former smokers, diabetic, or obese were 94.1% (16/17), 100% (5/5), and 93.3% (14/15), respectively. Subgroup analysis of these high risk subjects compared to subjects without risk factors demonstrated

Table 1 Patient demographics

Patient demographic	N (%)
Gender	
Male	11 (27.5)
Female	29 (72.5)
Age	
<50 years	20 (50.0)
<65 years	38 (95.0)
Smoking status	
Never	22 (55.0)
Current or former	18 (45.0)
Diabetic	
No	35 (87.5)
Yes	5 (12.5)
Weight status (base on BMI)	
Normal weight	11 (27.5)
Overweight	9 (22.5)
Obese	16 (40.0)
Extremely obese	4 (10.0)

Table 2 Fusion rates at 6 and 12 months

	Per subject fusion		Per level fusion	
Time (M)	6	12	6	12
Fused N (%)	23 (65.7)	34 (89.4)	38 (54.3)	71 (93.4)
Not fused N (%)	12 (34.3)	4 (10.6)	32 (45.7)	5 (6.6)

no significant differences ($p > 0.05$) in fusion rates at 12 months (not shown).

Clinical findings

All patient reported outcomes (NDI, VAS neck and arm pain, SF-36 MCS and PCS) demonstrated significant improvements in pain and function at 6 and 12 months as compared to baseline (Figs. 2, 3, and 4).

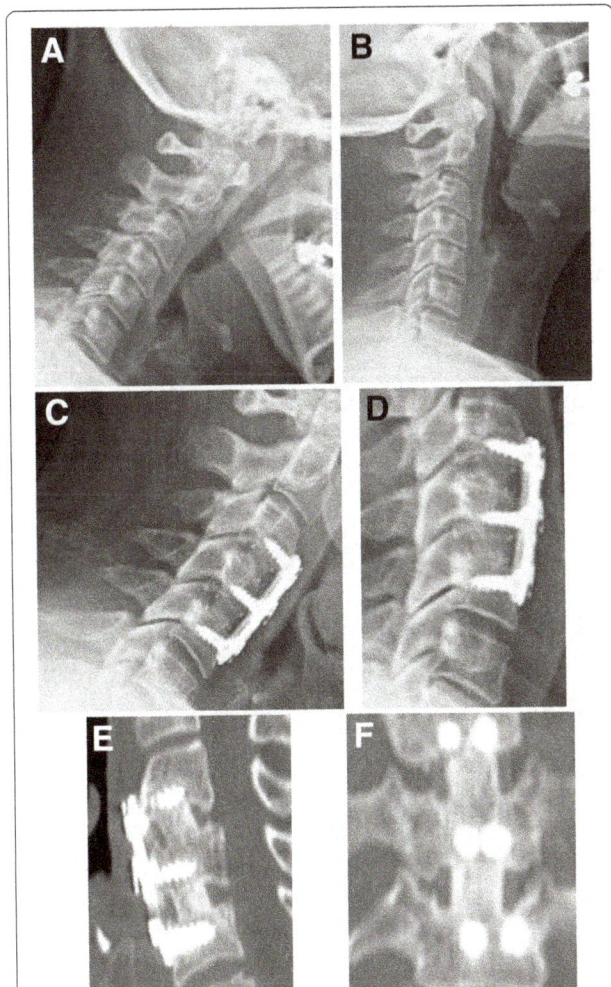

Fig. 1 Two-level ACDF using Trinity Evolution that was performed on a 44-year-old obese female at C3-4 and C4-5. **a** Pre-operative flexion radiograph. **b** Pre-operative extension radiograph. **c** Twelve month flexion radiograph. **d** Twelve month extension radiograph. **e** Twelve month sagittal CT. **f** Twelve month coronal CT

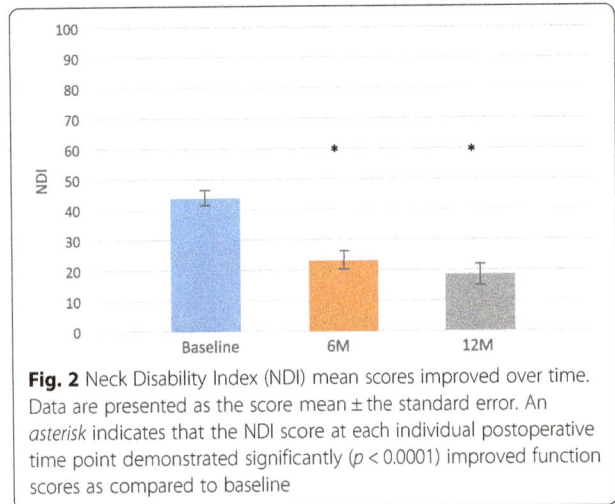

Fig. 2 Neck Disability Index (NDI) mean scores improved over time. Data are presented as the score mean ± the standard error. An *asterisk* indicates that the NDI score at each individual postoperative time point demonstrated significantly ($p < 0.0001$) improved function scores as compared to baseline

Safety

There were no adverse events or infections that were related to TE and no pseudoarthroses that required revisions. There was no neurological deterioration encountered (motor, sensory, or reflex) at any time as compared to baseline.

Discussion

The primary aim of this multicenter, open-label clinical study was to prospectively assess the safety and effectiveness of Trinity Evolution cellular bone allograft (TE) in two-level ACDF procedures using a PEEK interbody cage and supplemental fixation, which is the standard of care for each of our five practices. The use of TE did not raise any safety concerns, since there were no adverse events, infections, or reoperations. All measures of subject pain and function (NDI, VAS neck and arm, SF-36 overall and MCS and PCS subscales) significantly improved at both 6 and 12 months as compared to baseline.

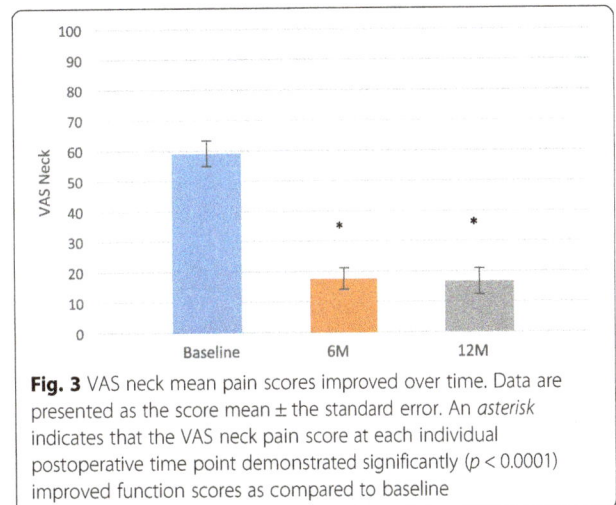

Fig. 3 VAS neck mean pain scores improved over time. Data are presented as the score mean ± the standard error. An *asterisk* indicates that the VAS neck pain score at each individual postoperative time point demonstrated significantly ($p < 0.0001$) improved function scores as compared to baseline

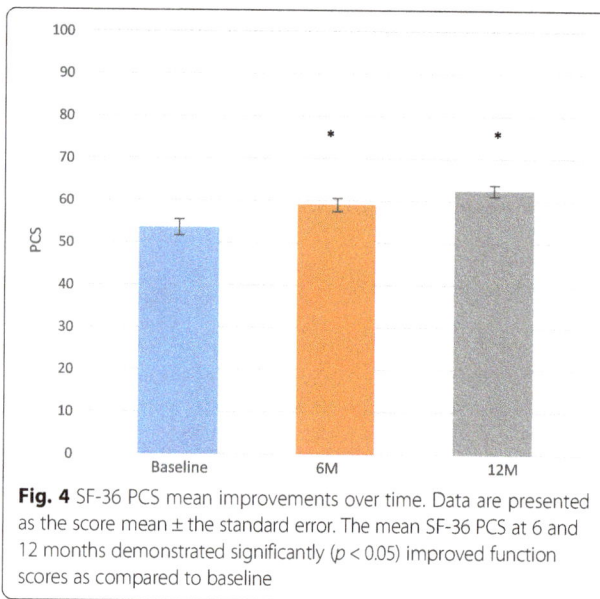

Fig. 4 SF-36 PCS mean improvements over time. Data are presented as the score mean ± the standard error. The mean SF-36 PCS at 6 and 12 months demonstrated significantly ($p < 0.05$) improved function scores as compared to baseline

One secondary aim of the study was to compare the fusion rates of groups at risk of pseudoarthrosis with normal controls. Smokers [7] particularly smokers who had a two-level ACDF [8] have been associated with increased rates of pseudoarthrosis. Although the sample size was small, there were no significant differences observed between normal and at risk subjects. TE may help overcome the biological factors that impede healing in these groups, but this evaluation was underpowered and a clinically applicable conclusion cannot be drawn.

Because surgeons have several bone graft materials available, a literature review was performed to compare these fusion results to studies that used a comparable approach and instrumentation (Table 3). Evaluation of both safety and effectiveness can help surgeons select a preferred bone graft among the several types including cellular bone allograft, non-cellular allograft such as demineralized bone matrix (DBM), recombinant BMP containing grafts such as INFUSE®, and autograft. Since TE is a cellular bone allograft that contains DBM, one way to assess the potential benefit of TE is to compare the fusion incidence to studies that used DBM. The Topuz et al. study [14] demonstrated a

69.6% fusion rate using DBM, which is twenty percentage points lower than the 89.4% fusion rate for TE. Another study used DBM in conjunction with a synthetic graft material [15], which is a potential confounding factor for accurate data comparison. The use INFUSE® was described in ACDF procedures [16–18]. Although the fusion outcomes using INFUSE are high, there is a substantial safety issue when using INFUSE for ACDF procedures. FDA issued a public health notification of life-threatening cervical swelling (https://wayback.arc-hive-it.org/7993/20170111190511/http://www.fda.gov/MedicalDevices/Safety/AlertsandNotices/PublicHealth-Notifications/ucm062000.htm) when INFUSE is used in the cervical spine. Table 3 also shows high fusion rate when autograft is used [15]. However, harvesting of autograft requires a second operative site which is associated with pain and morbidity that includes chronic harvest site pain, infection, increased operative time, and blood loss [19–23]. Thus, the results described herein appear promising because TE has the potential of increased arthrodesis rates as compared to allograft and TE lacks the safety concerns associated with INFUSE and autograft harvest.

Limitations to this study include a lack of a control group and thus TE treatment was not directly compared to autograft or non-cellular allograft treatments. Additionally, since the surgeons were not restricted with their use of operative approaches or fixation, either or both may have impacted outcomes. The impact of these factors on the outcome was not evaluated. Lastly, there was no sample size estimation in the protocol because there were no formal statistical hypotheses.

Conclusions

In conclusion, subjects who received Trinity Evolution in combination with a PEEK interbody device during a two-level ACDF procedure had a high rate of fusion success both overall and when stratified into high-risk groups, while having no serious adverse events related to the graft material.

Abbreviations
BMI: Body mass index; CaS: Calcium Sulfate; CT: Computed tomography; DBM: Demineralized bone matrix; IRB: Internal review board; MCS: Mental component score; PCS: Physical component score; PEEK: Polyetheretherketone; QMA: Quantitative motion assessment; SD: Standard deviation; SE: Standard error; SF-36: Short form 36; TE: Trinity Evolution; VAS: Visual analogue scale

Acknowledgements
Not applicable.

Funding
Orthofix funded the clinical study. The funding body was responsible for the design of the study and interpretation of data.

Table 3 Literature describing fusion rates after a two-level ACDF procedure using a PEEK cage and supplemental fixation

Reference	n	Graft	Follow-up time (months)	Fusion rate (%)
Xie, 2015 [15]	19	CaS/DBM	12	94.3
	20	Autograft	12	100
Tumialan, 2008 [16]	62	INFUSE	8–36	100
Boakye, 2005 [17]	9	INFUSE	12–16	100
Lovasik, 2016 [18]	34	INFUSE	12	100
Topuz, 2009 [14]	79	DBM	12	69.6

Authors' contributions

DEB, TAP, JSV, SKS, and PMA contributed to the surgical procedures and collection, analysis, and acquisition of data. EIW contributed to the data analysis and critical revisions. RH contributed to the data analysis. BLA contributed to the manuscript writing, literature search, and data interpretation. JTR contributed to the conception and design of the study and critical revisions. RJL contributed to the data analysis and critical revisions. All authors read and approved the final manuscript.

Competing interests

JTR, RH, and EIW are employed by and own stock in Orthofix, Inc., Lewisville, TX. In addition, JSV, TAP, DEB, SKS, RJL, and BLA are consultants of Orthofix, Inc., Lewisville, TX.

Author details

[1]Seaside Spine Medical Associates, 320 Santa Fe Dr., Suite 300, Encinitas, CA 92024, USA. [2]Triangle Neurosurgery, 1540 Sunday Dr., Raleigh, NC 27607, USA. [3]Tuckahoe Orthopaedic Associates, 1501 Maple Ave., Richmond, VA 23226, USA. [4]Denver-Vail Orthopedics, P.C., 8101 E. Lowry Blvd., Suite 260, Denver, CO 80230, USA. [5]Kansas University Medical Center, 3901 Rainbow Blvd Ste 2B, Kansas City, KS 66160, USA. [6]Orthofix, Inc., 3451 Plano Parkway, Lewisville, TX 75056, USA. [7]Atkinson Biologics Consulting, Highlands Ranch, CO 80129, USA. [8]PO Box 1671, Rancho Santa Fe, CA 92067, USA.

References

1. Lee S-B, Cho K-S, Kim J-Y, Yoo D-S, Lee T-G, Huh P-W. Hybrid surgery of multilevel cervical degenerative disc disease: review of literature and clinical results. J Korean Neurosurg Soc. 2012;52(5):452–8.
2. Martin GJ, Haid RW, MacMillan M, Rodts GE, Berkman R. Anterior cervical discectomy with freeze dried fibula allograft. Overview of 317 cases and literature review. Spine. 1999;24(9):852–8.
3. Nirala AP, Husain M, Vatsal DK. A retrospective study of multiple interbody grafting and long segment strut grafting following multilevel anterior cervical decompression. British J Neurosurg. 2004;18(3):227–32.
4. Suchomel P, Barsa P, Buchvald P, Svobodnik A, Vanickova E. Autologous versus allogenic bone grafts in instrumented anterior cervical discectomy and fusion: a prospective study with respect to bone union pattern. Eur Spine J. 2004;13(6):510–5.
5. Veeravagu A, Cole T, Jiang B, Ratliff JK. Revision rates and complication incidence in single- and multilevel anterior cervical discectomy and fusion procedures: an administrative database study. Spine J. 2014;14(7):1125–31.
6. Wang JC, McDonough PW, Endow KK, Delamarter RB. Increased fusion rates with cervical plating for two-level anterior cervical discectomy and fusion. Spine. 2000;25(1):41–5.
7. Glassman SD, Anagnost SC, Parker A, Burke D, Johnson JR, Dimar JR. The effect of cigarette smoking and smoking cessation on spinal fusion. Spine. 2000;25(20):2608–15.
8. Hilibrand AS, Fye MA, Emery SE, Palumbo MA, Bohlman HH. Impact of smoking on the outcome of anterior cervical arthrodesis with interbody or strut-grafting. JBJS. 2001;83-A(5):668–73.
9. Vaccaro AR. The role of the osteoconductive scaffold in synthetic bone graft. Orthopedics. 2002;25:s571–578.
10. Rush SM. Trinity Evolution: mesenchymal stem cell allografting in foot and ankle surgery. Foot Ankle Specialist. 2010;3:140–3.
11. Vanichkachorn J, Peppers T, Bullard D, Stanley SK, Linovitz RJ, Ryaby JT. A prospective clinical and radiographic 12-month outcome study of patients undergoing single-level anterior cervical discectomy and fusion for symptomatic cervical degenerative disc disease utilizing a novel viable allogeneic, cancellous, bone matrix (Trinity Evolution*) with a comparison to historical controls. Eur Spine J. 2016;25(7):2233–8.
12. Reitman CA, Hipp JA, Nguyen L, Esses SI. Changes in segmental intervertebral motion adjacent to cervical arthrodesis. A prospective study. Spine. 2004;29:E221–6.
13. Reitman CA, Mauro KM, Nguyen L, Ziegler JM, Hipp JA. Intervertebral motion between flexion and extension in asymptomatic individuals. Spine. 2004;29:2832–43.
14. Topuz K, Colak A, Kaya S, et al. Two-level contiguous cervical disc disease treated with peek cages packed with demineralized bone matrix: results of 3-year follow-up. Eur Spine J. 2009;18:238–43.
15. Xie Y, Li H, Yuan J, et al. A prospective randomized comparison of PEEK cage containing calcium sulphate or demineralized bone matrix with autograft in anterior cervical interbody fusion. Int Orthop. 2015;39:1129–36.
16. Tumialan LM, Pan J, Rodts GE, et al. The safety and efficacy of anterior cervical discectomy and fusion with polyetheretherketone spacer and recombinant human bone morphogenetic protein-2: a review of 200 patients. J Neurosurg Spine. 2008;8(6):529–35.
17. Boakye M, Mummaneni PV, Garrett M, et al. Anterior cervical discectomy and fusion involving polyetheretherketone spacer and bone morphogenetic protein. J Neurosurg Spine. 2005;2(5):521–5.
18. Lovasik BP, Holland CM, Howard BM et al. Anterior cervical discectomy and fusion: comparison of fusion, dysphagia, and complication rates between recombinant human bone morphogenetic protein-2 and beta-tricalcium phosphate. World Neurosurg. Epub ahead of print.
19. Dimitriou R, Mataliotakis GI, Angoules AG, et al. Complications following autologous bone graft harvesting from the iliac crest and using the RIA: a systematic review. Injury. 2011;42 Suppl 2:S3–15.
20. Kurtz LT, Garfin SR, Booth RE. Harvesting autogenous iliac bone grafts. A review of complications and techniques. Spine. 1989;14:1324–31.
21. Gupta AR, Shah NR, Patel TC, et al. Perioperative and long-term complications of iliac crest bone graft harvesting for spinal surgery: a quantitative review of the literature. Int Med J. 2001;8:163–6.
22. Sawin PD, Traynelis VC, Menezes AH. A comparative analysis of fusion rates and donor site morbidity for autogeneic rib and iliac crest bone grafts in posterior cervical fusions. J Neurosurg. 1998;88(2):255–65.
23. Summers BN, Eisenstein SM. Donor site pain from the ilium: a complication of the lumbar spine fusion. J Bone Joint Surg. 1989;71B:667–80.

Permissions

The contributors of this book come from diverse backgrounds, making this book a truly international effort. This book will bring forth new frontiers with its revolutionizing research information and detailed analysis of the nascent developments around the world.

We would like to thank all the contributing authors for lending their expertise to make the book truly unique. They have played a crucial role in the development of this book. Without their invaluable contributions this book wouldn't have been possible. They have made vital efforts to compile up to date information on the varied aspects of this subject to make this book a valuable addition to the collection of many professionals and students.

This book was conceptualized with the vision of imparting up-to-date information and advanced data in this field. To ensure the same, a matchless editorial board was set up. Every individual on the board went through rigorous rounds of assessment to prove their worth. After which they invested a large part of their time researching and compiling the most relevant data for our readers.

The editorial board has been involved in producing this book since its inception. They have spent rigorous hours researching and exploring the diverse topics which have resulted in the successful publishing of this book. They have passed on their knowledge of decades through this book. To expedite this challenging task, the publisher supported the team at every step. A small team of assistant editors was also appointed to further simplify the editing procedure and attain best results for the readers.

Apart from the editorial board, the designing team has also invested a significant amount of their time in understanding the subject and creating the most relevant covers. They scrutinized every image to scout for the most suitable representation of the subject and create an appropriate cover for the book.

The publishing team has been an ardent support to the editorial, designing and production team. Their endless efforts to recruit the best for this project, has resulted in the accomplishment of this book. They are a veteran in the field of academics and their pool of knowledge is as vast as their experience in printing. Their expertise and guidance has proved useful at every step. Their uncompromising quality standards have made this book an exceptional effort. Their encouragement from time to time has been an inspiration for everyone.

The publisher and the editorial board hope that this book will prove to be a valuable piece of knowledge for researchers, students, practitioners and scholars across the globe.

List of Contributors

Ersin Kuyucu, Baris Gülenç, Baris Gülenç and Mehmet Erdil
Orthopedics and Traumatology, Istanbul Medipol University, Istanbul, Turkey

Harun Mutlu
Orthopedics and Traumatology, Taksim Ilkyardım Training and Education Hospital, Istanbul, Turkey

Serhat Mutlu
Orthopedics and Traumatology, Kanuni Sultan Süleyman Training and Education Hospital, TEM Avrupa Otoyolu Göztepe Çıkışı No:1, Bağcilar, Istanbul, Turkey

Hong-hui Cao and Kang-lai Tang
Department of Orthopaedic Surgery, Southwest Hospital, The Third Military Medical University, Gaotanyan Str. 30, Chongqing 400038, People's Republic of China

Wei-zhong Lu
Department of Orthopaedic Surgery, The Traditional Medical Hospital of Chongqing, China, The Brach 4th Panxi Road, Jiangbei, Chongqing 400021, People's Republic of China

Hirotaka Mutsuzaki
Department of Orthopaedic Surgery, Ibaraki Prefectural University of Health Sciences, 4669-2 Ami, Inashiki-gun, Ibaraki 300-0394, Japan

Hiromi Nakajima and Shunsuke Nomura
Department of Agriculture, Ibaraki University, 3-21-1 Chuo, Ami, Ibaraki 300-0393, Japan

Masataka Sakane
Department of Orthopaedic Surgery, Tsukuba Gakuen Hospital, 2573-1 Kamiyokoba, Tsukuba, Ibaraki 305-0854, Japan

Amrit Shrestha, Peng Wu, Heng'an Ge and Biao Cheng
Department of Orthopedics, Shanghai Tenth People's Hospital, Tongji University School of Medicine, No. 301 Yanchang Middle Road, Jing'an District, Shanghai 200072, China

E. Rodriguez-Collazo
Chicago Foot & Ankle Deformity Corrections Center, Department of Surgery Adults & Pediatric Ilizarov Correction, Microsurgical Limb Reconstruction, Presence Saint Joseph Hospital, Chicago, Illinois, USA

Y. Tamire
Medical Science Liaison, Osiris Therapeutics, Inc., 7015 Albert Einstein Drive, Columbia, MD 21046, USA.

Uğur Tiftikçi and Sancar Serbest
Faculty of Medicine, Department of Orthopaedics and Traumatology, Kırıkkale University, Kırıkkale, Turkey

Hongtao Xu, Kai Kang, Wei Liu, Guorong Jin, Jiangtao Dong and Shijun Gao
Department of Joint Surgery, The Third Hospital of Hebei Medical University, NO. 139 Ziqiang Road, Shijiazhuang 050051, Hebei, People's Republic of China

Jian Zhang
People's Hospital of Ri Zhao, Taian Road, Rizhao 276800, Shandong, People's Republic of China

Dongmei Xin
Hospital of TCM, 35 Wanghai Road, Rizhao 276800, Shandong, People's Republic of China

Peng Huang, Yiguo Wang, Jiao Xu, Bo Xiao, Jianheng Liu, Luyang Che and Keya Mao
Department of Orthopaedics, Chinese PLA General Hospital, Beijing 100853, China

Bo Yuan, Shengyuan Zhou, Xiongsheng Chen, Zhiwei Wang, Weicong Liu and Lianshun Jia
Department of Orthopedic Surgery, Shanghai Changzheng Hospital, Second Military Medical University, Shanghai 200003, People's Republic of China

Qi Lai, Quanwei Song, Runsheng Guo, Haidi Bi, Xuqiang Liu, Xiaolong Yu, Jianghao Zhu, Min Dai and Bin Zhang
Department of Orthopedics, Artificial Joints Engineering and Technology Research Center of Jiangxi Province, The First Affiliated Hospital of Nanchang University, 17 Yongwai Street, Nanchang, Jiangxi 330006, People's Republic of China
Department of Orthopedics, Multidisciplinary Therapy Center of Musculoskeletal Tumor, The First Affiliated Hospital of Nanchang University, Nangchang 330006, Jiangxi, China

Nuri Aydin and Bedri Karaismailoglu
Orthopaedics and Traumatology Department, Istanbul University Cerrahpasa Medical Faculty, Kocamustafapasa Cad No:53, Fatih, Istanbul, Turkey

Jiukun Li, Xi Wang and Tao Pan
Department of Orthopaedic Surgery, The Sixth Affiliated Hospital of Sun Yat-sen University, 26 Yuancun Er Heng Road, Guangzhou, Guangdong 510655, China

Shuai Huang
Department of Orthopaedic Surgery, The Second Affiliated Hospital of Guangzhou Medical University, Guangzhou 510260, China

Yubo Tang
Department of Pharmacy, The First Affiliated Hospital of Sun Yat-sen University, Guangzhou 510080, China

Hisao Shimokobe, Hidehiro Nakamura and Naoto Shiba
Department of Orthopaedic Surgery, Kurume University School of Medicine, 67 Asahi-machi, kurume, Fukuoka 830-0011, Japan

Tatsuyuki Kakuma
Department of Statistics, Kurume University School of Medicine, 67 Asahi-machi, kurume, Fukuoka 830-0011, Japan

Masafumi Gotoh, Hirokazu Honda, Yasuhiro Mitsui and Takahiro Okawa
Department of Orthopaedic Surgery, Kurume University Medical Center, 155-1 Kokubu-machi Kurume, Fukuoka 839-0863, Japan

Ruoxi Liu, Xueling Yuan, Qi Quan, Haoye Meng, Cheng Wang, Aiyuan Wang, Quanyi Guo, Jiang Peng and Shibi Lu
Institute of Orthopedics, Beijing Key Laboratory of Regenerative Medicine in Orthopedics, Key Laboratory of Musculoskeletal Trauma & War Injuries PLA, Chinese PLA General Hospital, FuXing Road 28th, Beijing 100853, China

Jing Yu
Department of Kampo Medicine, Yokohama University of Pharmacy, 601 Matano-cho, Totsuka-ku, Yokohama-shi, Kanagawa-ken 245-0066, Japan

Yu Huang, Xuanwei Chen, Jianhua Lin and Hongjie Zhang
Department of Spinal Surgery, The First Affiliated Hospital of Fujian Medical University, Fuzhou, Fujian 350005, China

Jin Lin
Department of Basic Medical Science, Fujian Medical College, Fuzhou, Fujian, China

Yulan Lin
Public Health School, Fujian Medical University, Fuzhou, Fujian, China

Adam C. Shaner, Babar Shafiq and Lynne C. Jones
Department of Orthopaedic Surgery, The Johns Hopkins University, 600 N Caroline Street, Baltimore, MD 21287, USA

Norachart Sirisreetreerux
Department of Orthopaedic Surgery, The Johns Hopkins University, 600 N Caroline Street, Baltimore, MD 21287, USA
Department of Orthopaedics, Faculty of Medicine, Ramathibodi Hospital, Mahidol University, 270 Rama VI Rd, Ratchathewi, Bangkok 10400, Thailand

Erik A. Hasenboehler
Department of Orthopaedic Surgery, The Johns Hopkins University, 600 N Caroline Street, Baltimore, MD 21287, USA
Department of Orthopaedic Surgery, The Johns Hopkins University/Johns Hopkins Bayview Medical Center, 4940 Eastern Ave., #A667, Baltimore, MD 21224-2780, USA

Bo Yang, Fengchun Wang, Yanhua Lou, Juan Li, Lei Sun, Lei Gao and Feng Liu
Department of Orthopaedics, Tai'an Central Hospital, Tai'an, Shandong 271000, China

Tengbo Yu, Yanling Hu, Hao Tao, Kai Wang and Chengdong Zhang
Department of Orthopaedic Surgery, Affiliated Hospital of Qingdao University, Qingdao, Shandong 266000, People's Republic of China

Huazheng Pan
Department of Clinical Laboratory, Affiliated Hospital of Qingdao University, Qingdao, Shandong 266000, People's Republic of China

Tao Guo, Xiaobin Tian and Bo Li
Department of Orthopedics, Guizhou Province People's Hospital, Guiyang, Guizhou province 550002, China

Tianfu Yang
Department of Orthopedics, West China Hospital, Sichuan University, Chengdu, Sichuan province 610041, China

Yubao Li
Nanometer Analytical and Testing Center, Sichuan University, Chengdu, Sichuan province 610041, China

Derong Xu, Qianyu Zhuang, Zheng Li, Zhinan Ren, Xin Chen and Shugang Li
Department of Orthopedic Surgery, Peking Union Medical College Hospital, No.1 Shuai Fu Yuan, Wang Fu Jing Street, Beijing 100730, China

Masataka Inoue, Takamasa Yoshikawa and Tadashi Inaba
Department of Mechanical Engineering, Graduate School of Engineering, Mie University, 1577 Kurimamachiya-cho, Tsu City 514-8507, Mie prefecture, Japan

Tetsutaro Mizuno, Toshihiko Sakakibara, and Yuichi Kasai
Department of Spinal Surgery and Medical Engineering, Mie University Graduate School of Medicine, 2-174 Edobashi, Tsu City 514-8507, Mie prefecture, Japan

Takaya Kato
Community-University Research Cooperation Center, Mie University, 1577 Kurimamachiya-cho, Tsu City 514-8507, Mie prefecture, Japan

Hongwei Chen
Department of Orthopaedics Surgery, Yiwu People's Hospital, NO.699, Jiangdong Road, Yiwu, Zhejiang Province 322007, China

Dengying Wu, Tianlong Pan, Jun Pan, Rui Zhang and Xuchao Shi
Department of Orthopaedics Surgery, The Second Affiliated Hospital and Yuying Children's Hospital of Wenzhou Medical University, NO.109, Xue Yuan West Road, Wenzhou, Zhejiang Province 325027, China

Qun Zhang, Wei Zhang, Zhuo Zhang, Licheng Zhang, Hua Chen, Ming Hao, Junhao Deng and Peifu Tang
Department of Orthopaedics, Chinese PLA General Hospital, No. 28 Fuxin Road, Beijing 100853, People's Republic of China

Ulf Krister Hofmann, Christian Walter and Falk Mittag
Department of Orthopaedic Surgery, University Hospital of Tübingen, Hoppe-Seyler-Strasse 3, 72076 Tübingen, Germany

Ramona Luise Keller
Faculty of Medicine, Julius-Maximilians University of Würzburg, Josef-Schneider-Str.2, 97080 Würzburg, Germany

Fan Xing Meng and Tian Sheng Su
Third Military Medical University, No. 30 Gaotanyan Street, Chongqing 400038, China
Department of Orthopedics, Chinese PLA Army General Hospital, Dongcheng District, Nanmencang No. 5, Beijing 100700, China

Jing Ming Hou
Department of Orthopedics, Chinese PLA Army General Hospital, Dongcheng District, Nanmencang No. 5, Beijing 100700, China
Department of Rehabilitation, Southwest Hospital, Third Military Medical University, No. 30 Gaotanyan Street, Chongqing 400038, China

Grzegorz Guzik
Orthopedic Oncology Department, Specialist Hospital in Brzozów-Podkarpacki Oncology Center, ul Bielawskiego 18, 36-200 Brzozów, Poland

Timothy A. Peppers
Seaside Spine Medical Associates, 320 Santa Fe Dr., Suite 300, Encinitas, CA 92024, USA

Dennis E. Bullard
Triangle Neurosurgery, 1540 Sunday Dr., Raleigh, NC 27607, USA

Jed S. Vanichkachorn
Tuckahoe Orthopaedic Associates, 1501 Maple Ave., Richmond, VA 23226, USA

Scott K. Stanley
Denver-Vail Orthopedics, P.C., 8101 E. Lowry Blvd., Suite 260, Denver, CO 80230, USA

Paul M. Arnold
Kansas University Medical Center, 3901 Rainbow Blvd Ste 2B, Kansas City, KS 66160, USA

Erik I. Waldorff, Rebekah Hahn and James T. Ryaby
Orthofix, Inc., 3451 Plano Parkway, Lewisville, TX 75056, USA

Brent L. Atkinson
Atkinson Biologics Consulting, Highlands Ranch, CO 80129, USA

Raymond J. Linovitz
Rancho Santa Fe, CA 92067, USA

Index

Osteonecrosis, 6-7, 9, 11
Osteotomy, 2-3, 5-7, 9-10, 108, 126, 157, 164

P
Partial Repair, 82, 88
Pedicle Screw Fixation, 46, 50-52, 58, 74, 80, 192
Physical Therapy, 1, 31, 82, 182
Placental Membranes, 26
Platelet-rich Plasma, 18, 123-124, 131
Polymorphism, 89-94, 96-98
Popliteal Cyst, 117, 121-122
Posterior Oblique Ligament, 36-37, 44
Postoperative Infection, 61, 64, 66-67
Prevention, 28, 48, 61-62, 66, 97

R
Risk Factor, 61, 65-66, 81, 86, 88, 94, 96-98

S
Scaffold, 18, 123-125, 130-131, 141, 199
Sclerotic Bone, 100, 163-164
Screw Fixation, 45-47, 49-52, 56, 58, 60, 74, 80, 114, 116, 156-157, 160-162, 192, 195
Semimembranosus Muscle, 118
Sesamoid Excision, 1
Shoulder Arthroscopy, 68
Snapping Hip Syndrome, 19, 25

Spinal Cord Injury, 54, 101, 178, 185-186
Spinal Destruction, 100
Spinal Fusion Surgery, 142, 146-147, 175
Spinal Tuberculosis, 99-100, 102-108
Spinal Tumor Resections, 187
Spinous Process, 46, 48, 54, 74-75, 77-79, 100
Subchondral Bone, 4-5, 97, 133-135, 139-140, 195
Subperiosteal Osteotomy, 164
Supine Position, 2, 7, 118
Surgical Treatment, 1-2, 4, 9, 25, 40-41, 44, 56, 100, 108, 160, 170, 187-188, 192
Synovitis, 4, 89, 118

T
Tearing Pattern, 81
Tendon Graft Placement, 12-13, 16-17
Tendon Quality, 68
Tibial Bone Tunnel, 13
Tibiofibular Joint, 110
Tissue-engineered Bone, 123-124, 129-132
Titanium Cable, 53
Topical Txa, 142-146
Toxicity, 139, 178, 186

V
Visual Analog Scale, 5, 45, 51, 53-55, 59, 83, 101, 117, 119

www.ingramcontent.com/pod-product-compliance
Lightning Source LLC
Chambersburg PA
CBHW082030190326
41458CB00010B/3320